BIOLOGICAL IMPLICATIONS OF THE NUCLEAR AGE

Proceedings of a symposium held at
Lawrence Radiation Laboratory
Livermore, California, March 5-7, 1969

Sponsored by
The Bio-Medical Division
Lawrence Radiation Laboratory

and

U. S. Atomic Energy Commission

Cochairmen

Bernard Shore
Frederick Hatch

December 1969

U. S. ATOMIC ENERGY COMMISSION Division of Technical Information

St. Mary's College Library
Winona, Minnesota

Available as CONF-690303 for $6.00 from

National Technical Information Service
U. S. Department of Commerce
Springfield, Virginia 22151

Library of Congress Catalog Card Number: 74-603800

Printed in the United States of America
USAEC Division of Technical Information Extension, Oak Ridge, Tennessee

December 1969; latest printing, February 1971

FOREWORD

I would like to welcome you on behalf of the Lawrence Radiation Laboratory.

The Bio-Medical Division here at Livermore was created in 1963 at the request of the U. S. Atomic Energy Commission. At that time we had essentially no capability in the biological field. With a certain amount of trepidation we agreed to start the effort. We were extremely fortunate in obtaining the services of Dr. John Gofman to head the group. Since the beginning the division has been a very essential and meaningful part of our operation.

We at the laboratory are concerned with all phases of nuclear explosions — the basic problems and the physics associated with these problems, as well as the applications to military and civilian purposes. We are also concerned with the effects of nuclear explosions. Of course, we are not the only ones who are making these studies, but we do have as our primary mission the design and understanding of the explosive itself.

Since the Bio-Medical Division was established here, and particularly since we have obtained the services of very fine people, we have developed a much better understanding of the biological implications of our work. This is especially true for Plowshare, which is a program for applying nuclear explosives to civilian purposes. It is also true for nuclear testing. The Bio-Medical Division has become an integral part of the Lawrence Radiation Laboratory, and I believe its program now has a special meaning and usefulness to the Atomic Energy Commission in other aspects of its work.

Michael M. May

Lawrence Radiation Laboratory
University of California
Livermore, California

PREFACE

In the spring of 1963, a research program was initiated at the Lawrence Radiation Laboratory at Livermore to study the impact of the release of radiation and radionuclides upon the biosphere — especially upon man — from nuclear activities, particularly with reference to the uses of nuclear energy for excavations and other Plowshare events, and weapons testing activities, and also relevant to reactor releases, reactor accidents, and nuclear war. A systematic attempt was to be made to anticipate the biological and health significance of radionuclides produced in future designs and applications of nuclear explosive devices.

Since 1963 the program of the Bio-Medical Division has evolved to include work in four major areas. These areas are (1) prediction before each event, on a global basis, of the ultimate body and organ burden likely to be delivered to man by external radiation and by each of the radionuclides likely to be produced in an event; (2) quantitation of the life history of the radionuclides produced in an event; (3) determination of any effects on man of radiation from internal and external sources; and (4) the development of countermeasures to minimize any radiation burden to man.

An essential part of the new program at Livermore was the construction of a building to house the Division's interdisciplinary attack by biochemists, biophysicists, chemists, ecologists, electronic and mechanical engineers, physiologists, physicians, and physicists on the problems of the nuclear age. This building was occupied in November 1968, and accordingly it seemed appropriate to dedicate it with a symposium devoted to the biological implications of the nuclear age.

Since there is an increasing public awareness and concern about these biological implications, we undertook a review with expert speakers on a broad range of topics relevant to this issue. Scientists doing research in this area were invited to attend, and it was hoped that the formal presentations and discussions would be valuable not only to them but also to the American public. To help disseminate this information and promote intelligent discussion, we are publishing the proceedings of the symposium.

The nuclear age is with us. It is easy, but foolish, to say, "Stop the nuclear age, I want to get off!" It is more intelligent, however, to examine its promises, its possible problems, and to understand what it will mean to us in the future.

Bernard Shore
Frederick Hatch

Bio-Medical Division
Lawrence Radiation Laboratory
Livermore, California

September 1969

ACKNOWLEDGMENT

The chairmen wish to thank Anne M. Goulden for editing the papers and coordinating the publication of the proceedings.

CONTENTS

Foreword iii

Preface v

The Atom's Expanding Role in the Medical World 1
    Glenn T. Seaborg

Perspectives

Objectives of Biomedical Research in Relation to
Atomic Energy 23
    John R. Trotter

Planned Applications of Peaceful Nuclear Explosives . . . 31
    Glenn C. Werth

Application of Basic Radiation Protection Criteria 63
    Herbert M. Parker

Release and Distribution of Radionuclides in the Biosphere

Estimation of the Maximum Dose to Man from the
Contamination of an Aquatic Ecosystem with
Radionuclides 75
    Arthur R. Tamplin

Estimation of the Maximum Dose to Man from the
Fallout of Radionuclides on Agricultural Land 95
    Yook C. Ng.

Radioactive Pollution of the Atmosphere 125
   Joshua Z. Holland

Reactor Releases of Radionuclides 133
   R. L. Junkins

United Kingdom Studies on Radioactive Materials
Released in the Marine Environment 145
   H. J. Dunster

Presence and Persistence of Radionuclides; Possible Countermeasures Against Harmful Consequences of Radionuclide Contamination

Persistence of Radionuclides at Sites of Nuclear
Detonations. 159
   John J. Koranda and John R. Martin

Radionuclides in Food 189
   John H. Harley

Status of Remedial Measures Against Environmental
Radiocontamination 201
   C. L. Comar and J. C. Thompson, Jr.

Effects of Radiation in Man and Animals; Relations Among Radiation, Viruses, and Other Environmental Hazards; Repair of Radiation Damage

Some Biological Effects of Radiation in Relation to
Other Environmental Agents 223
   Norton Nelson

Effects of Single or Fractionated X Irradiation and of
Bone-Seeking Radionuclides on Mammals: A Review . . . 231
   Leo K. Bustad

Factors Affecting the Radiation Induction of Mutations
in the Mouse 255
   William L. Russell

Late Effects of External Irradiations in Animals and the
Prediction of Low-Dose Effects 269
   Douglas Grahn

Radiation Repair Mechanisms in Mammalian Cells . . . 283
   J. E. Cleaver

Delayed Radiation Effects Among Japanese Survivors
of the Atomic Bombs 307
    Robert W. Miller

Radiation and Virus Interactions in Leukemogenesis . . . 319
    Henry S. Kaplan

Closing Remarks 327
    John W. Gofman

List of Attendees 329

Index 335

THE ATOM'S EXPANDING ROLE
IN THE MEDICAL WORLD

GLENN T. SEABORG, Chairman
U. S. Atomic Energy Commission, Washington, D. C.

I am pleased that you have decided on a symposium as one means of dedicating your new biomedical building. The ideas presented and the information exchanged at this symposium will ultimately prove more significant than just the typical dedication ceremony.

For my own remarks today I will depart somewhat from the central theme of the symposium and speak broadly about some of the recent progress being made in the medical applications of the atom. One reason for doing this is that I have been looking for an excuse to describe the great progress that has been made since I last gave a talk devoted to this subject about 5 years ago — at the Medical Alumni Association banquet of George Washington University in Washington, D. C.

Unfortunately this is a subject that is not widely discussed outside the medical profession. Nuclear weapons, nuclear power, the Plowshare program, and even the role of the atom in space, all these are getting a growing share of the public's attention. But the remarkable contribution of the atom to medicine receives less acclaim — and it deserves more.

To some extent this is strange. Although we know the great potential of nuclear energy and nuclear science in other areas, in medicine we know more than its potential. We are already experiencing its benefits every day — every day it is helping to save human lives and relieve human suffering in this country and throughout the world. And such benefits reveal a payoff on our investment in the atom that few people realize. This was particularly called to my attention by a letter I received a few years ago from a prominent physician who even then was employing nuclear medicine with notable success. Expressing his enthusiasm, he wrote: "I believe that on the basis of benefits to mankind, in the field of medicine alone the whole cost of the atomic energy project could be justified." Though one cannot truly put a dollar value on the saving of lives or the alleviation of suffering, I would be inclined to agree with this physician's statement.

In view of this important contribution, it is regrettable that most people have no idea of the extent to which the atom has influenced modern medicine or its effect on it today. I am thinking particularly of the extensive use of radioisotopes at this point. For example, over the past 30 years more than 100 different radioisotopes, available in quantity largely as the result of their production by neutron irradiation in nuclear reactors, are used around the world in the diagnosis and treatment of many diseases and disorders and in continuing research on them.

We have made an assessment of the general use of radioisotopes in hospitals and clinics in the United States which indicates that these amazing servants of mankind are now being employed annually in approximately eight million individual therapeutic treatments or in vivo and in vitro diagnostic procedures. Of these, about 50% employ ^{60}Co (primarily for therapy), 33% use ^{131}I (for diagnosis and therapy), and 7% use ^{99m}Tc (for diagnosis). (Incidentally, I was fortunate to be involved in the discovery of all these radioisotopes — with the collaboration of Jack Livingood in the case of ^{60}Co and ^{131}I and of Emilio Segre in the case of ^{99m}Tc.) The remaining 10% of these procedures employ a large variety of other radioisotopes. It is interesting to note that ^{226}Ra, which in the early days of radiology was essentially the only isotope available for radiotherapy, is now used in less than 1% of all these applications.

Important new advances are being made in nuclear medicine and its related fields, but before I go into the specifics of this progress I will point out some overall signs of progress. The entire field of nuclear medicine — the use of radioisotopes for diagnosis, treatment, and medical research and the application of teletherapy and brachytherapy — all this is growing at a remarkable rate. Reports of recent years offer some interesting information related to this growth. For example, we are told that there are about 2000 U. S. hospitals using nuclear medicine and that on the average each is employing between $25,000 and $30,000 worth of nuclear instrumentation. With about 100 new nuclear facilities being added each year, the annual market in hospitals for nuclear equipment is already approaching $6 million. Another $1 to $2 million can be added to this nuclear-equipment cost figure for medical clinics and physicians' offices, bringing the total annual market for nuclear instruments alone up to about $8 million. To this we can add $8 to $10 million annual sales for radiopharmaceuticals and $6 to $8 million for radiochemicals — bringing total sales figures for nuclear medicine up to about $25 million. (At this point I should make clear that my discussion of nuclear medicine today and the facts and figures

THE ATOM'S EXPANDING ROLE IN THE MEDICAL WORLD 3

I will present do not include the very large radiological use of machine X-ray sources.)

At the risk of sounding like Robert Benchley giving his infamous "Treasurer's Report" let me add just a few more statistics. It is predicted that by 1980, with Medicare to spur its growth, the total annual medical market for nuclear instrumentation alone will be $30 to $35 million and the total for the nuclear medicine market will approach $100 million. As a result of this, I can envision a scene, similar to that classic one in the film "The Graduate," in which the well-meaning old-timer gives the young-man-about-to-go-out-into-the-world his famous one word of advice — "Nuclear."

But I must get away from this financial-sounding approach to the subject and talk about the growth and progress of nuclear medicine in other terms.

GROWTH OF RADIOISOTOPE USE

I will begin with a look at the general growth of radioisotopes in medicine for diagnosis and therapy. It was estimated in a study conducted by the Stanford Research Institute for the AEC that a total of 400,000 doses of radioisotopes were administered to humans during the year 1959, exclusive of teletherapy and brachytherapy. In 1966 the institute conducted a similar study for the U. S. Public Health Service (USPHS), and its preliminary findings show that approximately 1,743,000 administrations of some 30 different radioisotopes were made during the year 1966, excluding the use of teletherapy and brachytherapy. This means that the number of administrations per year increased approximately fourfold during the 7 years between 1959 and 1966.

Today nearly every medical specialty has found clinical uses for radioisotopes. As noted in the USPHS report, "One of the first function studies performed in clinical medicine was the study of thyroid physiology using ^{131}I. This test has been widely practiced since its inception and was the most used function procedure reported in this survey. Of the 50 different function studies reported in 1966, the number of administrations for this procedure represents more than one-half of the total administrations." In other words, about one million "atomic cocktails" containing ^{131}I are now served annually in the United States.

MAJOR APPLICATIONS OF RADIOISOTOPES

Since I shall try to focus on new developments, time does not allow me to more than mention a number of well-known therapeutic and diagnostic applications and organ-function tests. Most of these are in routine use now though some must still be regarded as experimental in nature. In some cases the diagnostic or function tests are performed with the radioisotopes in the form of simple radiochemicals and in other cases they are present in more complicated radiopharmaceuticals.

Cobalt-60 (and to some extent ^{137}Cs) is used as a source of radiation to treat cancer and to help suppress the immune reaction involved in the transplanting of human organs; ^{131}I (and in some applications other radioactive iodine isotopes, such as ^{125}I), to diagnose various thyroid disorders, treat hyperthyroidism and functional metastatic thyroid cancer, diagnose kidney and liver disorders and make function tests of these organs, screen for pulmonary emboli by lung scans, locate brain tumors, and make blood-volume and cardiac-output studies; ^{14}C, to study metabolic aberrations underlying diabetes, gout, anemia, and acromegaly; ^{68}Ga, ^{85}Sr, ^{87m}Sr, ^{18}F, and ^{47}Ca are used for bone scanning in suspected metabolic disorders and malignancies; ^{51}Cr, to measure cell mass; ^{74}As and ^{197}Hg, to locate brain tumors; ^{90}Yb, for pituitary gland therapy; ^{198}Au, as a palliative in lung cancer; ^{197}Hg and ^{203}Hg, for renal function tests; ^{75}Se (selenomethionine), for scanning the pancreas to detect carcinoma; ^{22}Na and ^{24}Na, to measure exchangeable sodium and diagnose circulatory disorders; ^{32}P, to treat such blood disorders as polycythemia vera and chronic leukemias, and in some cases even bone cancer; ^{59}Fe (and ^{55}Fe), to measure the rate of formation of red-cell mass, red-cell survival times, and intestinal absorption rates; and ^{57}Co (and ^{60}Co), for vitamin B_{12} absorption tests. Combinations of radioisotopes are used in many applications, such as the measurement of red blood cells and plasma volume for the control of blood transfusions.

This is, of course, only a partial listing of a total that is growing at such a rate that it is almost impossible to keep a complete, up-to-date inventory. I have reserved for special discussion, the manifold new applications of ^{99m}Tc, using this as an illustration of the rewarding use of radioisotopes as constituents of radiopharmaceuticals.

Sometimes a choice between more than one radioisotope of an element is possible. This choice offers the possibility of minimizing the hazard to the patient by using the shorter lived isotope or one with more favorable radiation characteristics in a diagnostic or organ-function-study procedure. For example, ^{57}Co (half-life 270 days), the second most widely used isotope in function studies, is used with 50% greater frequency than ^{60}Co (half-life 5.3 years) for vitamin B_{12} absorption tests because of its shorter half-life and greater counting efficiency with most detectors. Similarly, ^{197}Hg (half-life 65 hr) is recommended by some physicians over ^{203}Hg (half-life 47 days) for kidney-function tests because of its shorter half-life. In some cases ^{125}I is finding favor over ^{131}I owing to the lower energy of its radiation.

HODGKIN'S DESEASE AND SOFT-TISSUE TUMORS

Research studies at the Medical Division of Oak Ridge Associated Universities with carrier-free ^{67}Ga have proven beneficial in localizing lesions of Hodgkin's disease. This localization has spurred a renewed interest in ^{67}Ga and other radioisotopes in the hope that they will serve as successful labels for soft-tissue tumors and metastases. The ability to detect small soft-tissue tumors in the trunk region of the body will be greatly benefited by the use of the depth detection scanning equipment currently being developed at the Lawrence Radiation Laboratory, Berkeley.

TECHNETIUM-99m—A VERSATILE SHORT-LIVED ISOTOPE

Technetium-99m (developed at Brookhaven National Laboratory and Argonne Cancer Research Hospital) has in recent years proved to be such a versatile tool that I believe it is worth some special attention as an example of recent progress in nuclear medicine. This short-lived radioisotope (half-life 6.0 hr) is used for the diagnosis of thyroid disease, liver disease, brain disease, and kidney disease, depending on its physical and chemical state. Technetium-99m is obtained from a radioisotope generator. The generator, or "cow," often consists of a tube of ion-exchange resin upon which has been deposited ^{99}Mo, an isotope that decays by beta-particle emission with a 2.8-day half-life. As the ^{99}Mo decays, ^{99m}Tc is formed and can be readily "milked off" by the appropriate chemical process whenever there is need for the isotope. Some measure of the value of ^{99m}Tc can be gleaned from the fact that at least 2000 diagnostic procedures are being carried out daily in the United States with this radioisotope, and it is now being used on a worldwide basis because of its nearly ideal properties as a diagnostic tracer. These properties include general availability, reasonable price, convenience, low radiation dosage to the patient, and a simple decay scheme consisting only of photons (with some accompanying conversion electrons) with an energy that is nearly optimum for external visualization techniques. Other generator-produced radioisotopes are currently in use or under experimental evaluation.

Another factor which has played an important role in nuclear medicine and which will play a much greater role in the future is the development of pharmaceuticals labeled with radioisotopes. The value of labeling with a radioisotope a pharmaceutical that exhibits specific behavior towards a particular organ is frequently overlooked as a means of carrying the tracer to a desired location. Such techniques allow the transport of radioisotopes having excellent physical properties to areas of biological interest even though the isotope in simpler chemical state would not behave in this fashion. This technique can also increase the application of already useful isotopes by further increasing their use and thus further reducing their cost. The development of several carrier compounds for ^{99m}Tc may be cited as an example of what may be accomplished with this approach. These labeled materials have resulted in the application of this radioisotope to some 10 different procedures. For instance, a sulfur colloid labeled with ^{99m}Tc developed at the Brookhaven National Laboratory has become an important and widely used agent for studies of the liver, spleen, and bone marrow. For such applications, this colloid has proved superior to colloidal gold, which was previously used for these purposes.

CYCLOTRON-PRODUCED SHORT-LIVED RADIOISOTOPES

Certain radioactive isotopes of biological importance have half-lives so short that it has heretofore been difficult to apply them in medical practice. These include ^{11}C, ^{13}N, ^{15}O, and ^{18}F. Approximately 10 other short-lived isotopes are of immediate interest for metabolic isotope studies. A short half-life is an advantageous characteristic since it permits the use of larger initial amounts of activity, which, in turn, results in good counting statistics with no increase in the overall radiation exposure. Furthermore, sequential studies can be carried out in short time intervals without interference from residual radioactivity. Various metabolic studies in animals and in man require the use of short-lived radioisotopes, some of which emit positrons. Positron emission is of particular interest since it makes possible three-dimensional localizations with coincidence scanning systems.

Such radioisotopes often can be produced only by bombardment with charged particles and are now becoming more available as the result of the commercial sale of compact and relatively inexpensive cyclotrons. As examples of this, compact cyclotrons have been installed with AEC support at Sloan–Kettering Institute for Cancer Research and at Argonne Cancer Research Hospital. These cyclotrons will enable the clinical investigators at these hospitals to conduct basic metabolic studies with readily available cyclotron-produced, short-lived ^{18}F and ^{87m}Sr. A variety of pulmonary studies will be possible with ^{13}N and ^{15}O. Additionally, thyroid function studies and blood metabolic studies become possible with the availability of such radioisotopes as ^{123}I and ^{52}Fe. It will now be possible to conduct studies with elements that are available in radioactive form only as short-lived isotopes and also studies that are feasible only with short-lived radioisotopes owing to the requirement that the activity must be adequate at the time of investigation and still produce a limited radiation exposure to the patient.

CLINICAL RADIOISOTOPE SCANNING TECHNIQUES

The increase in the diagnostic use of radioisotopes today in clinical medicine is due in large part to greatly improved radiation-detection techniques, particularly the continuing advances in the development of radioisotope scanners. These detectors are used to localize and measure radioactive materials that have been introduced into the body. The scan can indicate size and position of organs as well as suspected space-occupying lesions. In addition, functional abnormalities can be demonstrated by anomalous distributions or movements of the introduced radioisotope.

The earliest attempts at scanning were performed with Geiger counters and were of limited success because of poor collimation and low sensitivity. In 1950 investigators at the University of California at Los Angeles Atomic Energy Project used a directional calcium tungstate scintillation detector to show that a rabbit thyroid gland could be sharply delineated after administration of a small dose of ^{131}I. This rectilinear scanning device was a collimated scintillation counter that moved back and forth across the thyroid region detecting and recording in a quantitative way the presence of radioactivity. The first scanners were successful for the thyroid because the gland lies near the surface and takes up radioiodine preferentially over other tissue. It is the introduction of pulse-height analysis, large crystals, efficient multiaperture collimator designs, and a variety of developments in image-display techniques since that time that have made scanning so reliable a clinical procedure for other body regions and other radioactive isotopes.

These improvements still employ techniques that require some form of mechanical motion in the scanning process. This imposes a fundamental limit to the speed with which a scan may be recorded. To eliminate completely the need for moving the detector back and forth above the patient, an entirely different technique of scanning was developed at Lawrence Radiation Laboratory's Donner Laboratory at the University of California, Berkeley, in 1955 and has been termed the scintillation camera. This stationary camera was developed by Hal Anger and commonly is known as the Anger camera. These cameras visualize the entire distribution of radioactivity in their field of view simultaneously. Their capability for taking pictures in rapid sequence makes possible dynamic studies of organ function where the isotope distribution is changing.

Subsequently the autofluoroscope, an adaptation of Anger's early work, was developed at Roswell Park in Buffalo. The Anger camera uses a thin sodium iodide crystal which is viewed by an array of photomultiplier tubes. The scintillation in the crystal generates a set of output signals from photomultiplier tubes. The image displays are generally photographed by a time exposure of the oscilloscope screen. The newer version of the autofluoroscope utilizes a rank and file system of photomultipliers and light pipes. The inherently digital nature of this method makes it very suitable for core memory storage or analog display.

Special forms of radioisotope cameras have been developed to provide images of distributions of positron emitters. Positron cameras use coincident detection of the two simultaneous positron-annihilation photons, which makes conventional collimators unnecessary. Perhaps the most important property of the positron camera is its substantially uniform response to emitters at different depths in tissue, which allows the visualization of deep-seated tumors with the same sensitivity as those on the surface. Although the first positron scanner was developed in 1954, this technique has not been widely employed as a clinical system, in part because the positron-emitting radioisotopes (often short lived) were not as readily available as those used with conventional scanning. Positron scanning has been limited essentially to brain scanning, whereas conventional scanners are widely used to study a number of organs. Nevertheless, positron scanning does offer unique advantages and with the development of the positron camera and the new availability of short-lived positron-emitting radioisotopes, this technique should have increasing clinical use.

Recently a new investigative technique has been developed for producing images of the thyroid gland and other organs through the use of K-shell X-ray fluorescence. Although the iodine content of the average thyroid gland is only 0.04% by weight, this quantity is sufficient to act as the target for this scanning method. This technique incorporates the basic scheme of an X-ray fluorescence spectrophotometer, and therefore no radioisotope is introduced into the patient. Americium-241 is used as a gamma-radiation source. Both the ^{241}Am and the detector are housed in the same lead collimator block. The scanning subject is placed beneath the block, and the source–detector housing block scans the subject in a rectilinear pattern. When the gamma ray from the americium interacts with the K-shell electron of the iodine atom within the thyroid gland, a characteristic X ray is produced. The characteristic X ray is detected and discriminated from the remainder of the scatter X rays by a lithium-drifted silicon detector coupled to a multichannel analyzer. The information obtained can be recorded directly on film or as a numerical readout for subsequent evaluation.

The information obtained from this device, developed at the Argonne Cancer Research Hospital, is unique. It describes the distribution and relative concentration of stable iodine within the thyroid gland and will serve as a valuable addition to conventional thyroid scans and studies.

IN VITRO DIAGNOSTIC PROCEDURES

Recent years have seen a rapidly increasing use of radioisotopes in in vitro diagnostic tests. Such tests eliminate radiation exposure to the patient since biological material is withdrawn from the patient and is tested in the laboratory. An example of such a procedure is the triiodothyronine binding test, or T3 test, using ^{131}I (or ^{125}I in some cases), which has received considerable attention as an aid for evaluation of the thyroid. The USPHS estimates that more than 1,000,000 such tests were performed in 1966. Measurement of serum thyroxine, or T4, levels by another in vitro ^{131}I test has also shown promise.

Radioimmunoassays employing labeled antigens have provided an excellent system for identifying and determining the concentration of various hormones in the serum. An example of this type of in vitro diagnostic procedure would be the use of radioimmunological methods to measure very small amounts of insulin. This test has, for the first time, made it possible to measure insulin in small volumes of blood plasma or other fluids on a routine basis.

In the simplest version of this procedure, the insulin is assayed by mixing an insulin-containing sample with a fixed amount of insulin that has been labeled with ^{125}I. To this mixture, anti-insulin serum is added to bind the insulin. A second antiserum is added to precipitate the insulin bound to the antibody. The precipitate with the bound insulin is then separated by filtration and its radioactivity is determined.

Various modifications of this in vitro radioimmunoassay technique have made it possible to quantitatively measure a variety of other substances.

PROBES

Radioisotopic studies can also be carried on with probes inside living systems. The probe is used to locate and measure the radioisotope, which serves as a label for the part of the anatomy to be studied. This technique usually requires measurements that are restricted to a small volume and are best performed with semiconductor detectors. Developmental probes are now available with a diameter of less than 1 mm and we can expect to see even smaller ones available in the future. Miniaturized detectors are important for precise volume resolution and to minimize tissue damage and interference with organ function. As an example of this technique, such detectors are now being used experimentally to measure regional blood flow in the brain.

It is generally thought that blood flow within different parts of the cerebral tissue is related to the metabolism of the tissue itself. Measurements of blood flow in specific areas of the brain should, therefore, give information about the metabolism of the parts studied. Some knowledge of regional blood flow has come from studies of cerebral structures that are accessible to detectors at the surface.

However, since a number of important neurological diseases are caused by subsurface disturbances, more refined probe methods for quantitative measurements in the depths of the brain are being developed. In one such program, miniaturized probes are implanted within the brain. Blood volume and flow rate are determined following the inhalation of either ^{133}Xe or ^{85}Kr by the patient. This technique has made it possible to pinpoint areas suffering from reduced blood flow. These measurements reflect regional circulatory or metabolic disturbances important in a number of neurological diseases, such as Parkinson's disease.

WHOLE-BODY COUNTERS

Whole-body counters have been developed to measure and identify radioactivity in the body. In their first applications their high sensitivity made it possible to measure natural body levels of radioactivity as well as levels encountered in radiological health work where the activity acquired accidentally, as from radioactive fallout or nuclear accidents, was to be measured. Now their additional potential in medical diagnosis and research is beginning to be realized.

The most widely used type of whole-body counter was developed at the Argonne National Laboratory. In this apparatus the detector is a sodium iodide crystal housed inside a large heavy-steel shield. The subject being measured is placed inside the shield on a tilted chair or couch. A different type of whole-body counter developed at the Los Alamos Scientific Laboratory uses a cylindrical shell filled with a liquid scintillator. The subject is placed inside the cylinder and thus is surrounded by the detector. An array of 24 photomultiplier tubes, 18 in. in diameter, monitors the liquid within the cylinder, an arrangement that has an obvious geometrical advantage. The increased geometrical efficiency permits measurements to be made in a much shorter time than by using the crystal system. However, spectral resolution is much better with the crystal detectors. Sharp spectral resolution is an important advantage in medical diagnosis and, in general, for the measurement and identification of body radioactivity.

THE ATOM'S EXPANDING ROLE IN THE MEDICAL WORLD 11

Through the use of radioactive isotopes such as ^{59}Fe, whole-body counters have provided a useful adjunct to the study of iron absorption and metabolism in many types of anemia. With naturally occurring ^{40}K as the tracer, whole-body counters have been used extensively to assess lean body mass in normal development and body-wasting conditions. Whole-body counters offer the physician a more sensitive alternative to the classical balance-type study for turnover of such materials as calcium in normal and diseased states. They afford information on tissue distribution, kinetics, and body content of labeled materials, for example, ^{57}Co labeled vitamin B$_{12}$.

Mobile whole-body counters that employ localized shielding of the radiation detector have also been developed. These detectors have been transported to such places as Alaska and the Colorado plateau.

TELETHERAPY

Teletherapy is defined as the treatment of a disease with radiation (usually gamma radiation) from a source located at a distance from a patient. The Oak Ridge Associated Universities had a major role in developing the use of ^{60}Co and ^{137}Cs teletherapy devices as a substitute for, or supplement to, high-voltage X-ray machines. Those who use these teletherapy machines claim excellent therapeutic results, and certainly they have a very high operational reliability. The 1966 Public Health Service survey respondents reported that over 150,000 patients received a total of almost two million teletherapy administrations during the course of the year. Cancer was the only condition reported as treated by teletherapy, and the only radioisotopes used were ^{60}Co and ^{137}Cs.

Several unique radiation sources are under investigation as therapeutic tools. For example, the Lawrence Radiation Laboratory 184-in. cyclotron has been used to produce high-energy particles (both alpha particles and protons) to destroy selectively pituitary tissue of patients with diabetic retinopathy or acromegaly, leading to marked improvements in the cases where the condition is related to pituitary function. At the Argonne Cancer Research Hospital, very high energy electrons (40 Mev) from a linear accelerator are being used to treat deep-seated tumors.

There are persuasive reasons for believing that beams of heavy ions or negative pi-mesons, which will be available in the future, may be far more effective than gamma rays, and even more effective than neutrons and protons, in the treatment of hypoxic (lower than normal oxygen content) solid tumors.

BRACHYTHERAPY

Brachytherapy is the treatment of disease with sealed radioactive sources placed near or inserted directly into the diseased area. The most commonly used implant is radium or radon gas in needles and seeds. These can present problems of leakage and loss, and, because of this, new radioactive sources are constantly being evaluated for their potential applicability for treating cancer patients. Recently radiotherapists at Argonne Cancer Research Hospital have begun using high-specific-activity radiochromium wire for implantation purposes. Other radioactive metals have been used previously as cancer-therapy implants, but chromium wire is unique among them because it can be left permanently in the body. Radioactive ^{51}Cr has a convenient half-life of 27 days. Such a half-life is sufficient to ensure an effective dose of radiation but is not so long that the metal would have to be removed to prevent an overdose. At the Argonne Cancer Research Hospital, the wire is cut into $3/16$-in.-long pieces and then irradiated in an Argonne National Laboratory reactor to convert some of the chromium atoms into the isotope ^{51}Cr. These small pieces or seeds are introduced into the body by a special radioisotope implantation gun. The seeds are placed in an array or distribution within the tumor.

An exciting new possibility is ^{252}Cf, which has the useful property of emitting neutrons as part of its decay process. Neutrons may be more efficient in destroying oxygen-deficient cancer cells than are X rays and gamma rays. Needles containing ^{252}Cf have been prepared at the Savannah River Laboratory and are being evaluated in radiation experiments at the Brookhaven National Laboratory. This possible use of an internal isotopic neutron source in cancer therapy could be a major advancement. Heretofore, neutrons have been applied in cancer therapy only from external sources, such as nuclear reactors and cyclotrons. Neutrons from such external sources have had limited use because of the damage done to healthy tissues surrounding the tumor. Only about a microgram of ^{252}Cf is needed to give a neutron-radiation dose equivalent in ionization to the gamma-ray dose from a conventional 1-mg radium needle. Extensive dose measurements and animal studies will precede the planned treatment of human cancer patients with the ^{252}Cf. The Commission has provided ^{252}Cf for evaluation as a therapeutic agent to the Medical Department of the Brookhaven National Laboratory and to the M. D. Anderson Hospital in Houston.

EXTRA-CORPOREAL IRRADIATION

Among the persistent and unsolved problems confronting physicians today are those concerning management of leukemia. At the Brookhaven

THE ATOM'S EXPANDING ROLE IN THE MEDICAL WORLD

National Laboratory, solutions are being sought by a new and unorthodox technique of intermittent irradiation of blood in an exteriorized shunt (extra-corporeal irradiation). Results so far indicate that certain forms of leukemia may be favorably influenced by this treatment. By means of surgical connections to a plastic tube, blood is made to flow in a temporary external circuit from an artery to a vein. The external circuit is made sufficiently long to include passage through a high-intensity field of gamma radiation. Thus only exteriorized blood and plastic tubing is irradiated while the rest of the body remains untreated. The results obtained from this procedure are similar to those seen when certain drugs are used to treat leukemia, but with one significant exception. The drugs have potential and actual toxic side effects on other tissues of the body whereas in the irradiation of exteriorized blood only the cells in the blood are affected.

In addition to its application in the treatment of certain leukemias, extra-corporeal irradiation of blood for suppression of the immune response is being used to prepare recipient patients for kidney transplants and to help patients in whom the rejection of a transplanted kidney is threatened.

LOW-DOSE-RATE FACILITY

The Medical Division of the Oak Ridge Associated Universities has constructed a facility that will allow prolonged total-body irradiation of patients at low dose rates. The new facility will make possible a reevaluation of the effectiveness of chronic total-body exposure to ^{60}Co gamma radiation in selected patients having chronic leukemias or other blood diseases characterized by an overproduction of blood cells. The exposure room is constructed and furnished so that these long exposures are automatically controlled for uniformity of dose rate by sensing switches. In addition, the environment is that of a modern motel room so as to minimize the understandable anxiety inherent with confinement.

The first patient to be treated in the new low-exposure-rate total-body-irradiation facility was exposed almost constantly in a 1.5 r per hour ^{60}Co gamma-ray field for 100 hr during 5 consecutive days. He experienced no ill effects and slept well during his entire stay in the facility. His cardiac and pulmonary functions were monitored remotely by electronic devices to detect any signs of physiologic disturbances. None were found. Since termination of radiation exposure his blood platelets, which were about four times too abundant, declined gradually to normal levels.

The new radiation facility not only will be useful in studying therapy of chronic leukemia but also will provide the opportunity to test whether or not total-body radiation delivered at low dose rates produces undesired effects. This information is of significant interest to the National Aeronautics and Space Administration since astronauts could conceivably receive similar low-level exposures during space travel.

TRANSPLANTATION

There are a number of indirect contributions to medicine resulting from the demand for more and more-precise information about radiation effects on biological systems. One of the most important effects of a single large exposure of the whole body to radiation is the prompt but temporary suppression of the function of the bone marrow and lymphoid tissues. Bone-marrow transplants administered after a large exposure to radiation could be effective in promoting recovery, and it was largely the stimulus of this work on marrow transplantation that led to a renewed interest in human-organ transplantation. It is known that lymphocytes are involved in the body's immune response mechanisms. For example, when an organ is transplanted from one individual to another, the lymphocytes of the host initiate the tissue response, which most often results in rejection or failure of the graft. The intensity of this reaction is proportional to the genetic dissimilarity between the donor of the transplant and the host.

In addition to their part in tissue and organ rejection, lymphocytes serve another important function in keeping the body immune from diseases, and they perform a variety of other vital defensive functions. Therefore an irradiated person is extremely vulnerable to infection. His immune system is temporarily crippled. Since radiation destroys the blood-forming cells in the bone marrow, one mode of therapy is to replace these cells by transplantation of undamaged bone marrow. Unfortunately this involves the same immunological problems of graft rejection as in organ transplantation. Since the transplanted bone marrow contains many cells capable of forming antibodies against host tissue, serious damage to the host may follow. These difficulties have until recently allowed only limited success except in genetically alike individuals, such as identical twins or inbred strains of animals.

Scientists at the Oak Ridge National Laboratory and other laboratories have shown that transplanting bone marrow in inbred mice where there is no genetic barrier to overcome can halt or even reverse the process of a disease. In addition to offering a means of ameliorating radiation injury, researchers say that bone-marrow transplants may in the future become a form of therapy for as many as 20 presently fatal inherited blood disorders.

The years of basic research in transplantation immunology may be beginning to finally pay off. From this basic research, techniques have been developed for "typing" the tissue of the patient and potential donor, similar to the way blood is typed. In yet another technique called "matching," cells from a patient are mixed with cells from a variety of potential donors until a donor is found whose cells do not react with those of the patient. As a result of this, several successful bone-marrow transplants between persons who were not identical twins but brothers and sisters have been carried out. Although these limited studies are encouraging, they do not in any way indicate that all the problems have been solved. However, in June of 1969 the future of bone-marrow transplants may be further clarified when a group of specialists will meet to compare their findings and discuss how widely applicable this form of therapy may become.

RADIOISOTOPES AS POWER SOURCES

The heat from the decay of a radioisotope offers an exciting and entirely different opportunity to use nuclear energy in medicine. This heat can be used to provide electrical energy by the principle of thermoelectric conversion or to provide mechanical power by the principle of thermodynamic conversion.

In a healthy heart the rate of beating is controlled by a small node of specialized tissue called a pacemaker. In certain disease conditions an artificial pacemaker is required to deliver small electrical impulses to the ventricle at a preset rate. Up to the present time, surgically implanted pacemakers of this sort have been powered by batteries with an average life of 2 years; so repetitive surgery is required at approximately 2 year intervals. The AEC in collaboration with the National Heart Institute has been supporting the development of an isotope-powered pacemaker system with a lifetime of 10 years or more to reduce greatly the need for repeated surgery. To achieve the specified operating lifetime and at the same time minimize size, weight, and radiation characteristics, ^{238}Pu has been selected as the radioisotope fuel primarily because of its low shielding requirements, the small amount needed, 0.3 g, and its relatively long half-life, approximately 90 years. The nuclear battery for the pacemaker will operate on the principle of thermoelectric conversion. It will provide continuous d-c power that will be changed into suitable electric impulses by electronic means and used in the same manner as in conventional pacemakers.

Interest in artificial organs goes back a number of years; however, recent efforts at human-heart transplantation have focused public attention on the problem of organ replacement. The AEC has joined the National Heart Institute in exploring the feasibility of using radioisotopes to power pumps which could assist or replace the functions of a diseased or damaged heart. Any device for total cardiac replacement involves problems of blood clotting, compatibility with tissues, dissipation of excess energy, weight of the device, and a variable response to changing physiologic needs.

In the radioisotope-powered artificial heart, the heat from the decay of the radioisotope would be used by a thermodynamic converter to provide hydraulic or pneumatic power for the blood pump. The encapsulated heat source might be ^{238}Pu. Other components of the engine would include a heat exchanger using blood as the cooling medium and a control system to regulate the power output of the engine.

In addition to the engine development phase of this program, a concurrent evaluation of the possible early or late effects of irradiation and thermal dissipation from an implanted source is also being conducted in animals.

Up to this point I have been speaking mainly about nuclear medicine — about the applications of radioisotopes, nuclear medicine instrumentation and the use of radiation in therapy. There are, however, some additional bonuses that have evolved from the medical and biological investigators at our AEC laboratories, and to conclude I will touch on some of these briefly.

AGING

Shortening of the life-span appears to be one of the long-term effects of total body irradiation. It is nonspecific in the sense that no single cause of death seems to be responsible for life shortening. So far as can be determined, this life shortening parallels the natural aging processes, and it follows that what we learn about radiation-induced aging might apply to natural aging.

Research at the Oak Ridge National Laboratory has indicated that an important factor in aging is a decrease in the capability of the body to defend itself against foreign substances, such as infectious agents and pollutants. As a result of this research, it appears that aged mice raised in a clean environment are better able to respond to foreign substances than are those which have been exposed to infectious agents and pollution.

Although many experiments have been done on radiation-induced aging in small animals, such as mice, only a limited amount of such work has been done with larger animals that might be more closely related to human beings in terms of their response. Therefore the Atomic Energy Commission is supporting a research program at the University of California at Davis and elsewhere with a large colony of beagle dogs. Besides the portion of the colony subjected to long-term irradiation through the administration of radioisotopes, a significant segment of these dogs has not received any form of radioisotopes and serves as the control population. These control dogs are monitored throughout their life-span and represent a major resource currently being exploited for establishing the process of aging in an animal population more closely corresponding to man than the rodent. This study of the life-span in pedigreed beagles represents the only quantitative evaluation of age-related changes in animals other than laboratory rodents. As a part of the research program, each control dog receives a thorough physical examination, including radiographic survey, at least once each year. This extensive documentation of age-related changes will represent a unique contribution to human gerontology.

Human data bearing on the radiation-induced reduction in life-span (accelerated aging) are few. The largest study of humans is the research program carried out by the Atomic Bomb Casualty Commission in Japan. This study includes 50,000 selected exposed Japanese and their 50,000 matched controls. A subsample of 20,000 (10,000 in each group) of the above 100,000 people is being examined intensively on a biannual schedule because the patterns of morbidity and mortality rates are shifting in Japan as elsewhere. Data from these 20,000 people are finding value as base lines and controls for numerous other medical studies.

ZONAL CENTRIFUGE PROGRAM AT OAK RIDGE

As an outgrowth of the centrifuge development program to separate fissionable ^{235}U from the heavier nonfissionable ^{238}U at Oak Ridge, a whole series of improved centrifuge systems for separating subcellular particles has resulted. This program headed by Dr. Norman Anderson of the Biology Division, Oak Ridge National Laboratory, has made possible the separation of large quantities of relatively pure cell constituents. For example, it is now possible to separate the various molecules responsible for the replication, transcription, and translation of the genetic code.

Just as large quantities of cellular constituents can be separated from a suspending liquid, so can large quantities of nearly pure virus be separated from the culture medium. This has made the zonal centrifuge particularly valuable in virus research. For example, the centrifuge has been used in attempts to isolate the viruses responsible for hepatitis, polio, rabies, the common cold, animal tumors, and other diseases.

Plans and designs for several of the centrifuges are available to industry. Several pharmaceutical firms are using the zonal centrifuge to produce a very much purified influenza vaccine, some of which is now on the market. A major problem with conventional vaccines is that they are not pure but contain large amounts of extraneous material that leads to unpleasant side effects and limits the safe-dose size. Large-scale studies in man are now under way to evaluate statistically the reduction in dose size permitted by the use of centrifuge-produced vaccine and to determine the dosage required to achieve effective protection.

KARYOTYPE ANALYSIS

In the high-energy physics program, millions of photographs are taken of nuclear events as they occur in the bubble chambers. The tedious labor involved in reading this massive number of photographs has presented the physicist with major problems. As a solution an electronic scanner was developed to transfer the image on the film to a computer memory, following which the computer was used to perform the data analysis. This technique has been carried over to medical research, where such analysis would be of considerable benefit in differential blood counts, in analysis of tissue sections, and in evaluating changes in chromosome structure and number.

One of the most interesting and potentially most important medical applications of the electronic scanner—analyzer now being developed is for determining the frequency and type of chromosome changes in cells. Chromosomal changes have been identified as a response to various environmental factors including low levels of external radiation and internally deposited radioisotopes. Quantitative chromosome analysis has heretofore involved a long and tedious procedure of making enlarged prints of photomicrographs, manually cutting out each chromosome print, pairing and assigning the pairs to their positions in the chromosome karyotype order, and searching for visual evidence of abnormality. The difficulties inherent in trying to apply this new automatic chromosome analysis are such as to demand the highest degree of sophistication both in the electronic scanning system and in the computer analysis program. Progress to date at various centers, including the important effort here at Livermore, has been encouraging, and it is hoped that shortly electronic scanner and pattern-recognition machines will be available for widespread use in biomedical research and application.

DOPA

The importance of trace metals to health and disease has been appreciated by clinical investigators for a number of years. However, these investigators have been handicapped by the sensitivity of their analytical tools. Neutron activation analysis has proved helpful to those scientists by enabling them to make precise measurements of extremely small quantities of certain of these elements. The material to be analyzed is placed in a nuclear reactor and bombarded with neutrons so as to cause the elements of interest to become radioactive in a highly specific and identifiable way. Procedures developed at the Brookhaven National Laboratoty have provided better sensitivity and specificity for measurement of the trace metal manganese. The importance of manganese as an essential element lies in its extensive participation in both catalytic and noncatalytic biochemical processes for which this metal is specific.

Among recent investigations of manganese have been those involving studies of melanin-producing tissues. Since melanin formation is defective in the brains of patients with the neurological disease Parkinsonism, efforts were initiated to affect melagenesis and to determine its influence on the disease. One of the agents investigated by Dr. Cotzias and coworkers at the Brookhaven National Laboratory was the melanin precursor dihydroxyphenylalanine (DOPA). They found a surprisingly favorable response to the drug DOPA by patients suffering from Parkinson's disease. The results are very encouraging. About 250 to 300 patients have been treated with DOPA and carefully studied. Roughly one-half of these patients have become self-sufficient. Of the 50% who did not become self-sufficient, the amount of nursing care was significantly reduced.

One can predict that the studies to date on Parkinson's disease and the continuing investigation of drugs similar to DOPA will lead to further understanding of the nature of several crippling neurological diseases.

I have tried to review some of the techniques and advances in nuclear medicine, and, in addition, I have described some of the biological and medical spin-off resulting from work at the Atomic Energy Commission laboratories. It was not possible in the time at my disposal to cover all the material that has come to my attention, which, in turn, must be only a small fraction of the total now known. I am sure that some members of the medical profession who may read the text of these remarks, and perhaps many in this audience, will be familiar with techniques and new developments that I have not covered. This, of course, would be quite indicative of the wide and rapid progress being made in this important field.

I hope and expect we will continue to see the atom used so successfully in these humane endeavors and that the work carried out at the new Biomedical Laboratory here at Livermore will contribute to that store of knowledge needed to advance such important work.

PERSPECTIVES

The introductory session of the symposium is concerned with the peaceful uses of nuclear energy. In a little more than two decades, there has been a tremendous growth of such peaceful applications, and further growth seems a certainty.

The "sword" to be beaten into the "plowshare" and into other incisive tools of biomedical and industrial utility is well known to have two edges. The overriding concern of those involved in the applications of nuclear research and technology, in the health protection of workers and the public, and in the study of basic biomedical implications is that we shall continue to exploit nuclear energy and tools beneficially, with a minimum of present and future hazards to man and his environment.

Dr. Michael May's Introduction to Dr. John R. Totter

Our first speaker is Dr. John R. Totter, Director of the Division of Biology and Medicine for the U. S. Atomic Energy Commission. Dr. Totter spent a couple of years in the 1950's with the Atomic Energy Commission and then joined its Division of Biology and Medicine in 1962, becoming its director in 1967. Prior to coming to the Atomic Energy Commission, Dr. Totter served with distinction in research in the fields of amino acids, bioluminescence, and associated areas at a number of universities in this country and also at the University of Uruguay. His latest position prior to joining the AEC was that of Professor of Biochemistry at the University of Georgia. He is well known to all of us, and we are particularly fortunate to have him here today. I specifically asked him to speak to us about the programs and the goals, both immediate and long-term, of the Division of Biology and Medicine. Without any further introduction, I turn this meeting over to Dr. John Totter.

OBJECTIVES OF BIOMEDICAL RESEARCH IN RELATION TO ATOMIC ENERGY

JOHN R. TOTTER
Division of Biology and Medicine, U. S. Atomic Energy Commission
Washington, D. C.

It is an honor to be asked to speak at the dedication of the new building that houses AEC's latest large addition to its national laboratory biological and medical program.

In the early years of this decade, atmospheric testing of nuclear devices by the United States and the USSR reached a rate that caused some to be concerned that biological damage might result and perhaps might even be reflected in measurable genetic or somatic effects in humans if it were to be long continued. It seemed wise at that time to attach to a weapons laboratory a biomedical division whose director would sit in council with the men whose responsibility was the fashioning and testing of new nuclear explosive devices.

The Lawrence Radiation Laboratory (LRL) at Livermore was chosen to be the site of this new division; and with the enthusiastic cooperation of its then director, Dr. John Foster, and of Dr. Ed McMillan, LRL's Director-in-Chief, it was established in 1963. Under Dr. Foster and now under Dr. May, with the guidance of John Gofman and Bernard Shore, the biomedical program has flourished, and we are assured that the division has been able to influence device construction in such a way that the production of certain potentially troublesome isotopes has been minimized.

The immediate work of the division has changed somewhat with the nuclear test-ban treaty, but its ultimate goals remain the same. There is, of course, the Plowshare program — peaceful nuclear explosives — which has occupied an important fraction of the people engaged. This program may well grow rapidly in importance, and its goal of negligible dispersal of radioactivity associated with the use of nuclear explosives remains of great importance both to the Division of Biology and Medicine and to the Laboratory here.

I was asked to speak about the objectives of biomedical research in relation to atomic energy. The ultimate objectives can be stated in a few words, namely: to learn how to live with radiation and radioactivity inexpensively and surely and with a minimum of hazard or disturbance to people anywhere, and, through applications of atomic energy to biology and medicine, to bring additional benefits to the public.

The accomplishments to date with respect to the first of these objectives can also be stated relatively simply: We have learned to live with radiation and radioactivity but not cheaply, not yet surely enough, and with what appears to be altogether too much disturbance to quite a number of people. And no one appears to believe that this situation will be much changed either quickly, cheaply, or without much intellectual and physical labor.

This is not to say that the accomplishments have been small. Quite the contrary. Twenty years ago everyone in the field of biology, with whom I discussed the future of our understanding, underestimated the progress as enormously as I did.

Twenty years ago the unraveling of the genetic code seemed as remote as the planet Pluto and was certainly not a thing to be accomplished in this century. The knowledge of the amino acid sequence of a protein was also relegated to the twenty-first century, but a few weeks ago the synthesis of a protein — a much more difficult task — was announced by two laboratories. Neither of these triumphs could have occurred for many years without the research and technological advances that grew out of the search for an atomic bomb. Many of the crucial steps in achieving these triumphs were first brought to light in the biomedical programs of the national laboratories.

It is easy to be more specific about the biomedical needs of the atomic energy program. I will discuss first practical requirements related to two phases of the AEC's responsibilities. In the explosives program the production, fabrication, and use of plutonium carries with it considerable potential hazard. Plutonium is perhaps the most toxic metal known which is produced in a relatively large scale. The fabricators of plutonium fuels for the Systems for Nuclear Auxiliary Power Program (SNAP) and other devices can invent and put to use new fuels and fuel forms much faster than the effects of these fuels on biological systems can be determined. With our most useful test animal — the dog — an experimental period of 12 to 15 years is required to explore the long-term biological response to internally deposited radionuclides. The problem of plutonium toxicity is both difficult and pressing. The design of experiments on plutonium toxicity that can provide us in a very few years with definitive information that may be used in connection with any conceivable kind of plutonium-containing fuel to which humans may be exposed in any manner is certainly one of the toughest jobs facing us now. We must also look ahead to other possible SNAP device fuels, such as ^{170}Tm, ^{171}Tm, and ^{210}Po, although the total likely potential exposure at this time does not appear to be so formidable.

Neither should we forget the radiobiological needs related to the nuclear reactor program at the Space Nuclear Propulsion Office. We are now studying effects of fissioned uranium particulates on skin, gastrointestinal tract, and lung tissue by both theoretical and experimental approaches.

A carefully planned research program on the acute and long-term radiotoxicology of various internally deposited radionuclides encompassing different routes of exposure, different chemical and physical forms, and different energies and total doses has been in progress for some years. These studies also look at the age at exposure and at whether the radionuclide is given in single dose or over a period of time. This overall effort is now producing handsomely.

The six or seven laboratories that have been able to keep sustained programs on large animal colonies going for many years without major disruption due to intercurrent diseases in epidemic form and without suffering from an epidemic of boredom on the part of the investigators are to be highly congratulated. An examination of their methods and their success leads to a conclusion one might have anticipated, namely, that a study of what appears superficially to be a simple practical problem can be carried out in such depth and with such scientific rewards that even the most skeptical scientist can be kept happy and productive.

The Division of Biology and Medicine (DBM) genetic program has been little changed in the last few years. It continues to be productive, especially now in the field of dose-rate influence — a fact that has eased somewhat the fear that mutations were always and inevitably linearly related to the dose by the same constant however and whenever given.

It does not seem likely that the genetics program will be much diminished for some time to come since the research is protracted because of the nature of the tests used and because the variables to be tested are numerous.

Exciting developments in this area are probably to come in the fields of molecular genetics — a field that is no monopoly of the AEC, although we have several strong groups that are making significant contributions.

Related to this, of course, is immunogenetics, a field in which the AEC has supported several strong contenders. Already the stimulus to this field from cell-transplant studies, largely conducted in the DBM program, has resulted in practical applications in human heart and kidney transplants. It is expected that steady progress will be made in our ability to treat radiation-accident cases with foreign bone marrow — still our most hopeful method of treatment of those accident cases which happen to receive radiation over nearly the whole body in the range of one to two lethal doses.

In the areas of interest to AEC which involve movement and transport of radionuclides, there seems to be a limitless need for new knowledge. Our previous knowledge of the movement of most elements in the air, in the ocean, and on the land was fragmentary before the advent of radionuclides to act as tracers. The contributions to atmospheric science and to oceanography made by studies of the movements of radionuclides are enormous, and the potential for further discoveries has scarcely been touched.

Terrestrial ecology, likewise, has undergone a rejuvenation with this new tool — so much so that one of its major subdisciplines is called radioecology.

It is obvious that the AEC must be able to document the movement of all radioactive isotopes by whatever method the movement occurs. The growing nuclear industry will bring with it many new problems with respect to alteration of the environment — some that we may not clearly foresee as yet. One which now draws much attention is that of thermal alteration. Research on this is slow and just beginning, but imagination concerning its possible ill effects is operating at supersonic speeds. At any rate the complexity of the problem posed by relatively large-scale thermal change provides as wide a scope for the ecologist to convert it to a beneficial influence as it does for the forecaster of doom.

In the area of biochemistry or molecular biology, there is clearly much to be done. This field, of course, finds much support from other government agencies since it provides basic information needed not only to understand and combat the effects of radiation but also to understand the underlying processes in physiology and in the pathology of all diseases from those of metabolic origin to cancer and aging. The advances in this field will surely be the most exciting and of the most lasting importance. One day we may find that this effort will provide the key to reversing damage or restoring to their unharmed state tissues or organs or whole bodies that have been subjected to doses of radiation now considered to be severalfold the lethal amount. Certainly we can see no alternative route likely to lead to that end. Whether or not that end is reached, however, the researcher in the basic field always has an unbounded optimism — amply supported by the history of science — that even though he may not reach a specific long-range goal, the new knowledge derived from his work will be of ultimate benefit.

Of course, one can predict with some assurance that the solution of enough of the complex problems posed by living organisms to provide us an easy means to reverse the effects of radiation will not come quickly. We therefore expect that the need for AEC's support of basic chemical research into living things will expand and continue into the indefinite future.

Up to this point I have indicated something about the major parts of the AEC biomedical program as it looks to us now. I believe it is evident that the AEC will continue to require a biomedical program and one which should expand to fulfill the increasing needs foreshadowed by a burgeoning nuclear power industry.

It is necessary, however, to look at AEC's requirements in the context of other national needs and desires. The availability of these objectives must be assessed in the light of the fact that our programs in various fields fully occupy the attention of a significant fraction of the scientific competence available in that field. If other national goals take precedence over AEC's needs, then undoubtedly some compromise has to be made. We will either have to reduce some of the AEC programs in order to release competence required for other purposes or will have to bend the direction of the programs so that the goals of other agencies may be met.

The AEC has a long history of collaborative effort with the Department of Defense and more recently with other agencies. In biology and medicine we have collaborative programs through interagency agreements with several institutes of the National Institutes of Health (Department of Health, Education and Welfare), Housing and Urban Development, National Aeronautics and Space Administration, and the Department of Defense.

Several years ago a joint program between the National Cancer Institute and the Biology Division at Oak Ridge National Laboratory was set up followed by similar programs with other national institutes. When Battelle–Northwest assumed responsibility for the Hanford Laboratories, a new kind of contract was devised for the operation of the installations which permits multiple agency support and provides a ready means for other agencies to make use of special competence available at Richland.

Still more recently the Atomic Energy Act was amended to permit more latitude for AEC in conducting work for other government agencies. The trend in this direction is accelerated by the makeup of the national laboratories where one can find strong, well-developed basic research in the physical and biological sciences allied with the highest quality engineering and production staffs. The very nature of the captive Atomic Energy Research and Development Program lends itself admirably to the present day needs of several government agencies new and old, which had never in the past required the services of so vast and varied a complex as is represented at our major laboratory and production facilities.

I will discuss briefly a few of the areas in which there are signs pointing to a most interesting future.

In the field of genetics, heavily supported by AEC because of the mutagenic effects of high-energy radiation, there are portents that suggest that the day of simple pharmacologic testing of chemical additives is nearing an end. There is a growing belief that perhaps some of the preservatives or other additives, purposefully or accidentally added to prepared or natural foods, may be just as mutagenic as ionizing radiation. Where would one turn for the large-scale testing in mammals to determine whether or not a chemical in food is mutagenic? Only the AEC has really conducted such tests on a large scale. In Europe some nations have started barring chemicals that have been used for years. Currently we hear about the uneasiness of the U. S. Food and Drug Administration over the great increase in intake of sugar substitutes.

Modern man has greatly lengthened his average life span by finding ways to reduce the stress on himself as an organism. He has succeeded in these endeavors largely by diverting the stress to his environment. Because the environment is a much larger reservoir, he has managed for several generations to remain almost scot-free from the consequences. Now, however, we are becoming increasingly apprehensive lest the insults to our surroundings lead to retaliation on a massive scale. The knowledge that humans are great gamblers does nothing to reduce that apprehension — and we have no sure way of knowing just when or how the dice will fall.

In fundamental environmental research the AEC has one of the very few integrated programs to be found in the United States. A large fraction of the available talent is AEC supported. One has only to compare the rosters of AEC's contractors with the U. S. International Biological Program's first committees to realize how broad and inclusive is our program in environmental research. This talent is not, of course, waiting for leadership from AEC to plunge into the problems of pollution. We do look forward to the possible linking of this kind of fundamental research to the engineering and production facilities and expertise in the AEC programs just as is already happening with the molecular biology segments of the DBM-supported efforts.

In this respect I recall what Dr. Dunham, former director, Division of Biology and Medicine, 1955 to 1967, often pointed out, namely, that molecular biology was after all only intracellular ecology.

I am confident that the small beginnings already evident will eventually enlarge and develop to the point where we find a suitable part of the AEC scientific and engineering staffs making valuable contributions to the more general needs of the nation — helping to solve problems and applying the solutions in areas where we have so far only conducted studies.

This new segment of the AEC's programs at Livermore as you will see is broadly based with developing projects in many of the areas that I mentioned. I am confident that it will take its place with our older biomedical laboratories and contribute fully to meeting both AEC's needs and those related to our wider national problems.

Dr. Seaborg will speak on some of the advances provided by the DBM programs in the past. The talk will not resemble at all the one I have just given. I am also confident that when some successor of Dr. Seaborg, 20 years or so from now, tells of the advances of the next two decades, he may scarcely mention the success in meeting the needs I have outlined. One takes for granted that the necessary effort required to meet them will be expended. The exciting things will be those which may have little relation to present programmatic requirements but will represent the triumph of someone's mind over the "tyranny of necessity." In view of the record I have for prophecy, which was mentioned earlier, my petition for a license as a "forecaster of assurance" was denied by higher authority. You are invited to have your own dreams.

PLANNED APPLICATIONS OF PEACEFUL NUCLEAR EXPLOSIVES

GLENN C. WERTH
Lawrence Radiation Laboratory, University of California,
Livermore, California

ABSTRACT

The basic objective of the Plowshare program at the Lawrence Radiation Laboratory is to explore possible industrial applications of nuclear explosives. The approach is through the development of an understanding of the effects of nuclear explosions on the environment, including the fracturing and movement of the rock, the disposition of the radioactivity, the effects of the seismic waves on structures, and the effects of the use of these explosives on man. Potential applications of nuclear explosives are conveniently defined by the depth of emplacement of the explosive. Deep emplacement produces the nuclear chimney, an underground cavity surrounded by fractured rock not extending to the surface. A promising application is the stimulation of gas production by breaking up rock in gastight reservoirs. The Gasbuggy experiment demonstrated the feasibility of the idea, and several other projects are in various stages of planning or preparation. Other possible applications include the breaking up of ore bodies for leaching, the in situ retorting of oil from shales, and terminal gas storage. Intermediate emplacement produces the "retarc," a cone of fractured rock extending to the surface. Proposed applications include the breaking up of ore bodies near the surface for leaching, the production of aggregate, and dam building. Shallow emplacement produces the crater, and a row array of such explosives has been demonstrated to produce a ditch. Applications include the construction of harbors and canals, including the proposed sea-level Panama Canal project now under study by the U. S. Atomic Energy Commission. One important aspect of the Plowshare program is the development of testing experience leading to the development of a capability to predict the effects of nuclear explosions under a variety of conditions. Through such work commercial application of nuclear explosives, fully responsive to the protection of public health and safety, is anticipated.

The U. S. Government has an enormous investment in the technology connected with nuclear explosives. This technology encompasses the designs of the explosives, the materials that have gone into them, the fabrication procedures, the testing procedures, and the engineering and manufacturing procedures. In 1957 this Lawrence Radiation Laboratory proposed to the U. S. Atomic Energy Commission that, in view of this substantial investment of the national resource, some small effort should be devoted to exploring the possibility of whether or not these explosives could have value to the nonmilitary economy, namely, to industry and for civil purposes. That is the basic concept behind the Plowshare program. Now we have some 200 scientists and engineers at the Laboratory engaged in this effort.

The goal of the program is to develop a basic understanding of the effects of nuclear explosions on the environment, including the fracturing and movement of the rock, the disposition of the radioactivity, the effect of the seismic waves on structures, and, most important, the effect of the use of these explosions on man. And therein, of course, lies the common interest with the biomedical program. When Plowshare plans an experiment on the Nevada Test Site, or plans joint experiments with industry or other government groups, we predict the levels of radioactivity and carry out experiments only if the levels are consistent with established guides. We are very pleased that the Bio-Medical Division here at the Laboratory is looking behind those guides and learning more about the processes on which they were based. By such work here and elsewhere should come a better understanding of the adequacy of these guides. The weapon programs as well as Plowshare will, of course, honor any revisions of such guides.

In discussing the proposed applications of nuclear explosives, we have divided the applications into three categories defined by the depth of emplacement of the explosive. These categories are shown in Fig. 1. If the explosive is placed deep in the ground, a nuclear chimney is formed. If the explosive is placed at an intermediate depth, rock is broken to the surface. On the other hand, if the explosive is placed at a more shallow depth, craters are produced. Basically, the main applications derive from the ability of the nuclear explosive to break and move rock.

The basic processes of chimney formation are displayed in Fig. 2. The explosive is lowered down a drill hole, and the drill hole is cemented up. The energy of the explosion generates a shock wave that, as it propagates away from the center of detonation, vaporizes the rock. As it continues to move outward, it loses its energy, and then only melting of the rock occurs. With further loss of energy, the shock wave fractures the rock and finally simply propagates as a seismic wave without producing permanent changes. Left behind in the so-called "cavity" is the vaporized rock at a very high pressure. This cavity expands, reducing the pressure until it balances the stresses that exist in the rock. This pressure may approximate the weight of the overburden rock, but in some cases it may be higher, depending on the

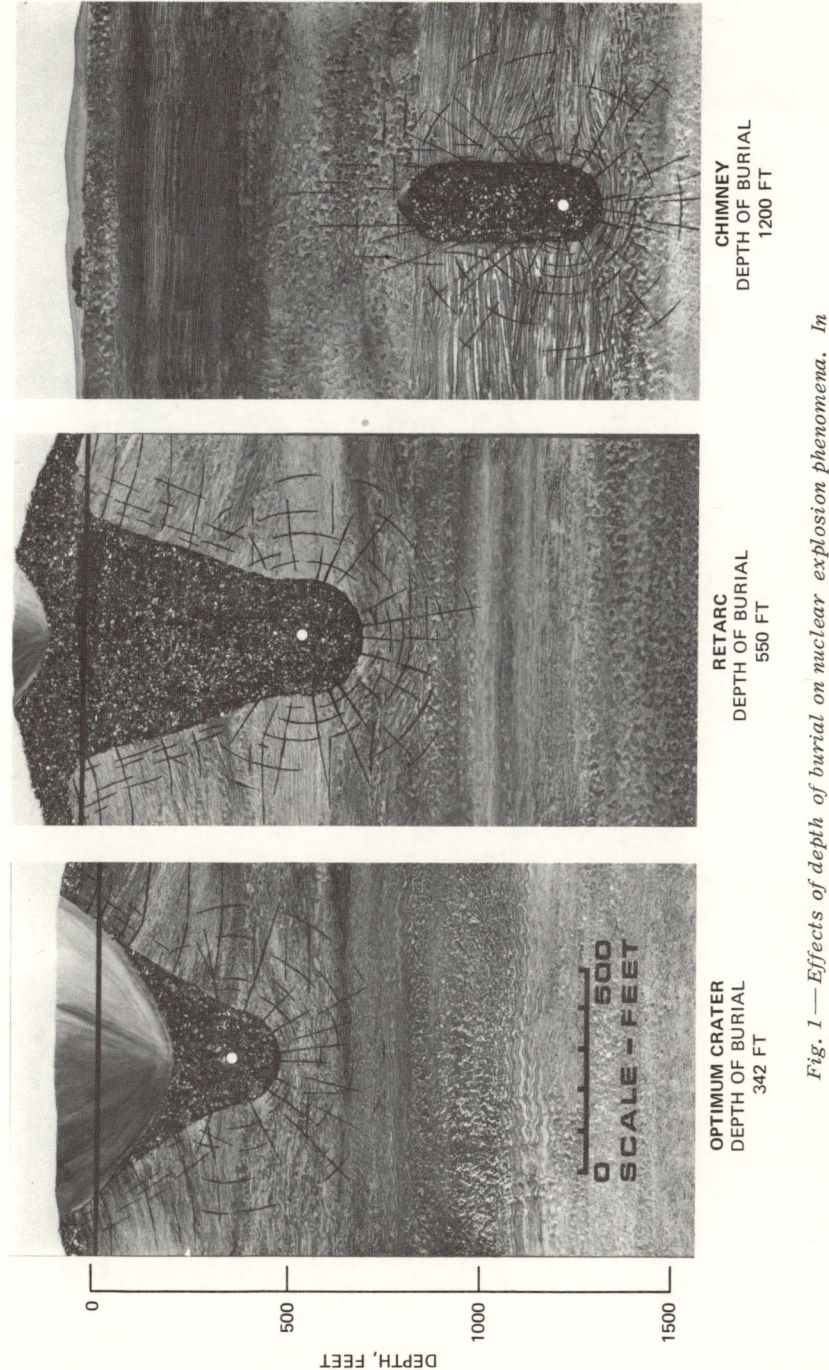

APPLICATIONS OF PEACEFUL NUCLEAR EXPLOSIVES 33

Fig. 1.—*Effects of depth of burial on nuclear explosion phenomena. In each case a 20-kt explosive was buried in dense dry rock.*

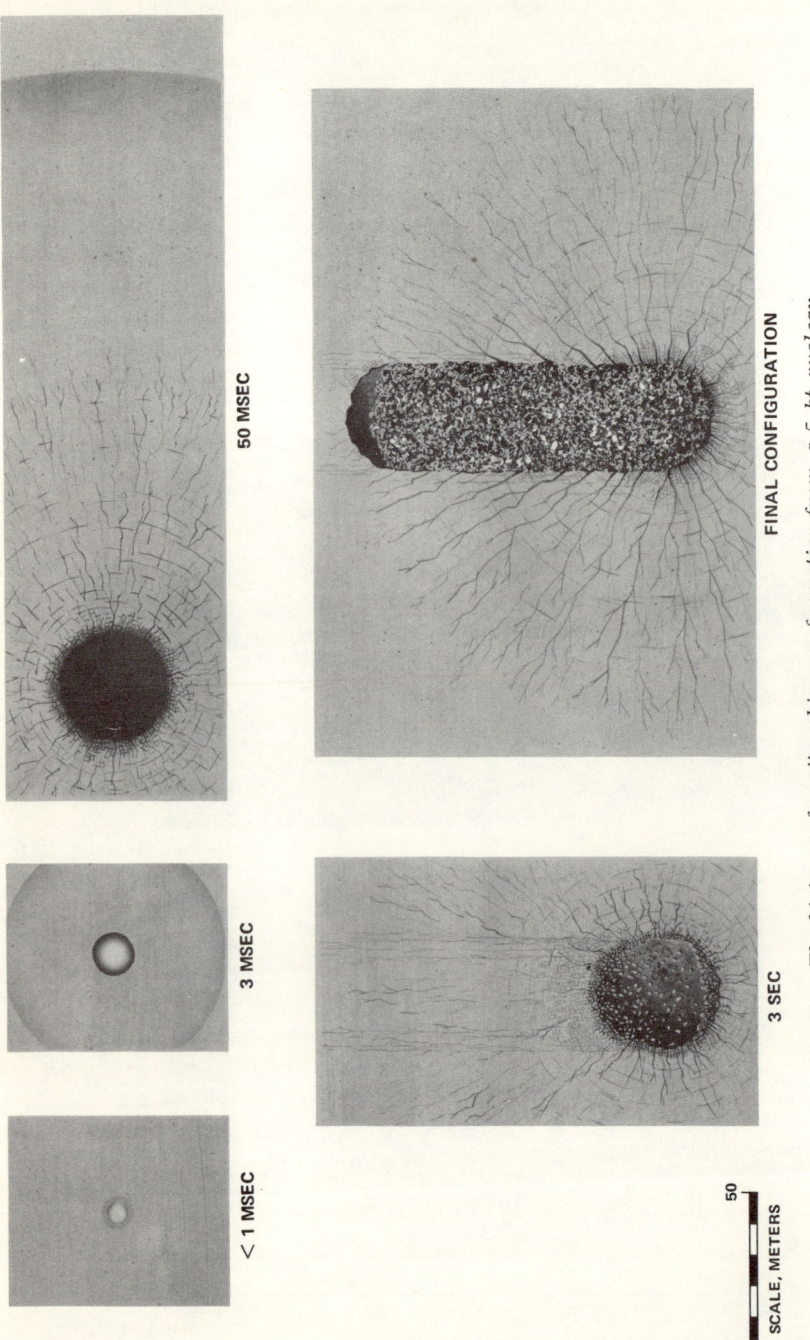

Fig. 2—*The history of cavity-chimney formation from a 5-kt nuclear explosion in granite.*

tensile strength of the rock. The molten rock drips down to the bottom of the cavity. Since the outgoing shock wave has weakened the rock, the roof falls in, and, as it falls in, it produces the final configuration of the chimney. In most situations the height of the chimney is controlled by the extent of the fracturing.

On the first underground explosion, Rainier, we mined down into the lower cavity boundary to find out what happened to the radioactivity. In Fig. 3 the frozen rock is dark; the light regions are rocks that fell out of the ceiling of the cavity. Some 90% of the particulate radioactivity is trapped in the solidified glass rock. Many people have inspected this cavity region of Rainier, and it is still a highlight of visits to the Nevada Test Site.

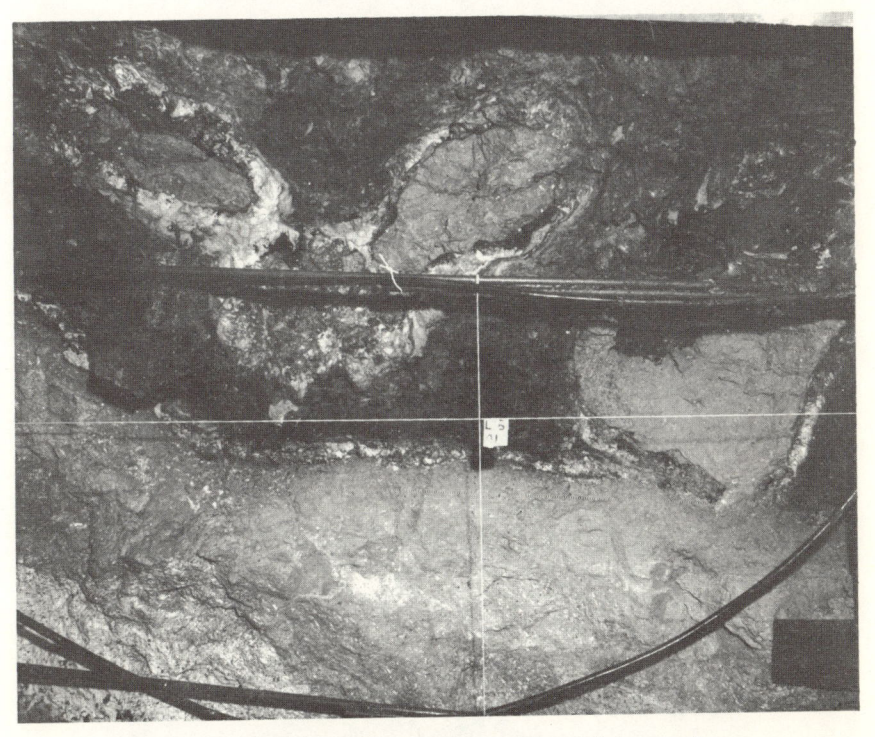

Fig. 3—The melt at the bottom of the Rainier cavity.

The chimney region has been explored in the Hardhat event, which was 5 kt in hard brittle granite. The preshot rock is shown in Fig. 4, and the broken rock in the postshot chimney is shown in Fig. 5. Some of the radioactive gases are located in the chimney region, and, before any such chimneys can be used, they must be flushed out. This broken

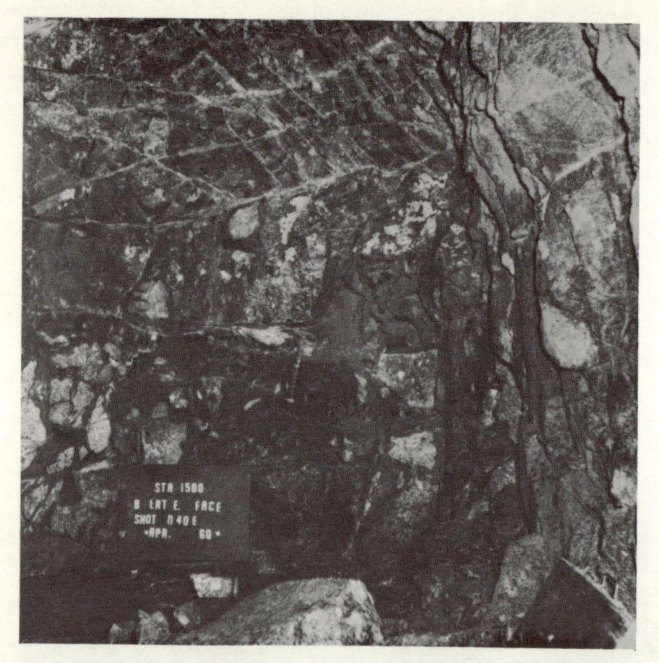

Fig. 4—*Rock at the end of a preshot drift for Hardhat.*

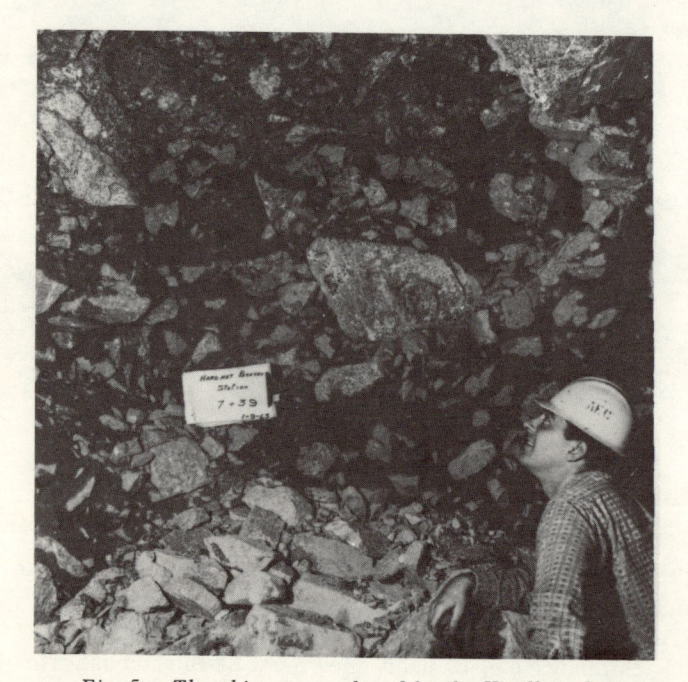

Fig. 5—*The chimney produced by the Hardhat shot.*

APPLICATIONS OF PEACEFUL NUCLEAR EXPLOSIVES 37

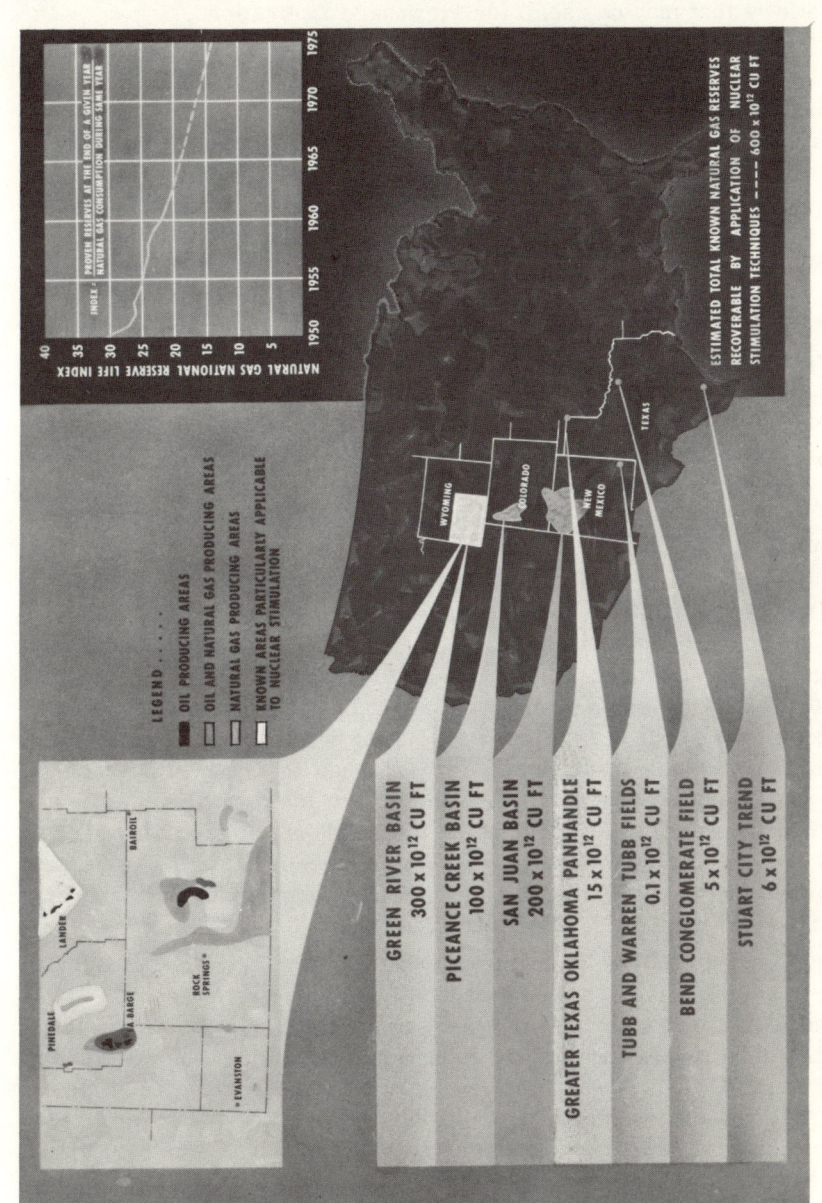

Fig. 6.—An estimate of the total U. S. natural gas reserves recoverable by the gas-stimulation technique. The graph gives the natural gas national reserve life index.

rock in the chimney and the surrounding spherical fracture region are the effects that may be useful for Plowshare applications.

The application that is of most interest to industry is gas stimulation, namely, the use of a nuclear explosive to break up the rock in a natural gas reservoir where the rock is so impermeable that the gas does not flow easily to the wellhead. The reason that U. S. industry shows such an interest in gas stimulation is indicated in Fig. 6. The natural gas national reserve life index in the graph is calculated by dividing the proved reserves in the ground by the annual rate of gas consumption and gives a measure of the number of years of gas supply left, assuming no increase in consumption and no new fields. Currently the index is down to around a 15- to 20-year supply. When you consider the number of major cities in the United States which are heated by natural gas, and the fact that natural gas cannot yet be economically transported from abroad (though some progress is being made with tankers for liquified gas), you understand the reason for the interest in Plowshare by the major gas producers. It is a tough application — certainly not a straightforward one that we would have suggested as a first effort. But it is the one industry wanted, and they cite the reservoirs of gas in Colorado, Wyoming, New Mexico, and Texas where this nuclear gas stimulation might be applicable.

An example of this concept was the Gasbuggy experiment in New Mexico. The Pictured Cliffs gas-bearing sandstone is at a depth of 4000 ft below the surface and about 300 ft thick. It is a very tight rock. It does have about a 10% porosity, but its permeability is very small; therefore the gas flows very slowly through the rock. Over geologic time, gas in the reservoir has flowed into the natural fractures and from there now flows to the wells. The principle of gas stimulation is that, instead of gas from a 6-in.-diameter well, a nuclear explosion allows production from a chimney 160 ft in diameter or rather from a fractured region 1000 ft in diameter.

This was the experiment proposed by the El Paso Natural Gas Company and executed Dec. 10, 1967. There was not enough gas in place to make it an economic operation for the company, but they suggested doing an experiment at 4000 ft before tackling one at 12,000 to 20,000 ft. At 4000 ft we can make many more measurements of the effects of the explosives than would be possible at greater depths, and thus more can be learned about gas stimulation. There was no question at any time that Gasbuggy would be an economic venture — it was simply an experiment to learn about the effects of nuclear explosives in that environment. The main purpose of Gasbuggy was to determine the extent of the fracturing and the increase in production. On drilling back in and tapping into the top of the chimney, we found gas to be produced as shown in Fig. 7. Production could be maintained at a rate of

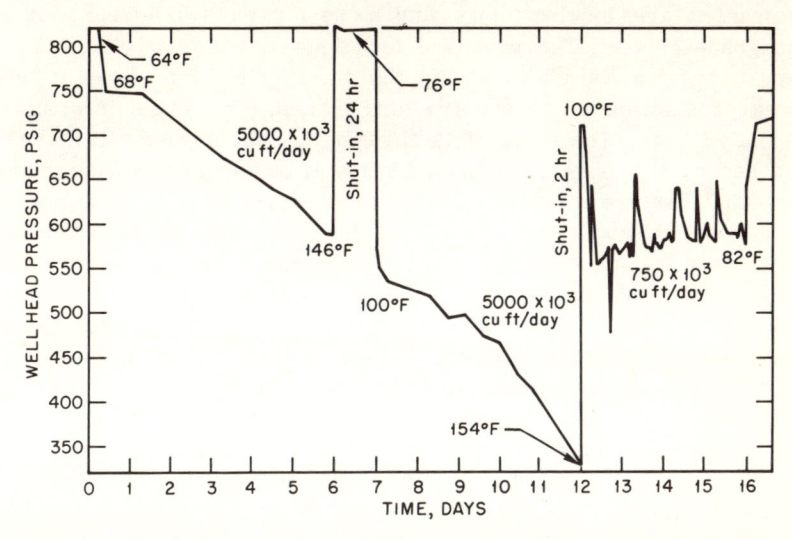

Fig. 7 — The results of the postshot gas-flow test on the Gasbuggy project. Production figures on the curves are in thousands of cubic feet per day.

750,000 cu ft/day. Although there were only a few days of production, this rate of gas production was 15 times what it would have been from a normal well in that location. Thus production from the reservoir was stimulated. Later production data (July 1968 to July 1969) show that we have produced 240 million standard cubic feet; however, the bottom hole pressure is dropping. It could be that in the very tight rock we are rapidly draining the natural fracture system. Nonetheless, in a year of production some 240 million cu ft of gas has been produced from the Gasbuggy chimney. Over a 10-year period, a conventional well nearby produced only 81 million cu ft. We have had a substantial increase in production.

One must conduct experiments in various kinds of gas reservoirs to understand gas stimulation. Gasbuggy is primarily a fracture-controlled reservoir. Dragon Trail, another experiment in the planning stage (with the Continental Oil Company), is a matrix-controlled reservoir; that is, the gas flows through the whole rock and not through the fractures in the rock. Another experiment in preparation is Rulison, in which the gas is contained in isolated rock lenses 50 to 100 ft thick. The Wagon Wheel and Wasp projects are under study for the Pinedale formation in Wyoming, and here the lenses are said to be over 100 ft thick.

Another potentially important application of nuclear explosives is the breaking up of ore bodies for leaching. The United States is the largest producer of copper in the world. With the rise of nationalization and the expropriation of foreign mining investments, our copper companies are looking more and more for ways to develop our own low-grade copper. The proposed technique is shown in Fig. 8. In our experiments in Nevada, we found that the rock has a tendency to break along preexisting joints and fracture planes. The copper is primarily deposited here. Therefore it is thought that the copper will indeed be exposed by the fracturing and that it will be possible to pass the acid through, dissolve and leach out the copper, pump it to the surface, precipitate it, and recirculate the acid. The precipitation of copper is a very old technique dating back to the Romans. Since the ore first has to be broken up, leaching has usually been done on the dumps or in old mines that still contain lower grade ore. But the nuclear explosive provides a technique for doing it underground, which avoids the huge waste dumps on the surface. It is becoming increasingly important not to clutter up our landscape with such dumps. We are hoping that copper companies will want to proceed with a copper-leaching experiment.

The storage of gas is another important possible application. We transport most of our gas from Louisiana and Texas into the northern tier of states. The pipelines are very expensive — up to 200 to 300 million dollars for a single pipeline. The gas companies are faced with providing storage on the terminal end of such pipelines and along the way because, during winter cold snaps that may last 2 or 3 days, the demand for gas increases sharply. To meet this demand the companies must either install another 200 to 300 million dollar pipeline or build a storage facility. They do both. One of the common techniques in the northern states, such as Pennsylvania and Ohio, is to pump the gas back underground into old, depleted natural gas fields for storage and then pump it out as needed. But those gas fields have been used up and other storage techniques must be found. The nuclear proposal is shown in Fig. 9. An impermeable formation must be found; in it the nuclear explosive will be used to produce a chimney that subsequently can be flushed to remove the residual radioactive gases. Then gas can be stored and used as needed.

The use of nuclear explosives to make available the oil contained in the oil shales of Colorado, Wyoming, and Utah is another important potential application. In the United States we had oil reserves of 31 billion barrels before the Alaskan finds. If the importation of oil into the United States stopped, we would have an 8- or 9-year supply left from production in the lower 48 states and southern Alaska. That is not very much oil when you consider how dependent on it our economy is. So the Alaskan oil finds are very important, but the transportation problem must be solved. The other possible new source of domestic oil is from oil shale, which, if developed by nuclear explosives, would yield 160 billion barrels and increase the U. S. reserve from 31 to over 200 billion barrels. We would then have a bountiful supply of oil and be independent of imports.

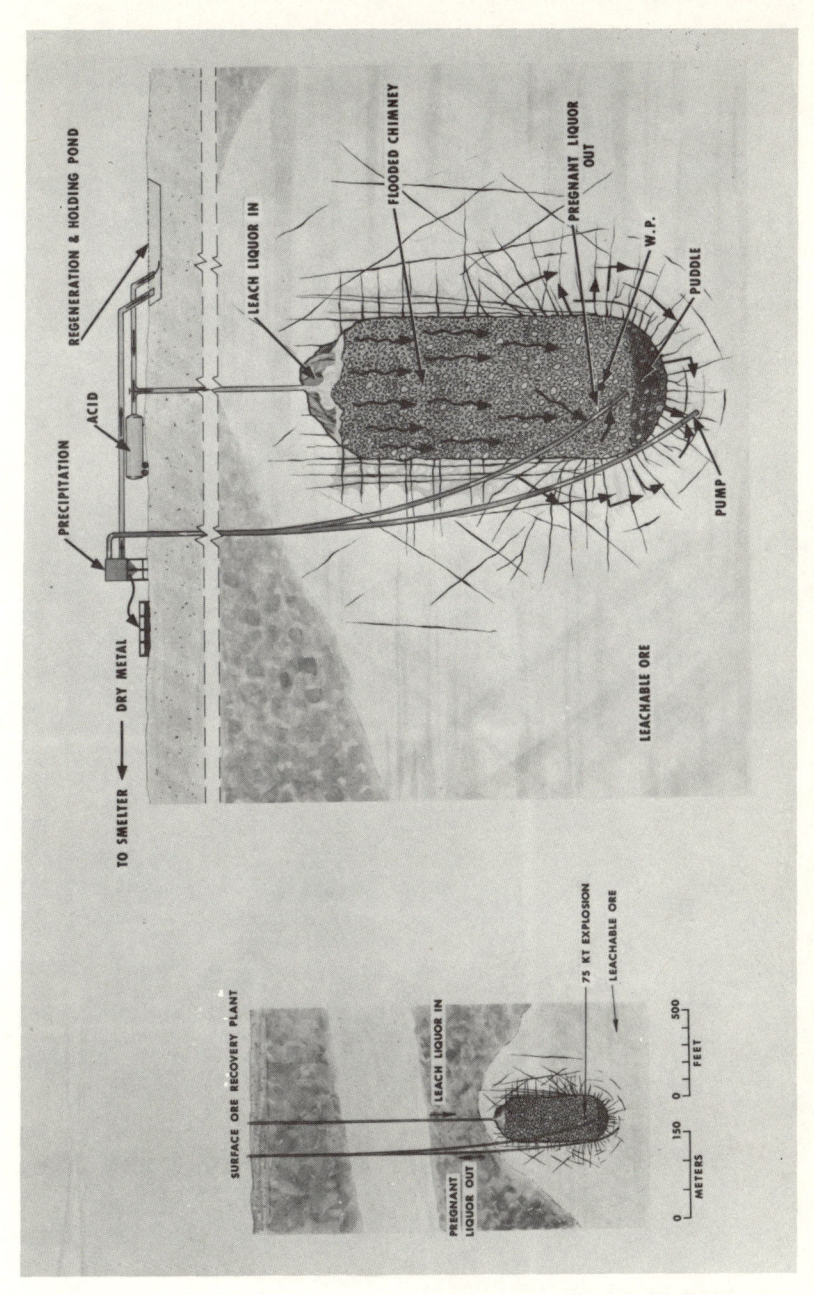

Fig. 8—The proposed technique for in situ leaching of copper ore.

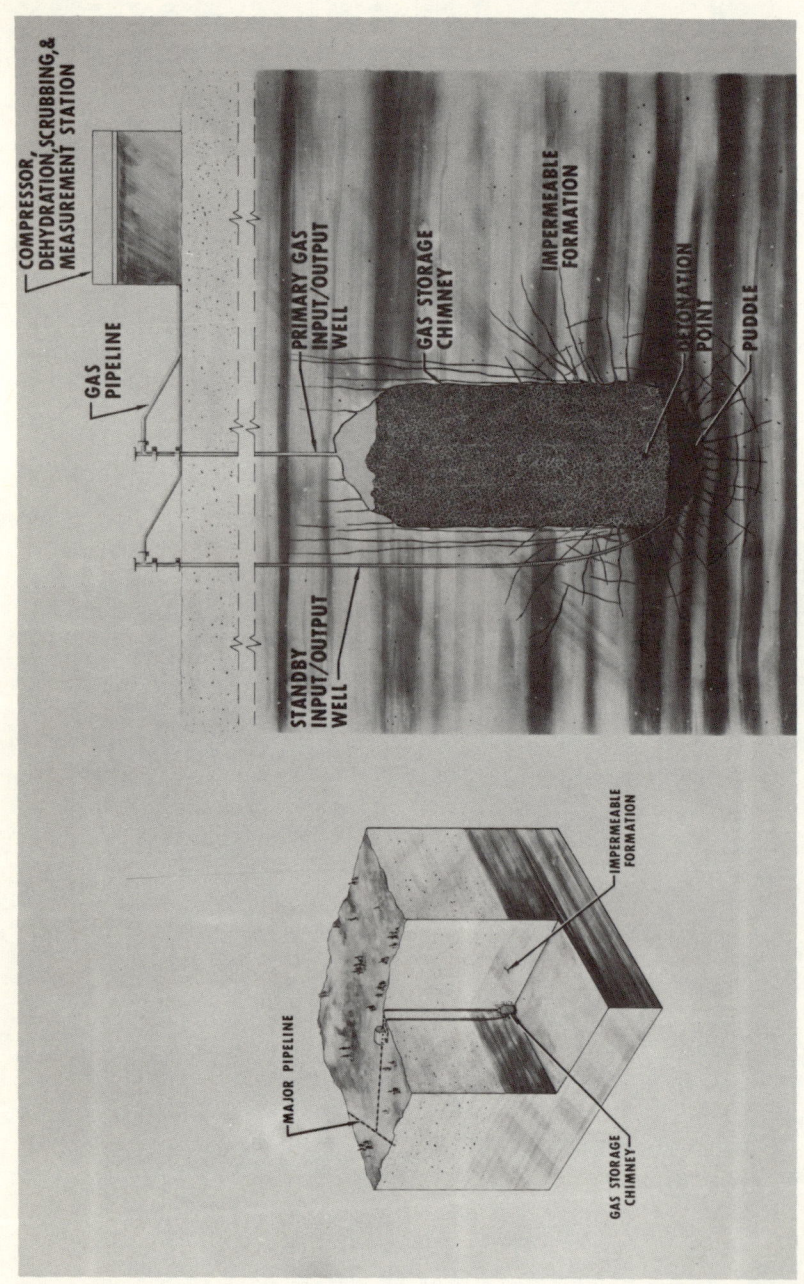

Fig. 9 — *The proposed technique for terminal gas storage.*

The idea in the oil-shale technique is again to break up the rock underground with the nuclear explosive so as to produce a chimney. Then, in one of several schemes, natural gas would be led down from the top, mixed with oxygen, and ignited. This starts the fire; then the gas is turned off because the combustion process is self-sustaining. The heat from that combustion is pulled down through the chimney (Fig. 10) and heats the oil shale in this region to about 750°C. The oil should bubble out as a mist that can be recovered from the gas stream. The residual carbon sustains the burn as it proceeds on downward. There are also other oil-shale techniques, such as passing through hot methane that raises the temperature of the shale so as to release the oil. What the nuclear explosion does is simply to break up the oil shale. This is a well-designed experiment in terms of its nuclear phase, but unfortunately the contract negotiations seem to be bogged down over patents, leases, and other nontechnical issues. We simply have to wait for removal of these stumbling blocks.

Bureau of Mines investigators, working with some of our people at Livermore, have studied the retorting phase. They packed appropriately sized blocks of oil shale into the 10-ton retort (shown in Fig. 11) and started the burn from the top down, simulating a very small pilot-scale nuclear chimney. They were amazed to get out 90% of the oil. They were able to penetrate and burn deeply into the big blocks, which means good recovery with very little requirement for air; that is, there was no packing or matting of the ash to impede the flow of air and hence the burn. These results are very encouraging. The Bureau of Mines has built a 100-ton retort that will be operational in a few months, and we shall be interested to see the results.

The second category shown in Fig. 1 is intermediate depth of burial. Since the surface is much closer, the reflected shock wave is stronger and causes the cavity to expand upward, throwing the rock into the air, and producing a broken cone of rock up to the surface. The name "retarc" has been given to this rock configuration. The sequence shown in Fig. 12 is for brittle rock, which after it is broken occupies a larger volume than before. If this were in alluvium or some other soft rock that occupies about the same space after fracturing as before, a subsidence crater would appear on the surface. Figure 13 shows the retarc formed by the Sulky explosion (100 tons) at the Nevada Test Site. The depth of placement was 90 ft; the mound was 20 ft high and 160 ft in diameter. An application of this technique might be to break up a copper-ore body that is near the surface. Cones of broken rock such as these extending to the surface would allow percolation of the leach solutions through the ore as shown in Fig. 14. Another possible application of a retarc is shown in Fig. 15. The explosive would be buried in the side of a hill to fracture rock and pro-

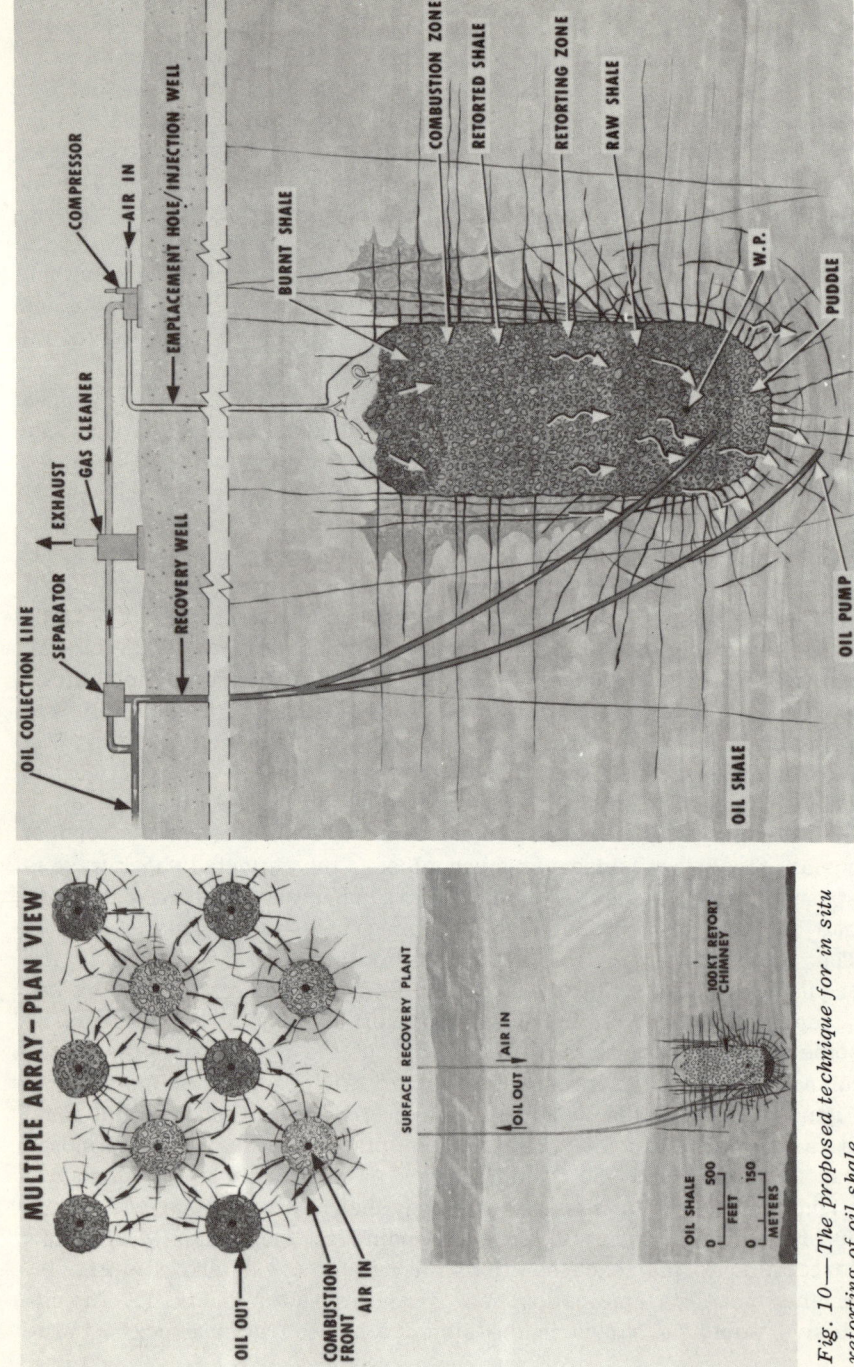

Fig. 10—*The proposed technique for in situ retorting of oil shale.*

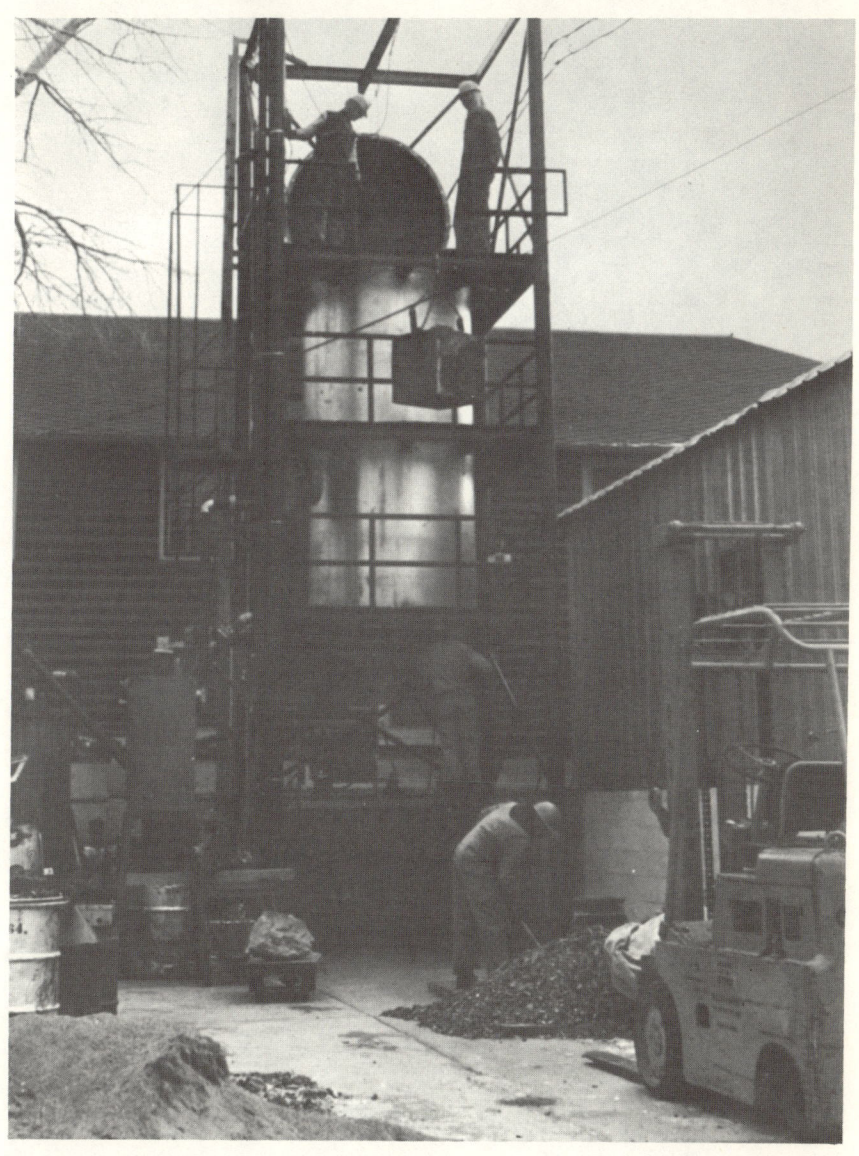

Fig. 11 — Loading the 10-ton retort for the oil-shale retorting experiment.

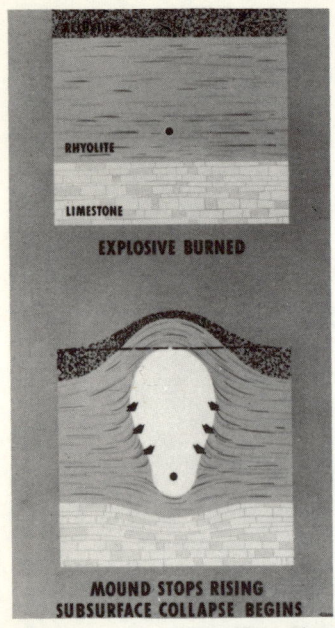

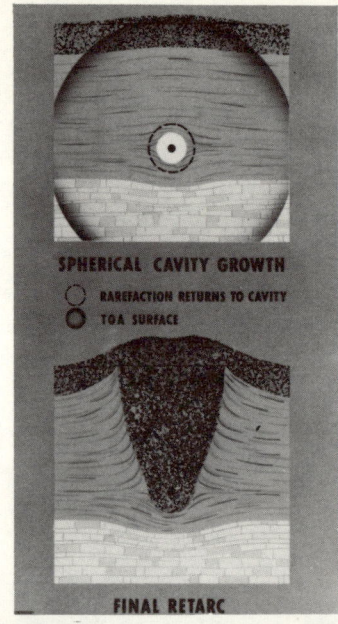

Fig. 12—The formation history of a retarc.

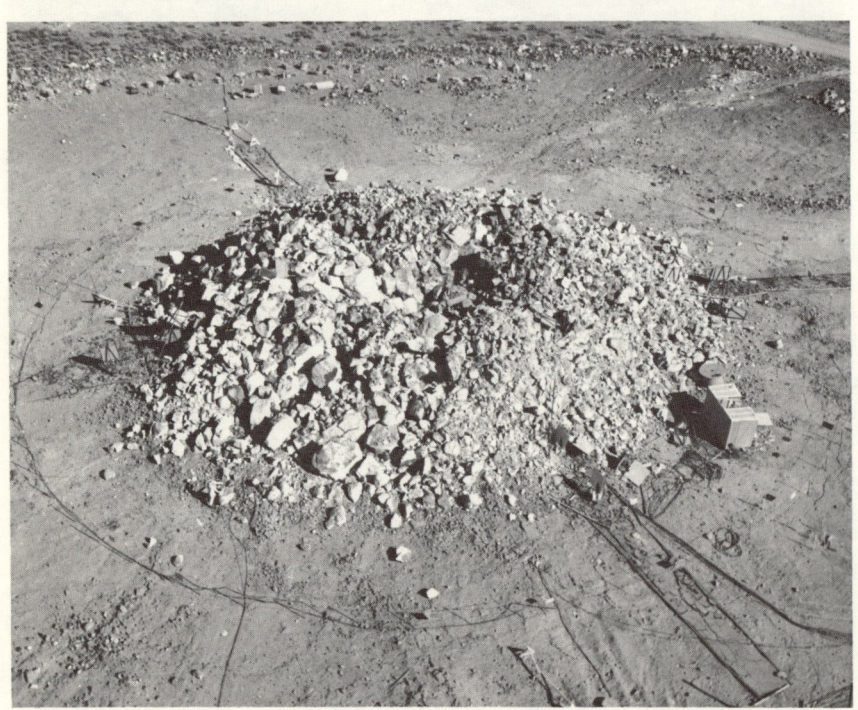

Fig. 13—The Sulky retarc.

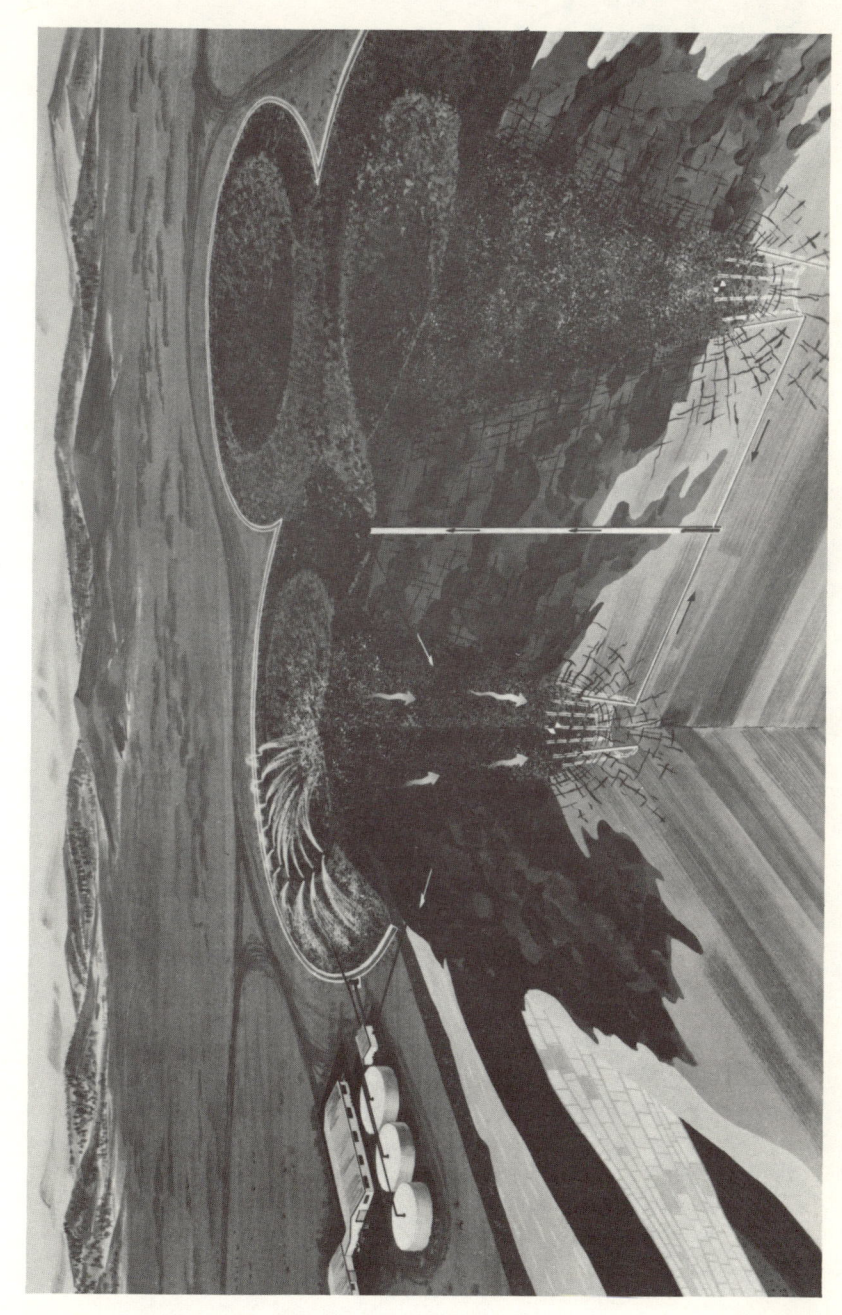

APPLICATIONS OF PEACEFUL NUCLEAR EXPLOSIVES 47

Fig. 14 — *A scheme for using retarcs for in situ leaching of ore.*

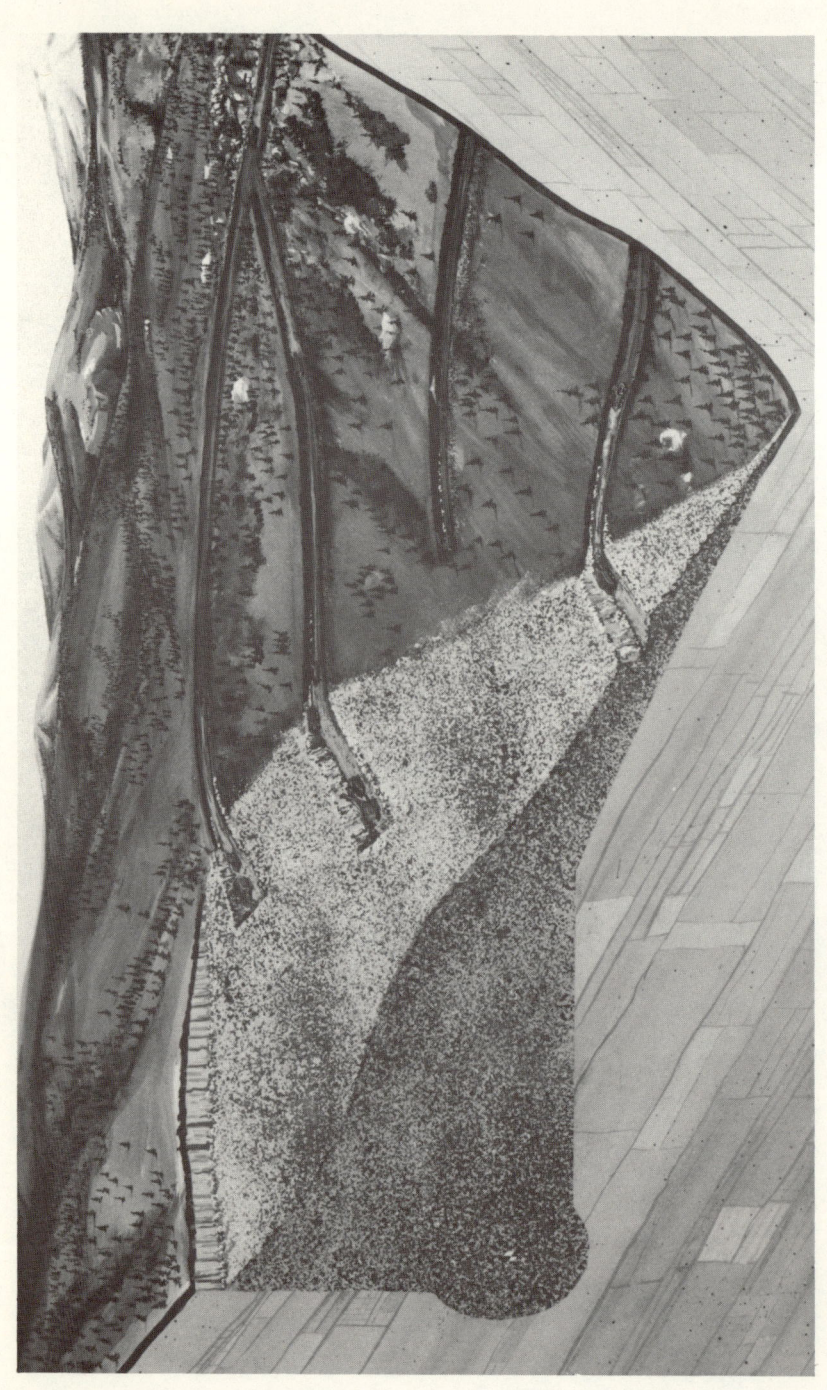

Fig. 15—A scheme for nuclear quarrying by retarc formation.

duce aggregate for use in an earth-filled dam, for road building, or for other needs.

Another and more difficult application of the retarc technique is in building dams. In a canyon with an appropriate cross section, an explosive buried on one wall will blow the rock across the canyon, filling up the canyon. The upstream face could subsequently be sealed. The process is illustrated in Fig. 16. There are engineering questions about this potential application because the weight of the water on the dam face will tend to settle the dam, and this may cause problems. We are very interested in what the USSR has done with high explosives to build dams by this technique. About 2 kt of high explosives were used to build the dam shown in Fig. 17. The USSR effected the sealing of the dam by putting silt and dirt in upstream and letting the water carry it down to clog up the pores of the dam. They claim this to be a very economical and quick way to build dams.

The third category shown in Fig. 1 is cratering. The cratering process (Fig. 18) is similar to the retarc formation process. Because the detonation is close to the surface, however, the rock above the shot point experiences high velocities and is thrown out, producing a crater. As this rock falls, it scavenges most of the radioactivity and holds it in the fallback region. Our understanding of cratering processes has been developed through a series of cratering experiments: Danny Boy, Sedan, Cabriolet, and Schooner. But our most exciting experiment in cratering is the Buggy experiment, a row-cratering experiment designed to produce a ditch that simulates a harbor or a section of a canal. Five explosives, each about 1 kt in size, were placed at a depth of 135 ft, 150 ft apart. The resulting ditch, shown in cross section in Fig. 19, was 855 ft in length, 65 ft in depth, and 254 ft across. An aerial view of the crater is shown in Fig. 20.

The big excavation project that we have been contemplating for many years is a nuclear-excavated sea-level canal between the Atlantic and the Pacific Oceans, either through Panama or Columbia. A Presidential Commission, established in 1965 to study the project along with the Atomic Energy Commission, has spent some 24 million dollars on site investigations. These studies, which include extensive biological studies, will be concluded in the next year and a half. It is too early to know what the results will be.

Those are the anticipated Plowshare applications at this time, but we are not merely thinking up applications here and going out to industry and saying, "How about putting a bomb down a hole and seeing what happens." That would not be a responsible Plowshare program, and we do not operate that way. Most of our 200 scientists and engineers are engaged in developing a basic understanding of the effects that I have briefly described here, that is, developing a detailed

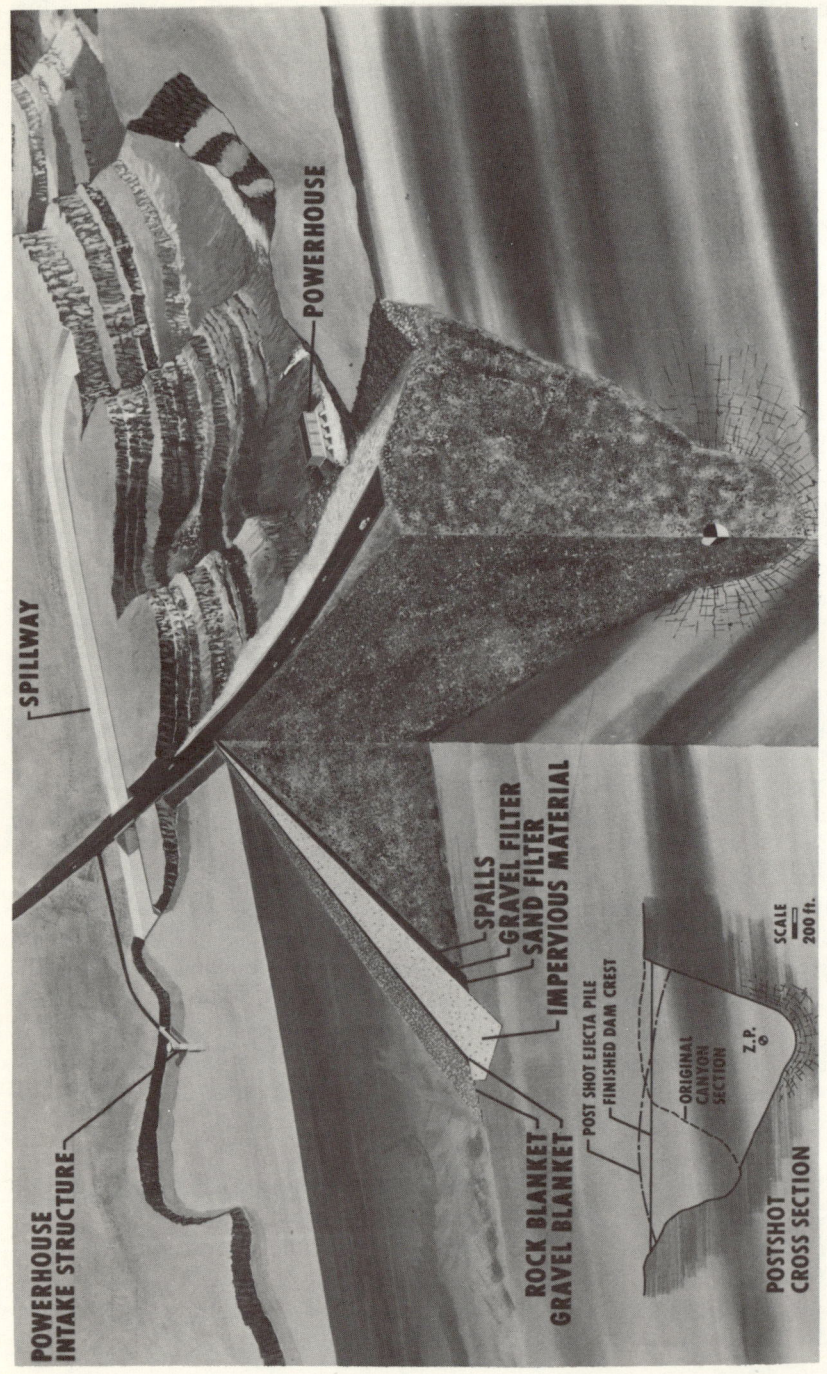

Fig. 16—*A scheme for construction of a dam by retarc formation.*

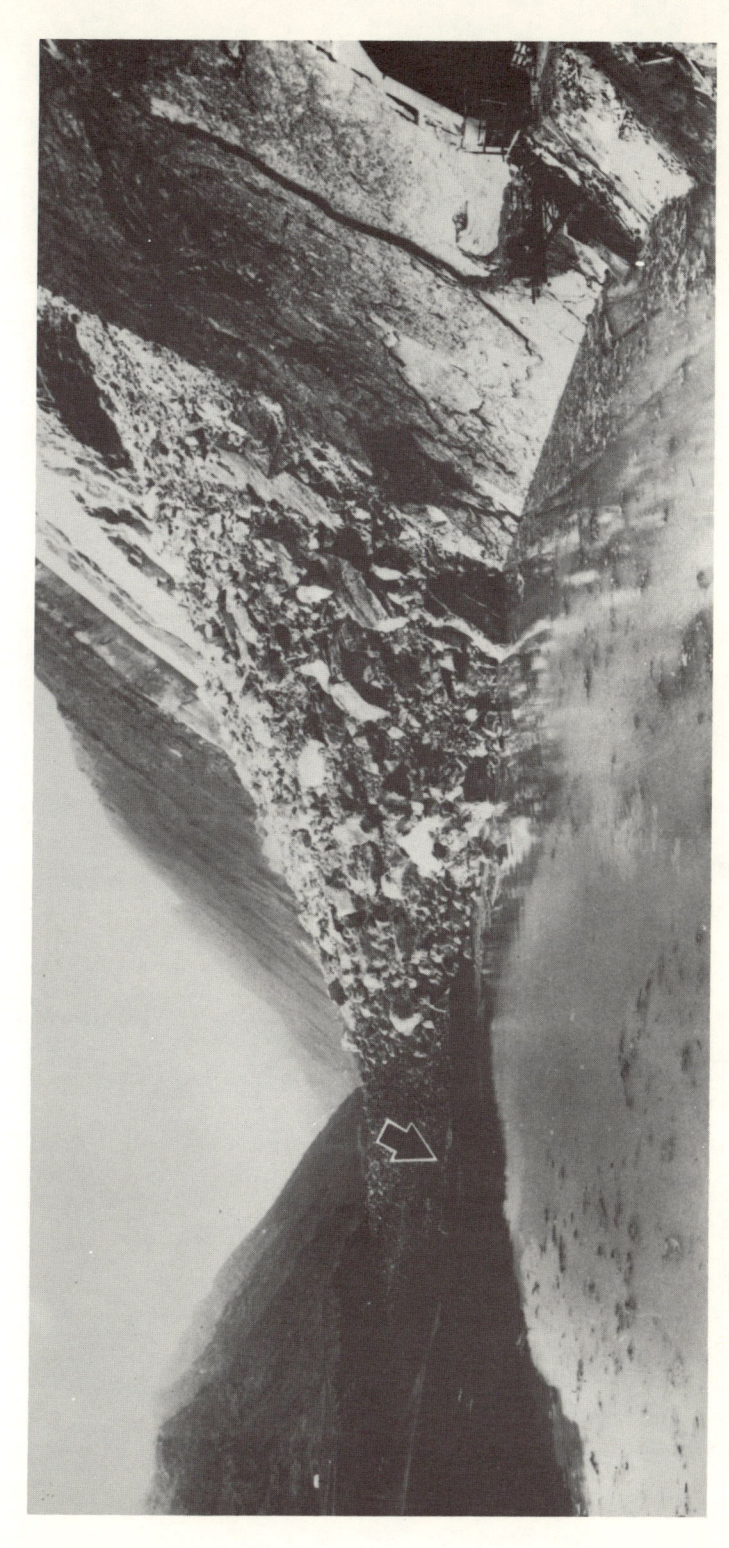

Fig. 17 — The USSR dam on the Vakhsh River, formed by ejecta from high-explosives detonations. (Reprinted from Engineering News-Record, p. 24, May 30, 1968, copyright McGraw-Hill, Inc.)

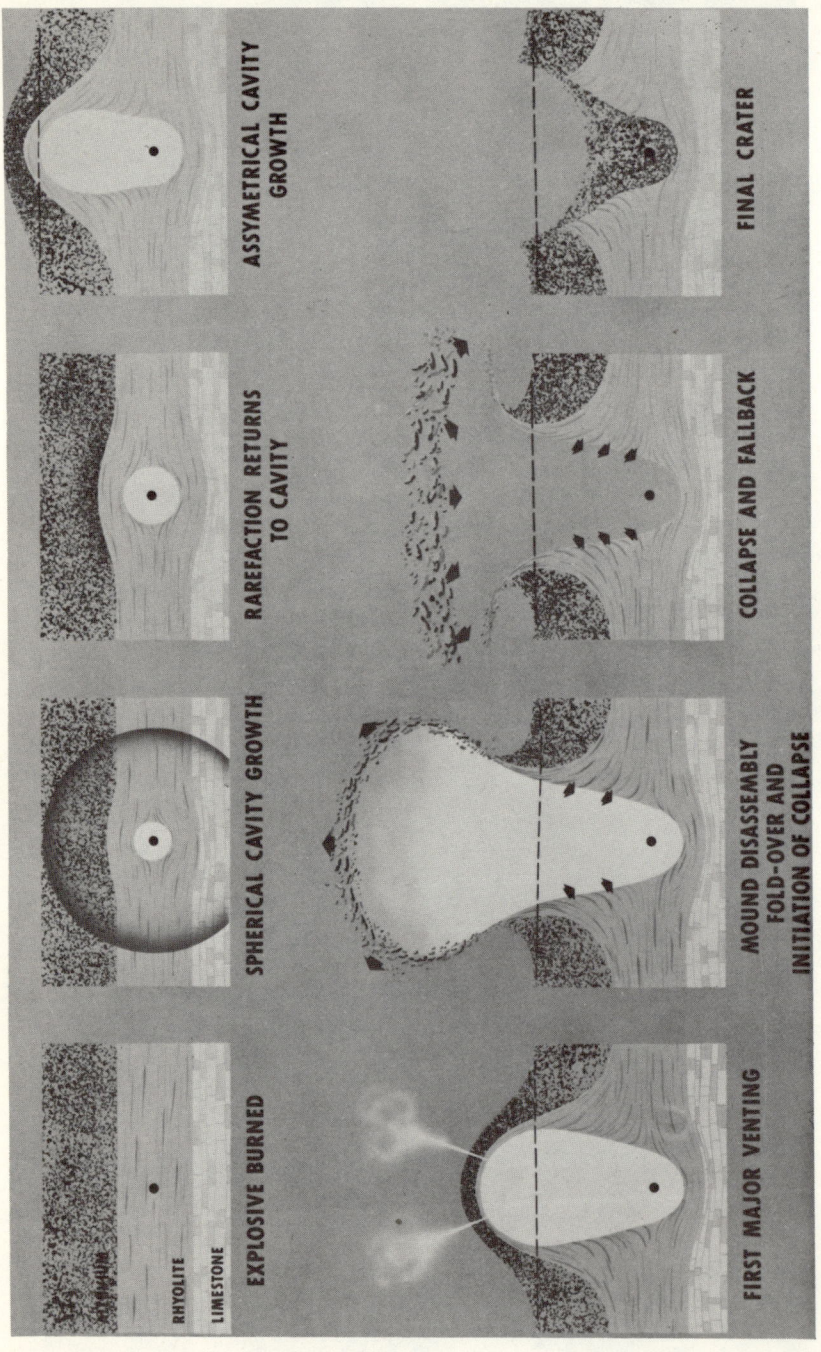

Fig. 18 — *The history of crater formation.*

APPLICATIONS OF PEACEFUL NUCLEAR EXPLOSIVES 53

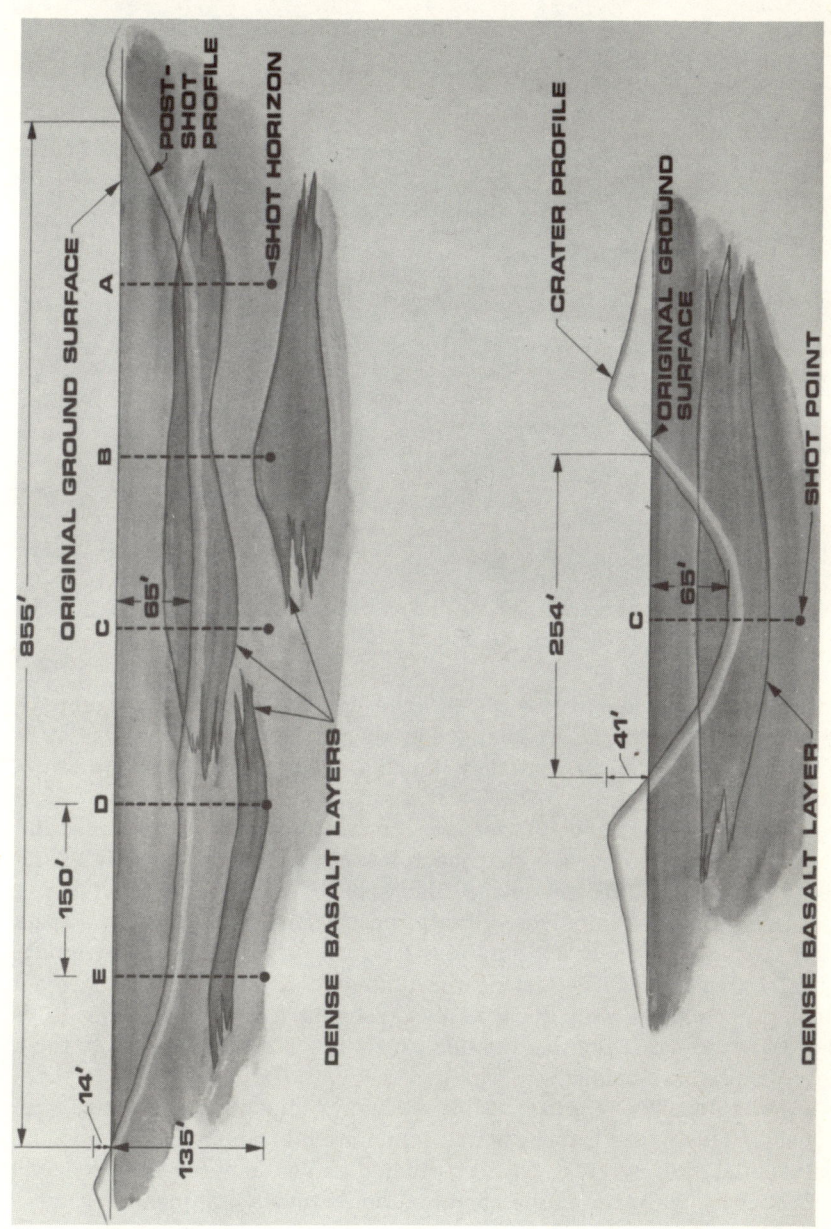

Fig. 19—Diagram of the Buggy experiment. Upper, longitudinal section. Lower, cross section.

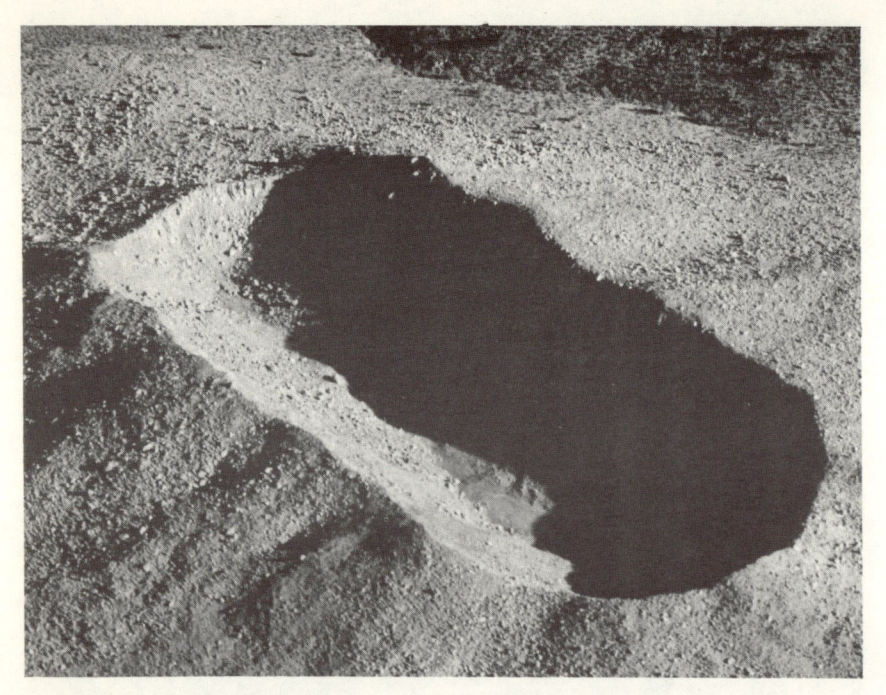

Fig. 20—*Aerial view of the Buggy excavation.*

understanding of the outgoing shock wave that vaporizes rock and melts it. Answers are sought to such questions as: How far do the fractures go? What controls the chimney height? What is the strength of the outgoing seismic wave? What is the size of the air blast wave? How are buildings damaged? These are the important questions, and the most important really are the questions concerning radioactivity. So the Plowshare program under the sponsorship of the Division of Peaceful Nuclear Explosives of the Atomic Energy Commission spends a great deal of effort, not only at the Lawrence Radiation Laboratory, but elsewhere, in investigating the distribution of radioactivity from nuclear explosions with the goal of developing a predictive capability. The Bio-Medical Division studies the fate of the radioactivity from these nuclear explosions.

I will describe a little of this work on radioactivity, starting with a description of the Gasbuggy gas stimulation experiment. At the gas-analysis laboratory (Fig. 21), we studied extensively the gas produced by Gasbuggy. We isolated the chemical constituents and measured their radioactivities so that we could learn about the radiochemistry of Gasbuggy. We found that the radioactivity, particularly the tritium, is lower by about a factor of 15 than we had anticipated. But we had very little way of knowing what to anticipate in Gasbuggy. We had two

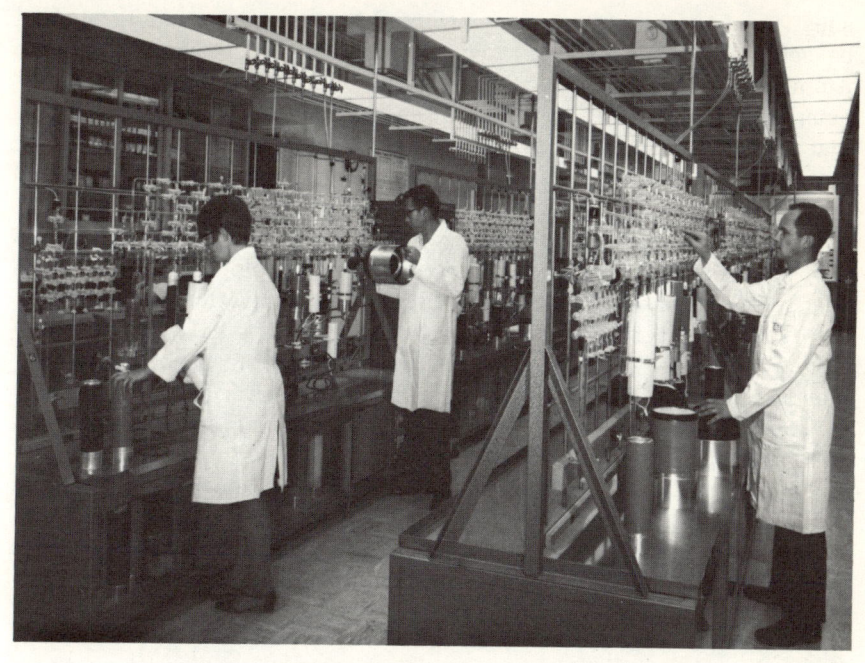

Fig. 21 — *The Plowshare gas-analysis laboratory.*

models. One suggested that, when the chimney fell in, the chemical reactions would cease because the temperatures drop; this apparently was not the case. There was continued exchange of tritium and hydrogen after chimney collapse, and more of the tritium went into the water than was anticipated. Consequently we had a pleasant surprise because, as gas is produced, the tritiated water can be easily removed and disposed of. Regulations of residual radioactivity have not yet been set for utilization of the gas. Of course, all gas wells within a 5-mile radius of Gasbuggy were removed from the normal distribution pipelines. Since no regulations have been set, it is hard to say whether we have adequately controlled radioactivity levels. Certainly one could produce gas and convert it locally to electricity, because that should require much less restrictive controls on radioactivity. However, the home consumption of gas is a different matter.

The explosive used for Gasbuggy was designed for military purposes. It is not a suitable explosive for gas stimulation because a low residual tritium explosive is needed. Further work is planned on Gasbuggy to reduce the radioactivity by flushing the chimney region. Reduction of radioactivity is also achieved by dilution with gas from other fields. There is no question of achieving zero radioactivity because gas already contains naturally occurring radioactivity. It is a question of levels, and we are concerned to see where those levels will be set. If they are set very low, then industry and Plowshare, and the Atomic Energy Commission have been wasting their time in considering the home-consumption market. If they are set at some values that can be attained in practice, we may very well have a technique that can significantly increase the natural gas reserves in the United States.

The ideal way of controlling the radioactivity from excavation projects is not to produce the troublesome isotopes. We have been designing and testing special explosives for excavation that minimize the troublesome fission products. In fact, we now have a most spectacularly "clean" explosive, which was used in the Schooner experiment at 35 kt. Additional work in making still further reductions in troublesome radioisotopes is possible, and we are continuing toward that goal. On excavation experiments extensive measurements are made of the distribution of radioactivity. The local fallout field is measured using a system of 50 remotely located sensors that can be interrogated from a central control point. One such sensor is shown in Fig. 22. Fallout trays can be remotely opened and closed on com-

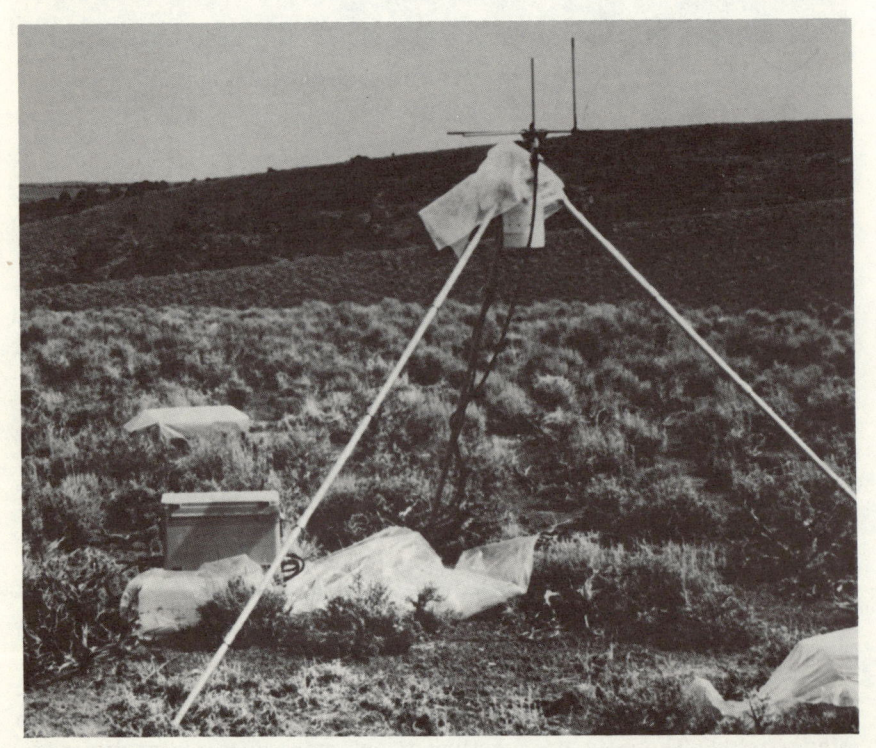

Fig. 22—A remote gamma sensor (on the tripod). The large package under the tripod is the power pack.

mand at each of these locations. Other radioactivity measurements are made on the base surge.

There is also extensive sampling of the airborne debris by aircraft. On a recent experiment we had quite an armada — some 17 different kinds of aircraft participating, flying some 41 different missions. A new development, which is quite exciting, is to drop from a small plane a package of 10 air samplers, which are timed to open at different levels in the cloud, thus obtaining 10 different samples as a function of height in the cloud. The samplers are shown in Fig. 23. On Cabriolet we dropped 422 samplers, of which 256 were recovered.

The fraction of radioactivity that is vented is a function of the shot depth and the water content of the material. If we know this fraction and the wind direction, we can compute the hot line. The computation compares very well with the field measurements. An example is shown in Fig. 24. So the prediction of the fallout based upon the amount of vented radioactivity, I think, is under good control. We have been working the last several years on the long-range diffusion of fallout — what happens out to time periods of 2 to 4 days. The results shown in Fig. 25 are for a reactor run on the Nevada Test Site, which released about the same amount of radioactivity as did the cratering shots, such as Cabriolet. Many of the samples were not taken directly in the hot line; so they lie below the curve. Predicting the concentrations along the 120-km path of collection is an important task. Rainout can also be included in the calculation.

Plowshare has also pioneered in the area of developing a relative significance index — rating the various isotopes according to their biological significance. These tables have to be updated, and the biomedical program is doing just that. From such work we can determine what radionuclides should be eliminated from future explosive designs.

With the map shown in Fig. 26, we can summarize the deeply contained engineering projects. We have executed Gasbuggy, the Rulison contract has been negotiated, and Dragon Trail has been fully designed. Studies are progressing on the two Pinedale projects with the El Paso Natural Gas Company and the WASP Company. Further experiments include Bronco on oil shale, Sloop on copper leaching, and Ketch on terminal gas storage. The Columbia Gas System storage experiment is looking for new sites in other states and perhaps elsewhere in Pennsylvania. As far as the canal is concerned, the two principal routes under study are 17 and 25, the latter being the route through Columbia. (See Fig. 1, Tamplin's paper, this volume.)

We are most pleased to have the biomedical program at the Laboratory because it is very useful to have investigators doing the background work on the guides on which we base our projects.

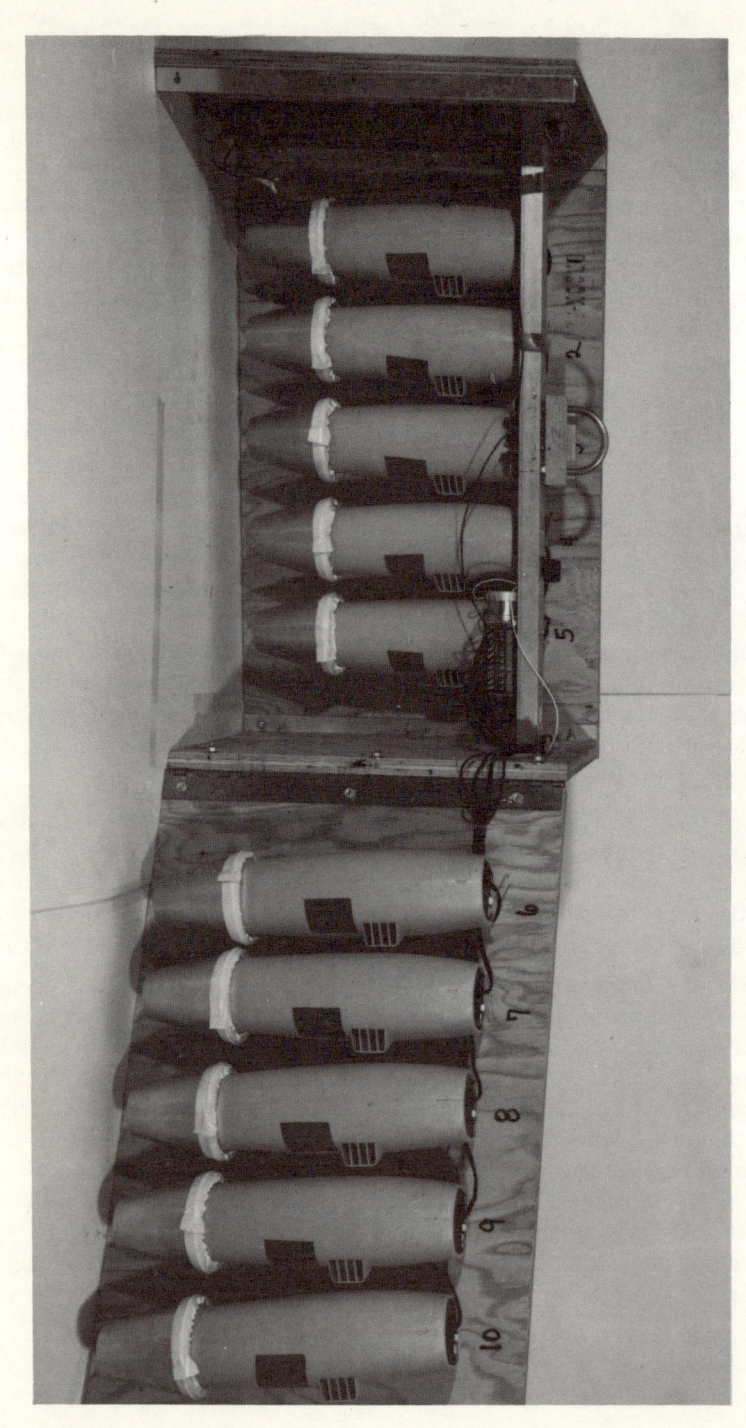

Fig. 23—The sampler assembly for the air-drop package.

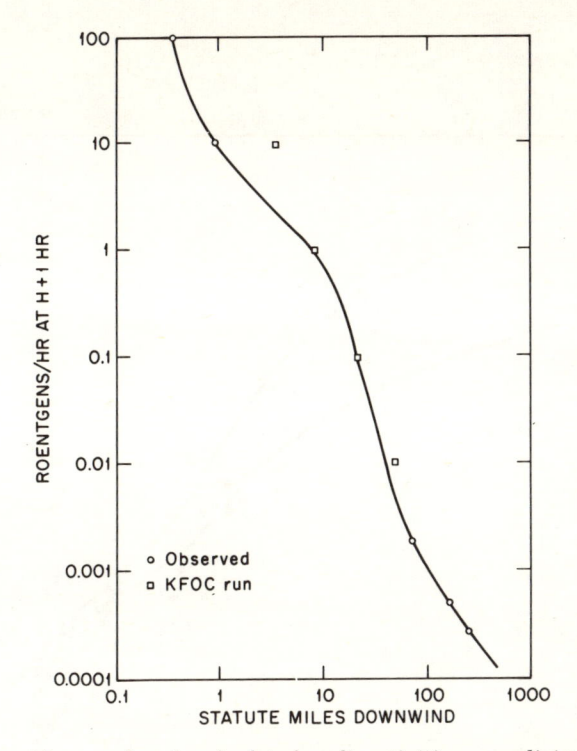

Fig. 24—Measured and calculated radioactivities vs. distance along the hot line from ground zero for a test shot. The KFOC is a predictive numerical computer model for close-in fallout.

DISCUSSION

PARTICIPANT: In addition to the consumption of the existing natural gas reserves, is there not an expectation for increased usage in the future in place of some of the uses of gasoline and fuel oils in order to decrease air pollution?

WERTH: Natural gas is much cleaner than fuel oil. In many cities, most recently in the Metropolitan New York area, the burning of high-sulfur fuel is no longer permitted. Therefore they are switching to natural gas. Of course, in the long-range future, the petrochemical industry looks at itself as a chemical industry. Petroleum gas and oil will be used as a base for chemicals more than for heating.

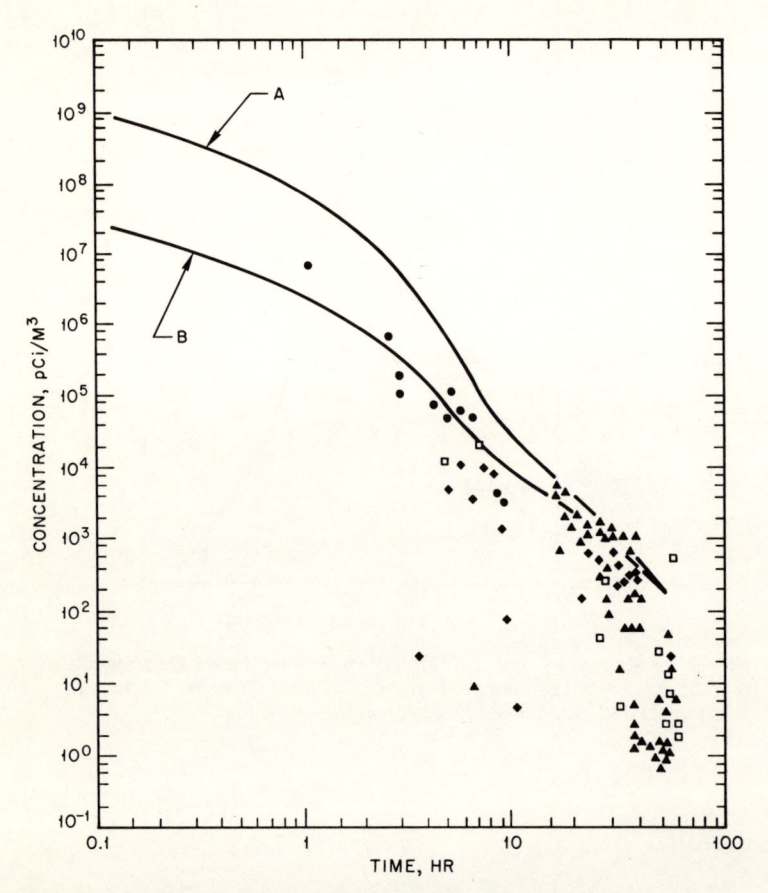

Fig. 25—Measured and calculated activities vs. time for a reactor release. The activities were collected on aircraft-mounted filters. Curve A, calculated concentration at cloud center. Curve B, calculated concentrations averaged over a 120-km path centered on the cloud center. The activity data are uncorrected for background. The points represent data obtained by aircraft of several participating agencies. Solid symbols, horizontal flights; open symbols, altitude spirals.

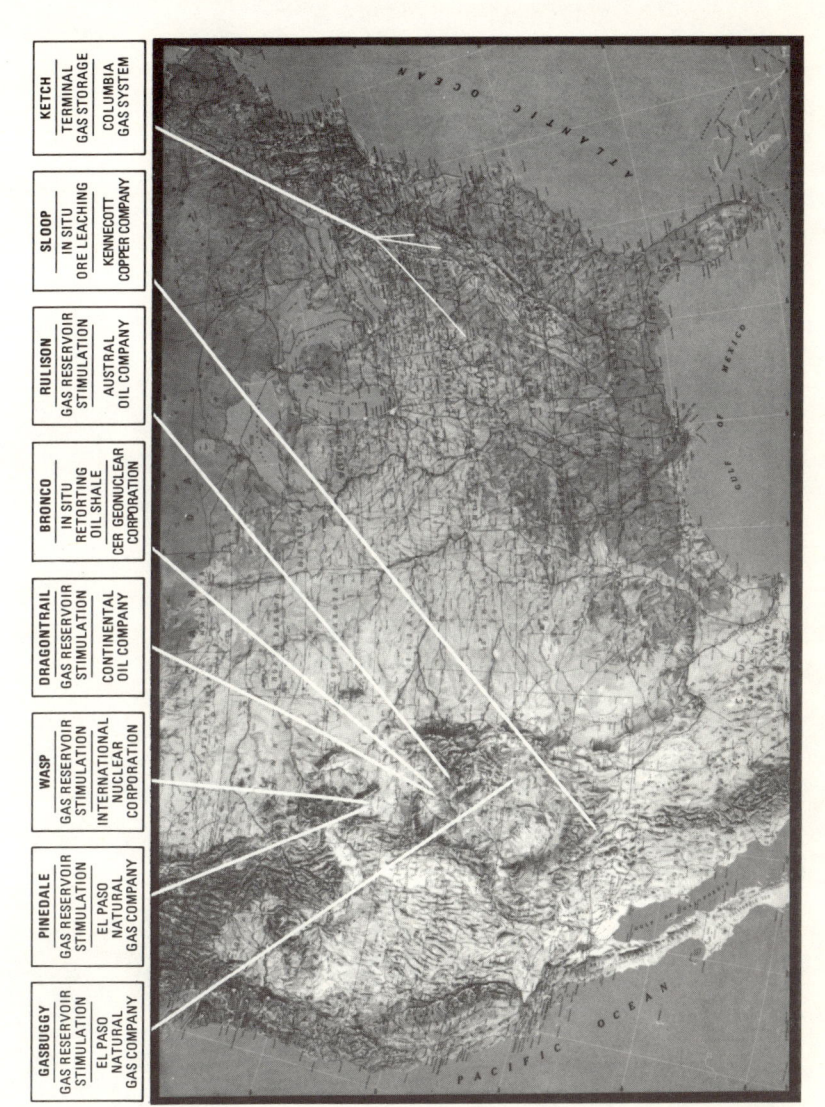

APPLICATIONS OF PEACEFUL NUCLEAR EXPLOSIVES   61

Fig. 26—Summary map of the deeply contained nuclear engineering projects.

APPLICATION OF BASIC RADIATION PROTECTION CRITERIA

HERBERT M. PARKER
Environmental and Life Sciences Division, Battelle Memorial Institute,
Pacific Northwest Laboratory, Richland, Washington

Nuclear energy has shown us its destructive forces in war, its harnessed powers in electrical generating facilities, its humane potentials in medicine, and most recently, its constructive capabilities in Plowshare programs. Are the radiation protection aspects of Plowshare applications ready to meet the needs of the rapidly developing programs? A look at the radiation protection guidance currently on hand says "yes." The problem seems to be: What radiation protection guidance should be applied? There is a need to establish a clear and unified policy relating to the application of radiation protection guidance to Plowshare.

The development of nuclear energy programs was accompanied by effective radiation safety programs. An exceptionally good radiation safety record resulted. The constructive application of nuclear energy to Plowshare programs should be accomplished with a similar radiation safety performance record. The safe history of the nuclear industry, the long-term potential benefits, and the varied applications for developing Plowshare technology may all be at stake if authoritative and sound radiation protection methods are not incorporated in all Plowshare experiments and applications. Well-balanced plans to assure radiation safety for all Plowshare programs are a necessity.

As with any safety program, the commonly undiscussed balance between the benefits to be gained and the risks to be incurred needs to be made so that the appropriate radiation protection guidance can be used. The difficult questions for selecting radiation protection guidance for Plowshare are: Who will make the benefits vs. risks balance? And then once made, who will accept the balance? It is too much to anticipate a balance that will be accepted by everyone. What, then, is the reasonable course of action?

Apparently only professionally concerned groups, such as the National Committee on Radiation Protection and Measurement (NCRP), Federal Radiation Council (FRC), or the International Commission on Radiological Protection (ICRP), are in a position adequately divorced from the controls and influences of government, trade unions, and the public to provide the necessary benefit—risk balance, and hence to provide the appropriate radiation protection guidance. However, we are unfortunately not considering protection, and the risk vs. balance in only a scientific frame of reference. In trying to put out practical radiation guides, we get involved with all sorts of socioeconomic and other considerations, about which we as radiation protectionists may not be the best qualified to decide. We certainly should not be heard alone and must admit that everyone else in the society properly has a voice at some stage.

To provide guidance is not to be confused with determining performance. The U. S. Atomic Energy Commission and the U. S. Public Health Service both have major roles in assessing and evaluating environmental conditions resulting from Plowshare activities. They both have the important role of determining just how well Plowshare programs meet the prescribed radiation protection guidance.

DISCUSSIONS

Presently available radiation protection guides include the publications of the NCRP, ICRP, FRC, and the International Atomic Energy Agency (IAEA). All these recommendations are based on limiting and controlling the radiation dose to the individual, be he a radiation worker or a member of the general public. All concentration limits that are derived are ultimately based on controlling radionuclide intake and depositions so as not to exceed some prescribed dose limit.

The basic theme of protection guidance by all the responsible agencies is acceptance of the concept that there is no threshold in the relation between exposure to radiation and the biological effects. The response is considered to be a monotonic, and in most cases an approximately linear function of absorbed dose. The actual circumstances in which these concepts have been proved to operate are so far very limited.

One or more of the NCRP or FRC guides may be translated into recommendations for Plowshare radiation protection guidance. For example, some may suggest that the prescribed guides for the public exposee, who is defined as the maximumly exposed member of the general public, or for the general public can yield recommendations

BASIC RADIATION PROTECTION CRITERIA

directly applicable to Plowshare radiation protection. Others may advocate the use of the dose limits for the radiation workers as Plowshare control limits. A few may advocate dose limits even higher than the annual limits recommended for radiation workers because of the relatively short duration of the Plowshare radiation exposures. I would suggest that only the guidance for the public exposee and for the general public can be unequivocally identified as applicable for Plowshare radiation protection guidance, since the populations to be exposed can hardly be considered as radiation workers.

Several factors need to be considered in selecting the proper radiation protection guidance for Plowshare. The principal factors of concern are the size of the group to be exposed by a Plowshare program and the extent to which the group can be monitored and moved to control its exposure. These factors may not always be the same for each Plowshare program. This is perhaps the most troublesome and often least appreciated aspect of some current deliberations on this subject. By accepting the concept of different guidance for different Plowshare programs, the risk vs. benefit balance can be made more justly. Before developing the potential of this approach, a short review of the basis for the various radiation protection guides for the workers, the public exposee, and the general public may be helpful.

The NCRP Committee No. 1 report on Basic Radiation Protection Criteria is yet unpublished and will make no sensational departures from previous recommendations. Here is an unofficial commentary on the considerations that the committee is thinking about.

For the radiation worker, dose limits were established such that a lifetime of occupational exposure within the dose limits would not result in deleterious effects that would be objectionable to the individual or to his physician. The public exposee is identified as the maximumly exposed individual of the general public. His exposure is limited to 0.5 rem per year primarily to avoid exposure of the fetus, although his general state of health and age are important factors also. For the general public the radiation-dose guidance is based on genetic-mutation considerations and is derived from the report of the National Academy of Sciences Committee on Biological Effects of Atomic Radiation (BEAR Committee) issued about 10 years ago.

Guidance for the occupational exposure to radiation is given by the equation, Dose = $5(N-18)$, where the dose is in rem and N is the age of the individual. This expression determines the acceptable occupational dose that may be delivered in a well-distributed pattern of both low dose and low dose rate to the whole body. The critical organs, in determining the whole-body limit, are the gonads and the red bone marrow. It is important to remember that the pattern of exposure needs to be relatively uniform with no short periods of high exposure followed by long periods of little or no exposure. However, the NCRP may recommend that a doubling of exposure to 10 rem, perhaps, in an isolated year would be possible, as long as it was not frequently repeated.

The exposure controls for the nonradiation worker are defined in two ways. The public exposee, or individual, should have his radiation exposure limited to 0.5 rem per year; however, the general public as a whole should receive exposure at a rate not exceeding 5 rem in the first 30 years of life, or about 0.17 rem per year. The rate of accumulation of this exposure should be relatively uniform. It would not be a good practice to exceed the rate of 0.17 rem per year.

The foregoing criteria, which are based largely upon the BEAR Committee report, did not take into account information obtained more recently on repair of, or recovery from, radiation damage. We now know quite a bit about recovery, both in genetic and somatic frames of reference. Recovery does occur, and its extent is sensitive to total dose, dose rate, and to the linear energy transfer rate (LET) of the radiation.

High LET radiation (e.g., alpha particles) may permit little or no recovery; but this is not of present concern since Plowshare is almost exclusively a problem of low LET radiations. For these (e.g., X rays, gamma radiation, and beta radiation—with the possible exception of tritium), there is great advantage in keeping each exposure at low dose and low dose rate in order to maximize recovery.

The newer knowledge about recovery tends to make everyone feel more comfortable. By retaining the criteria promulgated earlier, we are, in fact, increasing our conservatism.

A more detailed review of the dose limits indicates that there are three categories of occupational limits: (1) the critical organ, (2) the limiting organ situations, and (3) definable special cases. The 5(N-18) dose guidance is applied to the critical organs. A dose of 15 rem per year is defined as the maximum permissible for the limiting organs. Special definable cases are treated individually. Two cases of common interest are potentially pregnant women, whose dose is to be limited to 0.5 rem per year, and the fingers of the hands and the forearm. The fingers may receive up to 75 rem per year; whereas the transition area, the forearm, is permitted up to 30 rem per year.*

Now, to return to the concept of different guidance for different Plowshare programs. If a small group of individuals is to be involved in a Plowshare program and if this group can be totally monitored and their dose controlled by actions taken after the Plowshare event, should

---

*These comments on how limits may be changed should not be confused with authoritative actions to do so. In fact, some of these suggestions have been altered since this paper was presented. (Note added in proof.)

this become necessary, then control of exposures to near the public exposee limit of 0.5 rem per year seems appropriate. Through individual monitoring, the actual radiation exposure to each individual from all sources is known, and the exposure to each radionuclide should also be considered. If a large group of individuals is to be involved, such that individual monitoring or subsequent control is not feasible or possible for any reason, then the general public guidance should be used, and individual exposures should be limited to 5 rem per 30 years, or about 0.17 rem per year.

Some may advocate the concept that the short duration of the exposure for Plowshare detonations provides increased latitude and tends to permit higher doses than those normally recommended for the general public. Such an approach is not to be recommended because even short-term radiation levels, equal to or approaching those established as acceptable for radiation workers, may have some deleterious effect on special groups within the general population, particularly those in early pregnancy.

The very wide variations between the makeup of a worker population and a general population support the appropriateness of the public exposee or the general public limit guidance. Not many would advocate the exposure of pregnant women, children, the elderly, sick or chronically ill to doses comparable to those permitted safely to a select group of radiation workers or to a group whose exposure was monitored and was controllable to a reasonable extent.

One can estimate crudely what exposure levels from any new source will be acceptable to the general population. The environmental background in this country from cosmic rays and natural radionuclides ranges from a minimum of about 100 mrem per year in Florida to a maximum (for a major populated area) of about 400 mrem in Denver. There is no tendency for people to migrate eastward to avoid the higher radiation level. On the other hand, the estimated per capita exposure from medical diagnostic X radiation is 55 mrem per year, and there is public pressure to reduce this exposure. It seems to me, therefore, that any new type of radiation source in the environment (i.e., all Plowshare additions) would not be acceptable to the informed public if it contributed more than, say, 50 mrem per year.

What about considerations arising from possible multiple sources of exposure? Others have recommended reduction factors for the general population limits of 10 or 100 to 0.05 rem per year or 0.005 rem per year in the assignment of acceptable dose accumulation rates to particular radionuclides to make allowance for multiple radiation source contributions. Let us think about such calculations. They do not affect the basic dose guidance for Plowshare. They are a type of "allowance factor" to be applied in calculating doses to be permitted from particular radioisotopes. If, for a given Plowshare program, three radionuclides were present for ingestion and each of these had the whole body as the critical organ, then allowing $1/3$ of 0.5 rem per year or 0.17 rem per year for each radionuclide would be in order; however, the basic guidance has not changed. If some other unrelated source of exposure could be identified, then an appropriate allowance also should be made for it. However, a practical analysis of the recommendations to use reduction factors of 10 or 100 arbitrarily for all Plowshare programs immediately runs into difficulty. Although keeping radiation exposure at the lowest practical level is our prime and absolute objective, it is, however, not appropriate to prescribe mandatory control limits with unneeded conservatism. One should consider multiple radiation source exposures of the general public only as they become definitely identified.

The problem of dose allocations from multiple sources of radiation exposure is not yet a necessary part of protection criteria. We would all be happy if all contributions—from nuclear power generation, isotope applications, medical usage, Plowshare, etc.—were small enough that the aggregate simply was far below the established limits. Today this appears to be true, but we should be laying the groundwork for the possible need for "pie cutting" later on.

Guidance at 5 rem per 30 years or less also seems advisable when considering the use of Plowshare products by the general public. Consider the tritium contamination in Plowshare-assisted natural gas wells. The distribution of this natural gas and its small amount of tritium to homes over wide areas of the country can lead to the exposure of a very large population under unmonitored conditions. This is clearly a general population exposure in its fullest sense.

One might consider the benefit—risk balance made by a family with respect to natural gas associated with Plowshare programs. I dare speculate that many a family would make the benefit—risk balance at a higher cost of gas and the absence or near absence of tritium. Similar considerations enforce and support actions to very seriously keep radiation exposures as low as practical. There is more in the benefit—risk balance than company profits and technical safety. Each family will have its own criteria for measuring benefits and risks and hence the general acceptability of Plowshare-linked products. One should be reluctant to break with the long-standing guidance on exposure of the general population in any Plowshare program. It would seem prudent to advise exposure control limits no more restrictive and no more liberal than those used for some time now. Any change would call for a complete review of the technical basis for change by the NCRP and the FRC.

We cannot arbitrarily decide what cost will be attributed to Plowshare radiation protection activities due to the ecological studies to support dose estimations. Each situation may be unique, and adequate information needs to be collected before, during, and after each program to demonstrate that a completely safe program within the dose guidance is attained. The conditions of each Plowshare program will determine the cost required to provide adequate, but not excessive, radiation protection.

SUMMARY

Evaluation of each Plowshare program should be made individually, providing the necessary studies and population considerations, so that one may use the correct dose-limit guidance for determining acceptable conditions. The AEC and the Public Health Service need to give careful attention to collecting and analyzing environmental exposures and dose data so that we may learn from experiences and assure safe conditions. We need to maintain the good record of the nuclear energy program by not making unsafe errors in estimating the consequences of any Plowshare programs.

Plowshare can be performed safely. To do so requires good judgment, sound application of existing radiation protection guidance, and sufficient funding to meet the needs of practical safety programs. A safe approach using the public exposee or the general population dose control limits, as the situation may demand, is necessary to help assure the rapid development of Plowshare programs. A high priority should be assigned to developing methods to apply the existing radiation protection guidance so that Plowshare programs may proceed safely. There seems to be no doubt but that the peaceful applications of nuclear energy in Plowshare programs will develop as rapidly as funding and commercial opportunities present themselves.

DISCUSSION

HOLLAND: Something occurred to me recently that perhaps others have realized for a long time. The linear hypothesis, which is very fine for extrapolating downward from high doses, is very treacherous for extrapolating upward from low doses. In other words, if it is true that the dose—response curve is not straight but starts slowly then rises more steeply at some point and if this steep rise should occur near or somewhat above the level of natural background radiation, then any arguments based on small increases or doubling of the natural background dose cannot conservatively be based on the linear hypothesis. Is this true?

PARKER: Yes, it is correct. We have preached this linear hypothesis as being the safest, knowing really that when you get right down to the mathematical cases it is not necessarily the most conservative in the region going down from the limits of our observation to zero. It is overwhelmingly probable that it is, in fact, excessively conservative, but that is another issue. It is not proof. Going in the other direction, as you say, the whole thing breaks down. We preached that if it is not linear, then at least it is monotonic—so we avoid any argument about drawing a straight line through points. But we know perfectly well that these relations are not monotonic if we go to high enough doses. Our attention is focused on one kind of biological effect, and at high enough doses another effect can intervene and kill the person we are considering. You could be doing this with a brilliant study of leukemia and realize that all your people are dead if you go up far enough. The leukemia incidence would certainly go down markedly with increased dose in that frame of reference because the people would be killed before they got old enough to have leukemia.

TAMPLIN (LRL): I noticed that you still use 1% life shortening per 100 r. How do you treat the beagle data that was done at the University of California at Davis?

PARKER: What you say is this—the evidence for life shortening in man in a controlled situation is absolutely zero—there is not any evidence. So we will say there may or may not be life shortening in man. You go back to the general overview, the animal experimentation. If you look at enough biological experiments, you can almost always, I believe it is fair to say, find one that denies whatever you proved by a previous one. So it does not concern you greatly that any one particular experiment might not fit a pattern. I do not believe any responsible person thinks there is an absolute law that says that life shortening in all species of mammals goes at the rate of 10^{-4} life spans per roentgen. I use that number because those who have looked at this more closely come up with it as their best guess. This is for the low LET radiations. If you want a figure for high LET radiations, you will find that some people will multiply this by either 3 or 4. When I offered you a number of 83 days, I hope you did not ascribe any significance to the 3 and will not ascribe too much to the 8.

TAMPLIN: One of the reasons I think the beagle data may be more pertinent (and I may be impertinent in saying this) is that they are a longer lived species than the rat or the mouse on which the 1% figure was based. At a 100 r dose, the beagles showed a 12% reduction in life span. If I can study the rat and get a 1% reduction over 3 years, and if I study something like the beagle, I get a 12% reduction over 15 years, then if I consider man, with a 60-year life span, do I get more than a 12% reduction per 100 r, perhaps 20 or 30%? I wonder why the longer lived species (beagle) was not given more weight in making the decisions.

PARKER: I cannot answer that specifically on the beagle experiments. I am quoting those in NCRP who have spent their careers on this aspect. Their figure is something like a shortening of $2\frac{1}{2}$ days per roentgen for man.

TAMPLIN: When the female mouse showed a 5% reduction in life span, the female mouse was discredited because she was unusually sensitive to radiation. Now the beagle seems not to be considered, perhaps because they were females.

PARKER: The formal conclusion that will be reported is that no number can, in good conscience, be quoted for man. The numbers I gave as 83 and 890 are stylized calculations from that particular base.

CRAWFORD (LRL): You talked about the 0.5 rem to the public as a life-shortening effect. If you get that much every year for many years, do you notice anything?

PARKER: No. I think I stated that very clearly. There is no reliable evidence of a numerical estimate of life shortening in man at the NCRP levels.

CRAWFORD: In the light of John Totter's discussion earlier of the involvement of DBM in the total environment problem, would you contrast the use of MPC's in radiation safety with the use of air quality standards in air pollution.

PARKER: I do not mean to evade the question, but I think most of us feel the attention to the radiation component as a sort of insult to man is absolutely out of proportion to the attention paid to many other equally important deleterious vectors. To detail an answer further would take too long.

GRENDON: In regard to the 0.5-rem exposure to the public that you said was based on life shortening, that was actually based on the genetic aspect, I believe.

PARKER: No, it is not.

GRENDON: I thought the 0.17-rem value was based on a statistical consideration in trying to determine the 0.5 rem in a population sample.

PARKER: That is the difference between NCRP's thinking and FRC's thinking. As far as we (NCRP) are concerned, we accept the opinion of the distinguished genetics committee of the BEAR studies [Committee on Genetic Effects of Atomic Radiation report, in The Biological Effects of Atomic Radiation, Summary Reports, National Academy of Sciences—National Research Council, Washington, D. C., 1960. The recommended exposure first appeared in Recommendations of the International Commission on Radiological Protection, Adopted Sept. 9, 1958, Pergamon Press, Inc., New York, 1959], which allowed 5 rem in 30 years (a generation). That is where the 0.17-rem value came from.

GOFMAN (LRL): A very important distinction should be made in answering T. Crawford's question. He asked "if you give people this dose, does something happen?" The real answer to his question is that nobody has looked in any significant manner to find out. The answer is not that nothing happens; the answer is nobody has done the proper study.

CRAWFORD: The reason I asked was because air quality standards, which are being reset for California, are set up at levels at which there are physiological effects. Then we return to the point being made earlier about risks vs. benefits. Should you look at the total pollution problems as criteria for the choice of building a fossil-fuel plant or a nuclear-fuel plant?

PARKER: I think the nation is moving slowly toward a greater realization of the additivity of these different effects.

ABRAHAMSON: Two comments. First, there is the tendency by some people at the trough, as it was put earlier, to look upon the 0.5 rem a year as a legal limit up to which they as individuals can release radioactivity. This is particularly noticeable to those who look at routine releases from reactors. Second, your comment about perspective, that radiation is receiving more attention than other contaminants, which may or may not be of much consequence. I think this is a very dangerous argument. Irresponsible waste management in the past must not be used as the reason for propagating this same attitude toward radioactive wastes, the characteristics of which are quite different.

PARKER: I do not know very many people that are promulgating a lax attitude toward radioactive waste disposal. I see many who are doing precisely the reverse. I think the next point of reference is to spend as much money on measuring the effects of the other pollutants as has been properly spent on measuring the radiation effects and see what shows up as a first approximation to the damage. I do not know the answer. If one knew the answer there would be no need to do the work. I would be astounded if it did not turn out that the radiation component is relatively small compared with the whole picture.

ically observed in the environment are known. The metabolic behaviour of all important radionuclides is known for the predominant transfer processes involved.
RELEASE AND DISTRIBUTION OF RADIONUCLIDES IN THE BIOSPHERE

What are the sources, species, and quantities of man-made radionuclides entering the biosphere? How are they distributed, and by what mechanisms might they become a hazard to man? What predictions can be made regarding future growth in releases to the environment? How shall the releases be measured and monitored to provide useful data for protection of workers and the public? These questions are dealt with in this session.

ESTIMATION OF THE MAXIMUM DOSE TO MAN FROM THE CONTAMINATION OF AN AQUATIC ECOSYSTEM WITH RADIONUCLIDES

ARTHUR R. TAMPLIN
Lawrence Radiation Laboratory, University of California, Livermore,
Bio-Medical Division

ABSTRACT

A method is described for estimating the maximum internal dose that could result from the radionuclides released to an aquatic environment. With this analysis one can identify the nuclides that could contribute most to the internal dose and determine the contribution of each nuclide to the total dose. The calculations required to estimate the maximum dose to an infant's bone after the construction of a sea-level canal are presented to illustrate the overall method. The results serve the basic aims of preshot radiation safety analysis and of guidance for postshot documentation. The usefulness of the analysis in providing guidance for device design is further pointed out.

We have developed a practical state-of-the-art approach for predicting the dosage to man from each and all the radionuclides produced in the detonation of a nuclear device. This approach is presented in a series of reports.[1-6] In his paper, Y. C. Ng describes this series of reports and discusses the background of the studies.

The contamination of aquatic environments can logically be broken into three categories: groundwater, surface water, and marine. Part VI of Report UCRL-50163 deals with the contamination of groundwater.[6] This paper will treat both the surface-water and marine aspects.

There are essentially three ways through which these aquatic systems can be contaminated by the debris from a nuclear explosion: (1) direct contamination by an explosion in or near the water such as in the construction of harbors or canals, (2) transfer of the debris to the aquatic system as fallout in the atmosphere, and (3) transfer of the debris to the aquatic system by erosion and runoff or by stream-bed erosion. The atmospheric transport of the radioactive debris[1] is discussed in Part I and the aquatic transport[6] in Part VI of Report UCRL-50163.

This paper presents our approach for estimating the dosage to man that could result from this aquatic contamination. We can determine with this analysis that

1. The radionuclides that could contribute most to the internal dose in man can be identified.

2. The maximum internal dose to tissues and organs of man can be estimated.

3. Contributions of individual nuclides to this dose can be determined.

The biological exchangeable pool concept has been used for the analysis.[7] With this approach, the passage of a radionuclide through the biosphere is presumed to be governed by the same factors that govern the distribution of the related stable isotopes within the biological exchangeable pool. It must be assumed, of course, that the radionuclide is biologically no more available within the environment than the related stable isotopes.

The overall method will be illustrated by presenting the calculations required to estimate the maximum 30-year internal dose to an infant's bone. It will then be shown how the results can be used to fulfill the basic objectives relating to preshot radiation safety analysis, postshot documentation, and device design (see paper by Ng, this volume). Estimates of the maximum dose to the whole body and various other somatic organs have been made, but they will not be considered in this paper since the estimated bone dosage was shown to be the most critical in the example employed.

THE UNIT-RAD CONTAMINATION (F_A)

The basic relation used in this paper is F_A, the unit-rad contamination. F_A is the initial concentration of a radionuclide in water that would result in a 30-year integrated dose of 1 rad. Its units are, therefore, $\mu Ci/m^3/rad$. The basic assumptions in the derivation of F_A are that the radionuclides equilibrate instantaneously within the biological exchangeable pool exclusive of man and that man exists totally on a diet of aquatic origin. These assumptions, in keeping with the objectives, maximize the internal-dose estimate from any aquatic contamination. The equation used to determine F_A is similar to that used in Part II of Report UCRL-50163 to calculate F_1, the unit-rad deposition on terrain. The equations for F_1 were derived by Burton.[8] The equation for F_A is derived in an identical fashion by substituting aquatic values for terrain values:[4]

$$F_A = \left(\frac{37.1}{Q}\right)\left[\frac{C_A}{C_B^*}\frac{T_B(T_A - T_E)}{T_A T_E}\right]\left[\frac{1}{T_A(1 - e^{-20.8/T_A}) - T_E(1 - e^{-20.8/T_E})}\right] \quad (1)$$

where F_A = unit-rad contamination, $\mu Ci/m^3/rad$
Q = energy absorbed in the tissue per unit disintegration, Mev
C_A = stable-element concentration in the water
C_B^* = stable-element concentration in the tissue resulting from an aquatic diet
T_B = biological half-life in man's tissue, years
T_E = effective half-life in man's tissue, years
T_A = effective half-life in the water, years

Since T_A is determined by the radiological decay rate of the radioisotope and the rate of dilution of the aquatic system by uncontaminated water, it is quite site dependent.

If the only mode of decay in the water is radiological decay, then $T_A = T_R$, the radiological half-life. Since $T_B = T_R T_E / T_R - T_E$, Eq. 1 reduces to

$$F_A = \left(\frac{37.1}{Q}\right)\left(\frac{C_A}{C_B^*}\right)\left[\frac{1}{T_R(1 - e^{-20.8/T_R}) - T_E(1 - e^{-20.8/T_E})}\right] \quad (2)$$

When F_A values based upon Eq. 2 are used, the assumption that $T_A = T_R$ minimizes F_A and, hence, maximizes the estimates of dosage and hazard.

Actually, two values for F_A should be used, one for adults and one for infants. The F_A for infants is the most restrictive. It is determined by assuming that the infant instantaneously equilibrates with the environment. Since the newborn infant experiences rapid growth, he will come into equilibrium with his diet (the environment) much more rapidly than an adult. For the infant Eq. 1 thus becomes

$$F_A = \left(\frac{37.1}{Q}\right)\left(\frac{C_A}{C_B^*}\right)\left[\frac{1}{T_A(1 - e^{-20.8/T_A})}\right] \quad (3)$$

and Eq. 2 becomes

$$F_A = \left(\frac{37.1}{Q}\right)\left(\frac{C_A}{C_B^*}\right)\left[\frac{1}{T_R(1 - e^{-20.8/T_R})}\right] \quad (4)$$

The F_A values for the infant based upon Eq. 4 are used in this paper. These values can be corrected for the aquatic half-life by using the ratio T_C:

$$T_C = \frac{T_R(1 - e^{-20.8/T_R})}{T_A(1 - e^{-20.8/T_A})} \qquad (5)$$

Equation 5 can be approximated, except for radionuclides of very long half-lives, by

$$T_C = \frac{T_R}{T_A} \qquad (6)$$

DETERMINATION OF INPUT PARAMETERS

All the values for the parameters in Eq. 2, as well as the F_A values for adults and infants, are listed in the handbook portion[4] of Report UCRL-50163 for all radionuclides with half-lives greater than 12 hr. Whenever the value of a particular parameter was not known, a worst-case value was assumed that would minimize F_A and hence maximize the hazard estimate. For example, if T_E were not known, it was assumed that Eqs. 3 and 4 applied. In some cases values were based upon collateral data; each of these cases is discussed in detail in the appendix of the handbook.

The ratio C_A/C_B^* is critical in the determination of F_A. Therefore it is appropriate to discuss the selection of the values for this ratio at this point.

The Concentration in Water (C_A)

The values for concentrations of various elements in the ocean as reported in the literature often vary over orders of magnitude. Much of this difference can often be accounted for as a difference between the open ocean and the Continental Shelf or an estuarian area. The higher concentrations are reported for the latter, which are abundant with suspended material. Thus this difference is often accounted for as the difference between the "element in solution" and the total concentration. At the same time, in those cases where there is a wide range in the concentration in the water, the literature also demonstrates a proportionate range in the concentration in seafood. In other words, the element in solution appears to be in equilibrium with suspended material; hence the total concentration is representative of the biological exchangeable pool. Therefore in each case we have selected the higher values since in any peaceful application of nuclear explosives, such as in digging harbors or canals, the Continental Shelf or estuarian situation will be the area of interest.

For freshwater, the differences in concentration often represent differences in the source of the water. Therefore average values were selected for freshwater concentrations.

The Tissue Concentration from an Aquatic Diet (C_B^*)

Many elements, such as sodium and potassium, are under homeostatic control throughout an entire ecosystem. Consequently only small changes can occur in the concentration found in man's diet; these result in even smaller changes in the concentration in the tissues of man. For many trace elements this tight homeostatic control does not exist at the levels normally encountered in the environment, and man's diet and body concentrations will increase with increasing concentrations in the environment. Indeed, the concentrations of such elements as selenium or arsenic will increase to toxic levels. Many elements will be 10 to 100 times more concentrated in aquatic diets than in terrestrial diets; hence the body concentrations of these elements could also be expected to increase. Therefore the tissue concentration from an aquatic diet, C_B^*, has been determined by

$$C_B^* = C_B \, C^* \tag{7}$$

where C_B is the tissue concentration from a normal diet and C^* is the ratio of concentrations (aquatic diet/terrestrial diet).

The concentrations selected for the aquatic diet reflect those of the Continental Shelf and estuarian areas. They therefore account for the differences noted in C_A and lead to an appropriate C_A/C_B^* ratio. In keeping with the conservative aspects of the analysis, if $C^* < 1$, we set it equal to 1. This would account for those situations where a trace element is essential and the body can compensate for a lower intake.

Modified F_A for Mixed Diets (F_A')

The handbook[4] lists the values of F_A only for a population existing totally on an aquatic diet. These can be modified in a straightforward manner to handle any dietary mix by the relation

$$F_A' = C' F_A \tag{8}$$

where F_A' is the modified F_A and C' is a correction factor that includes a factor for the dietary mix and a correction of C^*. The value of C' is determined by the relation

$$C' = \left(\frac{I_A'}{I_A' + I_T'}\right)\left(\frac{C^* I_T}{I_A' + I_T'}\right) \tag{9}$$

where I_A' and I_T' represent the daily intake of an element from the mixed aquatic and terrestrial sources, respectively, and I_T represents the standard terrestrial intake used in calculating C^*. The $I_A'/I_A' + I_T'$ term in Eq. 9 determines the fraction of the daily intake from aquatic sources. The other term corrects C* for this dietary mix (this term should be limited to values between C* and 1). The handbook lists values for the concentrations in terrestrial plants and meats and in edible portions of marine and freshwater plants, invertebrates, and fish. Thus C' can be calculated for any dietary mix.

ESTIMATED MAXIMUM DOSE (EDA)

The estimated maximum dosage (EDA) from a particular radionuclide is obtained by dividing the aquatic contamination (μCi/m^3) by the F_A (μCi/m^3/rad). Alternatively, we can write

$$(\text{EDA})_i = \frac{(\text{ECA})_i}{(F_A)_i} \quad (10)$$

where (EDA)$_i$ is the estimated dose from an aquatic diet for radionuclide i (rads) and (ECA)$_i$ is the estimated contamination of the aquatic environment by radionuclide i (μCi/m^3). The total dose for a particular contamination is then determined by summing the doses from all radionuclides.

ESTIMATED AQUATIC CONTAMINATION (ECA)

The aquatic environment can be contaminated by three processes: (1) by fallout of atmospheric debris, (2) by mixing of the water with the debris in the crater created by the nuclear explosive, and (3) by transfer of the debris to the aquatic system through erosion and runoff.

During the process of forming a crater with nuclear explosives, the radionuclides produced are mixed with a certain mass M_C of rock material. A fraction of this mass, less than 20%, is released to the atmosphere as fallout debris, both close-in and long-range fallout. Up to 90% of the material is deposited in the crater or in the immediate vicinity of the crater where it is subject to processes 2 and 3.

Now, if it is assumed that a fraction f of this entire mass M_C of crater material comes into equilibrium with the aquatic system by any or all the above processes, then the estimated contamination is

$$(\text{ECA})_i = \frac{(fP_i^0)C_A}{fM_C(C_S) + V(C_A) + M_S(C_S)} \quad (11)$$

where P_i^0 = production of radionuclide i, μCi
C_A = concentration of the stable isotopes of i in the water system, g/m^3

M_C = mass of the crater rock material with which i is mixed, g
C_S = concentration of the stable isotopes of i in the rock mass, g/g
V = volume of the aquatic system, m³
M_S = mass of the bottom sediment of the aquatic system that is in equilibrium with the water, g

Equation 11 assumes that the radionuclides and stable elements in the debris are equally as available as the elements in the biological exchangeable pool of the aquatic system. In other words, the crater debris is considered equivalent to the bottom sediments and suspended and dissolved materials of the aquatic system. The determination of f from atmospheric fallout is discussed in Part I of Report UCRL-50163, and f for the other two processes is discussed in Part VI. The value suggested for M_C is approximately 10^{13} g per megaton of total yield.[9] This value appears reasonable when compared with data from the Sedan crater.[10,11]

The term M_S is related to the area of the aquatic system and the depth of the bottom sediment with which the water is in exchange equilibrium:

$$M_S = Ad\rho \tag{12}$$

where A is the area of the aquatic system in square centimeters, d is the sediment depth in centimeters, and ρ is the sediment density in grams per cubic centimeter.

THE AQUATIC HALF-LIFE (T_A)

When T_A is estimated, the rate of disappearance of the radionuclide from the combination of the aquatic system and its associated sediment mass must be considered. Neglecting radiological decay, this can be estimated by

$$\frac{dP_i}{dt} = -k(ECA)_i \tag{13}$$

where k is the rate of exchange of water in the aquatic system in cubic meters per year. Substituting Eq. 11 for ECA leads to

$$\frac{dP_i}{dt} \frac{1}{fP_i} = \frac{-k\,C_A}{fM_C(C_S) + V(C_A) + M_S(C_S)} \tag{14}$$

Thus T_A is obtained by dividing the above rate constant into 0.693

$$(T'_A)_i = 0.693 \left[\frac{fM(C_S) + V(C_A) + M_S(C_S)}{k\, C_A} \right] \qquad (15)$$

and then correcting for radiological decay

$$(T_A)_i = \frac{T_R\, (T'_A)_i}{T_R + (T'_A)_i} \qquad (16)$$

EXAMPLE: SEA-LEVEL CANAL

To illustrate how this predictive approach can be used to meet the objectives discussed by Ng (this volume), we will give estimates of the potential dose to man that could result from the construction of a sea-level canal across the Isthmus of Panama with nuclear explosives. We have selected Route 17, the Sasardi-Morti route for our example. Figure 1 shows its location.[12]

Dosage estimates will be made for contamination of the Gulf of Panama on the Pacific terminus of the canal. Since this represents a

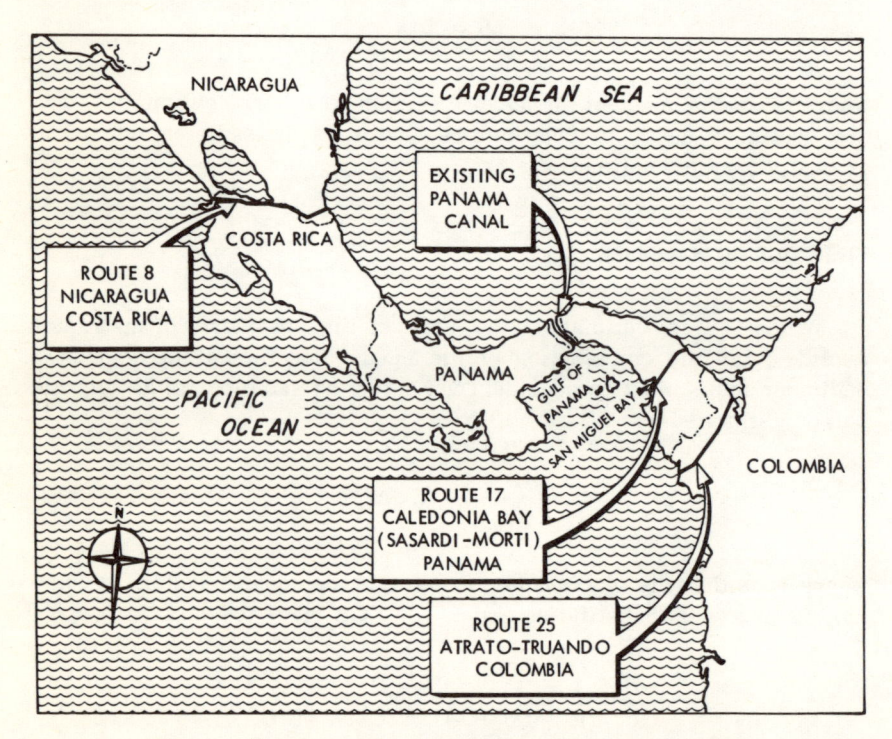

Fig. 1 — The four major potential sea-level canal routes.

comparatively small and somewhat isolated body of water, we anticipate these dosages will equal or exceed those for the Caribbean terminus.

Radionuclide Production

The detonation program for this route includes 14 separate cratering explosions.[13] Thirteen of the explosions will have yields of about 10 Mt each, and one will have a yield of 35 Mt, for a total yield of 165 Mt. The explosive devices will be thermonuclear in nature; hence there will be three sources of radionuclide production: (1) fission products, (2) activation products of the rock in which the device is detonated, and (3) activation products of device materials. In addition to these, tritium is produced. Tritium is considered separately later in this section.

Fission-product production will depend upon the fission-to-fusion ratio of the devices. At this time this ratio is classified. However, for purposes of illustration in the subsequent dosage estimates, we shall assume a fission yield from ^{239}Pu of 10 kt for the entire project. The fission-product yields listed by Weaver[14] are then used in the calculations. The 10-kt figure was chosen because it leads to a dosage estimate in the neighborhood of natural background, and it does not correspond to any real nuclear devices. Since the dosage estimate is directly proportional to the total fission yield, a limiting fission yield (LFY) for the project could be determined by

$$\text{LFY} = \frac{\text{allowable dose}}{\text{dose per kt of fission}} \qquad (17)$$

The activation products derived from rock materials depend on the fraction of the neutrons released by the device to the environment and their energy distribution. They also depend on the device design as well as on the amount of nonactivating neutron absorber (blanketing) placed around the device. In the subsequent dosage estimates, we shall assume that 10 moles of neutrons (6×10^{24}) are released to the environment per megaton of yield. Ng's data[15] on neutron activation of granite are then used for the radionuclide production estimates. Again, since the dosage is linear with the number of neutrons released, the limiting neutron release (LNR) can be determined by

$$\text{LNR} = \frac{\text{allowable dose}}{\text{dose per mole of neutrons}} \qquad (18)$$

Determination of the activation products from device materials requires access to the classified data on device design and, hence, will not be considered in this paper. The nature of these activation products and our approach toward estimating their production is discussed in Part III of Report UCRL-50163.[3] An approach similar to this can also be used to determine the limiting device activation dosage (LDA).

These three dosage estimates must then be combined to produce the total dosage estimate. The final dosage estimates will depend upon the device design and on the placement technique. The necessary guidelines for device design and placement can be supplied by comparing the dosage estimates with the total allowable dosage (TAD) by

$$TAD = \text{fission dose} + \text{neutron release dose} + \text{device dose} \quad (19)$$

The final device design and placement, as well as the total nuclear explosive yield, can thus be adjusted to meet the constraint imposed by TAD in Eq. 19. In addition, these dosage estimates will point out those radionuclides which represent the greatest hazard.

Determination of ECA

Since the Gulf of Panama lies at a terminus of the canal, contamination by all three processes — fallout, surface runoff, and crater flushing — would be expected. Hence all three processes will contribute to the value of f in Eq. 11. Two dosage estimates will be presented, one for $f = 1$ and one for $f = 0.1$. It is reasonable to assume that f would actually be somewhat larger than 0.1 since, in the construction plan considered here, some 30 Mt would be used to construct craters that would be contiguous with San Miguel Bay.[12] However, the dose changes by only a factor of 2 as f changes from 1.0 to 0.1.

With the value suggested, 10^{13} g/Mt, the total M_C in Eq. 11 is 1.65×10^{15} g for the canal project. A reasonable estimate for the volume of the Gulf of Panama (V in Eq. 11) is 10^{12} m^3. Since there is a salinity gradient in the Gulf (indicating less than complete mixing), this volume may be an overestimate.[16,17] However, choosing a smaller volume would not change the dosage estimates since the $M_C(C_S)$ and $M_S(C_S)$ terms in Eq. 11 dominate the expression for the majority of those radionuclides singled out as contributing the bulk of the total dosages.

The Gulf of Panama has a salinity gradient, indicating that it is not a well-mixed body of water and that only the bottom sediments of a narrow region of the shoreline would be in exchange equilibrium with the surface waters. Consequently it is reasonable to assume that a large fraction of the sediment that determines the value of M_S in Eq. 11 is contained in San Miguel Bay, which forms the actual terminus of the canal. San Miguel Bay is a rather shallow body of water with an extensive mud-flat area.[12] Its surface area is roughly 8×10^8 m^2. If it is assumed that the first 5 cm (2 in.) of sediment are in exchange equilibrium with the water and that the sediments are 50% water and 50% soil of density 2.5 g/cm^3, then M_S for the bay as given by Eq. 12 is 5×10^{13} g. If an equal value is assumed for M_S of the Gulf of Panama, a total M_S of 10^{14} g results. Pomeroy's data[18] suggest that the value selected for the San Miguel Bay is reasonable. Overall, this value of 10^{14} g would appear to be a reasonable, yet conservative, value for M_S. By conservative we mean that the actual value may be somewhat larger; hence this value may overestimate the dosage. However, a fourfold increase in M_S would lower the dosage estimates by only a factor of 2 when $f = 0.1$. (This occurs because the $f \times M_C$ term is 1.65×10^{14} g.) For the dosage estimates to be increased, both M_C and M_S would have to be overestimated in these calculations.

To summarize, the following values have been used to estimate ECA by Eq. 11: $f = 0.1$ and 1.0 (the actual value of f is expected to be approximately 0.1), $M_C = 10^{13}$ g/Mt, or 1.65×10^{15} g, for the canal, $V = 10^{12}$ m^3, $M_S = 10^{14}$ g, and $P_i^0 = 10$ kt of fission and 1650 moles of neutrons released to the environment for the entire project.

Determination of T_A and T_C

During the months January through March, persistent northerly winds blow across the Gulf of Panama.[16,17] As a result, the surface water is blown southward, and marked upwelling occurs in the Gulf. It is estimated that the upper 40 m of surface water is displaced in this manner. Consequently, in estimating T_A by Eqs. 15 and 16, k was set equal to the volume used for the Gulf, namely, 10^{12} m^3/year, and T_C was then determined by applying Eq. 6.

EDA for Infant's Bone

Only the dosage estimates for infant's bone are presented here since the calculations revealed that they were the highest among dosage estimates for the whole body and various tissues (kidney, liver, spleen, ovaries, testes, and gastrointestinal tract).

The dosage estimates for fission products are presented in Table 1, and those for neutron-activation products of granite are presented in Table 2. Only those radionuclides contributing the most to the total dosage are listed. Estimates are presented for both $f = 0.1$ and $f = 1.0$. The T_C values are presented only for the $f = 0.1$ cases. Only the radionuclides with half-lives of 1 week or greater are listed since these will be less compromised by the assumption of instantaneous equilibration in the aquatic foodstuffs. Furthermore, two columns are tabulated for the $f = 0.1$ case, one for $T_R < 150$ days and one for $T_R > 150$ days. The dosages listed under $T_R < 150$ days would still be compromised by this assumption and lead to dosage estimates that in some cases are high by an order of magnitude.

Table 1

THE EDA FOR INFANT BONE FROM FISSION PRODUCTS
IN THE CANAL EXAMPLE ($T_R > 7$ DAYS)

Radionuclide			Estimated dose, rads			
					$f = 0.1$	
Z	A	T_R days	$f = 1.0$	$T_R < 150$	$T_R > 150$	$1/T_C$
Sb 51	126	12.5	15.3	6.2		1.0
Sb 51	125	985	9.2		3.8	0.3
Cd 48	115m	43	4.7	2.0		1.0
Ru 44	106	365	5.8		1.4	0.5
Sb 51	124	60	3.0	1.2		1.0
Te 52	129m	33	1.0	1.2		1.0
Y 39	91	59	0.8	0.5		1.0
Ru 44	103	40	2.0	0.4		1.0
Cd 48	113m	5,110	0.7		0.3	0.1
Te 52	127m	105	2.4	0.3		1.0
Ce 58	144	285	0.4		0.3	1.0
Cs 55	137	11,000	0.5		0.2	0.1
Cs 55	136	13	0.4	0.2		1.0
Pm 61	147	985	0.09		0.06	1.0
Sn 50	125	9	0.1	0.04		1.0
Sr 38	90	10,200	0.4		0.04	0.03
Sr 38	89	50	0.3	0.03		1.0
Ag 47	111	7.5	0.2	0.02		1.0
Ce 58	141	33	0.04	0.02		1.0
Sn 50	123m	125	0.04	0.02		1.0
Ba 56	140	13	0.02	0.01		1.0
Sn 50	117m	14	0.02	0.006		1.0
Eu 63	156	15	0.005	0.004		1.0
Ar 40	95	65	0.004	0.002		1.0
Sn 50	119m	250	0.005		0.002	0.6
Sn 50	121m	9,130	0.004		0.002	0.1

Estimated Dosage from Tritium

Tritium is one of the major radionuclides produced in a thermonuclear explosive. Production estimates[14] range from 7×10^6 to 5×10^7 Ci/Mt. If the larger value is used, there would then be 8.3×10^{15} μCi produced in the canal project.

Setting $f = 1$ in Eq. 11 would lead to an ECA for tritium of 8.3×10^3 μCi/m^3. Since F_A for tritium is 640 μCi/m^3, the estimated dosage would be 13 rads. With $f = 0.1$, the estimated dosage would be 1.3 rads. Considering that T_A is 1 year, these dosage estimates should be reduced by a factor of 13. The dosage estimate for tritium in the Gulf of Panama would then, depending upon the actual value of f, be between 0.1 and 1.0 rad. The dosage from tritium would be higher in the rivers and in San Miguel Bay where the dilution volume is smaller. For example, Ko-

Table 2

THE EDA FOR INFANT BONE FROM GRANITE ACTIVATION PRODUCTS IN THE CANAL EXAMPLE ($T_R > 7$ DAYS)

Radionuclide			Estimated dose, rads			
		T_R,		f = 0.1		
Z	A	days	f = 1.0	$T_R < 150$	$T_R > 150$	$1/T_C$

	Z	A	T_R, days	f = 1.0	$T_R < 150$	$T_R > 150$	$1/T_C$
P	15	32	14	430	230		1.0
Cs	55	134	767	8		4	0.5
Co	27	60	1920	3		2	1.0
Eu	63	152	4530	3		2	1.0
Zn	30	65	245	4		2	0.7
Sc	21	46	84	1.6	1		1.0
Bi	83	210	8030	3.7		0.6	0.05
Mn	25	54	303	0.7		0.5	1.0
Ta	73	182	115	0.6	0.4		1.0
Sb	51	124	60	0.6	0.3		1.0
Dy	66	159	144	0.3	0.2		1.0
In	49	114m	50	0.24	0.16		1.0
Ir	77	192	74	0.7	0.15		1.0
Eu	63	154	5840	0.2		0.13	1.0

randa's data[19] demonstrate that kangaroo rats in equilibrium with plants growing on the ejecta from the Sedan crater are receiving doses ranging from 18 to 268 rads/year.

Interpretation of the Dosage Estimates

As was stated previously, these dosage estimates are dependent on the assumptions used in the calculations. Nevertheless, the radionuclides singled out by these estimates represent the most critical radionuclides. For some of the radionuclides listed in the tables, the estimated dosage results, at least in part, from "what we do not know." This is the case for antimony, which heads the list of fission products. But, as stated earlier, until actual data are available to replace the worst-case assumptions, these estimates represent the best assessment of the hazard and should be applied in preshot radiation safety analysis.

The question of biological availability should be asked in interpreting these estimates with respect to guidance for postshot monitoring. It was assumed here that the radionuclides would be no more available than their related stable nuclides. Although this is a reasonable assumption for cratering explosions, it has not been shown to be valid for all the radionuclides in Tables 1 and 2. It is therefore suggested that until such data become available all the radionuclides listed in

Tables 1 and 2 be included in postshot monitoring programs. Additional radionuclides should be added to this list from consideration of other tissues and from consideration of radionuclides produced by activation of the device materials.

With Eqs. 17 to 19, these dosage estimates can be used to supply guidance for device design and placement and for the total nuclear yield of the project. Since these dosage estimates are related to individuals existing totally on an aquatic diet, they represent the most conservative constraint on the contamination of an aquatic environment. These restrictions could possibly be relaxed on the basis of diet data of the individuals in the proposed canal area by use of Eqs. 8 and 9. Since the terrestrial environment would also be contaminated, Part II of Report UCRL-50163 would have to be used to estimate this portion of the dosage.[2]

It is important, however, to insert one final word of caution against using a less restrictive approach to the dosage estimates. It must be remembered that these are only estimates of the dosage. The actual dosage can only be determined by postshot monitoring. If less-restrictive estimates are employed and the design criteria are adjusted to the limit of the allowable dosage, then, owing to the perversity of nature, the postshot monitoring may demonstrate that tolerances are being exceeded.

REFERENCES

1. A. R. Tamplin, Prediction of the Maximum Dosage to Man from the Fallout of Nuclear Devices. I. Estimation of the Maximum Contamination of Agricultural Land, USAEC Report UCRL-50163 (Pt. I), University of California Lawrence Radiation Laboratory, Livermore, 1967.
2. Y. C. Ng and S. E. Thompson, Prediction of the Maximum Dosage to Man from the Fallout of Nuclear Devices. II. Estimation of the Maximum Dose from Internal Emitters, USAEC Report UCRL-50163 (Pt. II), University of California Lawrence Radiation Laboratory, Livermore, 1966.
3. C. A. Burton and M. W. Pratt, Prediction of the Maximum Dosage to Man from the Fallout of Nuclear Devices. III. Biological Guidelines for Device Design, USAEC Report UCRL-50163 (Pt. III), University of California Lawrence Radiation Laboratory, Livermore, 1967.
4. Y. C. Ng, C. A. Burton, S. E. Thompson, R. K. Tandy, H. K. Kretner, and M. W. Pratt, Prediction of the Maximum Dosage to Man from the Fallout of Nuclear Devices. IV. Handbook for Estimating the Maximum Internal Dose to Man from Radionuclides Released to the Biosphere, USAEC Report UCRL-50163 (Pt. IV), University of California Lawrence Radiation Laboratory, Livermore, 1968.
5. A. R. Tamplin, H. L. Fisher, and W. H. Chapman, Prediction of the Maximum Dosage to Man from the Fallout of Nuclear Devices. V. Estimation of the Maximum Dose from Internal Emitters in Aquatic Food Supply, USAEC Report UCRL-50163 (Pt. V), University of California Lawrence Radiation Laboratory, Livermore, 1968.
6. H. L. Fisher, Prediction of the Maximum Dosage to Man from the Fallout of Nuclear Devices. VI. Transport of Nuclear Debris by Surface and Ground-

water, USAEC Report UCRL-50163 (Pt. VI), University of California Lawrence Radiation Laboratory, Livermore, in preparation.
7. Y. C. Ng, The Biological Exchangeable Pool, in Program Book for the Advisory Committee for Biology and Medicine of the U. S. Atomic Energy Commission, USAEC Report UCRL-14739 (Pt. 2), pp. 19-32, University of California Lawrence Radiation Laboratory, Livermore, 1966.
8. C. A. Burton, A Graphical Method for Calculating the Dose in Man from Individual Radionuclides in Fallout, USAEC Report UCRL-14922, University of California Lawrence Radiation Laboratory, Livermore, 1966.
9. F. W. Stead, Distribution in Groundwater of Radionuclides from Underground Nuclear Explosions, in Engineering with Nuclear Explosives, Proceedings of the Third Plowshare Symposium, University of California, Davis, April 21-23, 1964, USAEC Report TID-7695, pp. 127-139, 1964.
10. M. D. Nordyke and M. M. Williamson, The Sedan Event, USAEC Report PNE-242F, University of California Lawrence Radiation Laboratory, Livermore, and U. S. Army Corps of Engineers, 1965.
11. S. M. Hansen, Results from Sedan Postshot Drilling, USAEC Report UCRL-50213, University of California Lawrence Radiation Laboratory, Livermore, 1966.
12. U. S. Atomic Energy Commission, U. S. Army Corps of Engineers, and Panama Canal Company. Isthmian Canal Studies—1964. Annex III, Construction of an Isthmian Sea-Level Canal by Nuclear Methods—1964, Appendix 2, General Construction Plan, USAEC Report PNE-2005, 1964.
13. E. R. Graves, R. S. Holmes, M. D. Nordyke, L. J. Cauthen, and M. M. Williamson, Isthmian Canal Studies—1964, Annex III, Appendix I, Nuclear Excavation Plan, USAEC Report PNE-2000, University of California Lawrence Radiation Laboratory, Livermore, 1964.
14. L. E. Weaver, P. O. Strom, and P. A. Killeen, Estimated Total Chain and Independent Fission Processes, Report USNRDL-TR-633, U. S. Naval Radiological Defense Laboratory, 1963.
15. Y. C. Ng, Neutron Activation of the Terrestrial Environment as a Result of Underground Nuclear Explosions, USAEC Report UCRL-14249, University of California Lawrence Radiation Laboratory, Livermore, 1965.
16. M. B. Schaefer, Y. M. M. Bishop, and G. V. Howard, Some Aspects of Upwelling in the Gulf of Panama, *Bull. Inter-Amer. Trop. Tuna Comm.*, 3: 79-111 (1958).
17. R. H. Fleming, A Contribution to the Oceanography of the Central American Region, *Proc. Pacific Sci. Congr. Pacific Sci. Assoc. 6th Congr., 1939*, 3: 167-175 (1940).
18. L. R. Pomeroy, E. P. Odum, R. E. Johannes, and B. Roffman, Flux of ^{32}P and ^{65}Zn Through a Salt-Marsh Ecosystem, in *Disposal of Radioactive Wastes into Seas, Oceans, and Surface Waters*, Symposium Proceedings, Vienna, 1966, pp. 177-188, International Atomic Energy Agency, Vienna, 1966 (STI/PUB/126).
19. J. J. Koranda, Residual Tritium at Sedan Crater, USAEC Report UCRL-70292, University of California Lawrence Radiation Laboratory, Livermore, 1967.

DISCUSSION

BROWN: In the case of antimony, it appears high on the list because of what you do not know about it; in contrast, in the case of strontium, it is high because of what you do know about it. Would you discuss which factors are least known about antimony?

TAMPLIN (LRL): For antimony the major uncertainty lies in the concentration of antimony in algae or seaweed, in other words, in edible marine plants. This leads us to a rather high value for C* which corrects the body concentration for the aquatic diet. The number we have used, the worst-case estimate, is probably high by something like a factor of 10. This would mean that when the real data come in you might expect the antimony to be valued at a factor of 10 lower. For most of the others on the list there was not a great deal of uncertainty in the numbers.

RIVERA: You have discussed estimates for bone of infants on an aquatic diet. This assumes that an infant is on a wholly aquatic diet. What has it eaten?

TAMPLIN: The fetus is a rapidly growing organ in the mother. After the infant is born, it is still sort of a rapidly growing organ of the mother if it happens to be nursing. The general conclusion is that the infant will see a diet that at any one particular time is more closely equilibrated with his environment than he is. We have used a worst-case assumption, I will admit that. But the result is that, if you look at it that way in most cases, the assumption only causes a factor of about 2 overestimate and in the worst kind of situation causes a factor of 10 difference in the dosage estimate. For most radionuclides that assumption does not make a serious difference.

RIVERA: If an infant gets a certain dose rate for a time, then it is no longer an infant.

TAMPLIN: But it has equilibrated with its environment. The only difference that our assumption makes is in the rate of equilibration with a contaminated environment and diet. Since the adult already has, for example, a large amount of strontium in him, it takes him a long time to get the activity of the strontium per gram of stable strontium equal to that in the environment. But with an infant who starts off with practically no strontium in him and over a period of a few years increases his total-body strontium content by a factor of 10, he comes much more quickly into equilibrium with that environment. And that is the only thing that this particular assumption says—that the child more rapidly looks like the environment. I think the adult, after 30 years, is only about 70% equilibrated with his intake as a result of the long half-life of the strontium in the bone.

FLEMING (LRL): I noticed that you had ^{113m}Cd. If I am not mistaken, we have no evidence that ^{113m}Cd is produced in fission. So what did you use for a yield?

TAMPLIN: That is a worst-case assumption—that all the radionuclides are assumed to be in the metastable state. In the absence of evidence to the contrary, that is not totally unreasonable. I understand Ng is revising some of the production estimates as data become available, and these revisions eliminate ^{113m}Cd.

PICKLER: What assumption did you make about the percentage of the diets made up of shellfish and the percentage made up of invertebrate fish?

TAMPLIN: I arbitrarily assumed that 60% of the diet came from plants, 20% came from invertebrates, and 20% came from fish flesh. This again is a worst-case assumption. It is weighted toward those aquatic materials that have the highest concentration factors.

COMAR: I did not understand whether the transfer coefficients of these various radionuclides to the infant through the food chain was taken into account in your calculation.

TAMPLIN: No, the assumption here was that the radionuclides behaved like stable nuclides in the environment.

COMAR: Did you base this on a comparison of the levels of the stable nuclide in the environment and levels in infants?

TAMPLIN: Yes. Equation 2 again.

COMAR: Another comment while we are waiting. Have you ever made any calculations using the transfer coefficients to see if you come up with about the same order of result? In other words, if you have a certain amount of radionuclide released, so much gets into fish, so much can be consumed by the mother, and so much gets into the infant. Do values calculated in that way agree with the values calculated in this method?

TAMPLIN: They would have to if we used the same assumptions going through it that way that we used in our method. One of the reasons we went the way we did was because, when you try to look at these things in detail, you generally do not find all the data you need, and therefore you have to make assumptions. What we tried to do was to make a set of assumptions that were not totally unreasonable in terms of the concentrations the radionuclides would achieve. This approach is quite similar to the one used by the National Academy of Sciences in treating aquatic contamination, except that we look at the individual tissues; and we do not use the critical organ from ICRP. But we simply make the assumption that the radionuclide behaves like the stable nuclide. The term C_A over C_B (in Eq. 2) simply relates the concentration in the environment, in this case water, to the concentration measured in the whole body. In this case, if the concentration in an aquatic diet is higher than the concentration in the terrestrial diet, then we jack up C_B to account for a higher intake. For most things, this is not an unreasonable assumption.

COMAR: Intuitively, I have a little difficulty understanding why you would get your values for yttrium which is so poorly absorbed by the biological system.

TAMPLIN: The only reason yttrium comes out high in these equations is because the ratio of concentration of yttrium that has been found in the body related to the concentration of yttrium that is found in the environment is higher than one would obtain by using the transfer coefficients in the ICRP tables. I think everybody knows that eventually ICRP is going to update its tables; and in some cases we found that the ICRP values have been off. One of the values that will come out much higher in our calculations than if you use the ICRP is ruthenium. The data that are now coming in on ruthenium in man and in the environment suggests there is actually a factor of about 100 above the ruthenium values that you would get out of the ICRP tables.

PARTICIPANT: What factors are involved in the error?

TAMPLIN: It looks like a combination of two factors — the uptake and the half-life. The biological half-life in the body of ruthenium seems to be too low in the ICRP tables, and the fraction taken up seems to be too low also.

FOSTER: People using this specific activity approach usually run into a couple of major problems, one of which is lack of information on elements not typically found in the body. Plutonium is the extreme example. The other one is in estimating the dose to the GI tract where there is no equilibrium between food intake and the body. I wonder how you handle those two problems in your equation.

TAMPLIN: We have scanned the world literature for concentrations in all sorts of plants, animals, soil, man, and all the various aquatic plants and animals. On the basis of this, we do end up with a certain amount of data that gives us a concentration of the various stable elements in the tissues and organs of man. In the absence of that type of data, then we go to the animal data. We are able to find the concentration in beef and in plants. All these approaches using collateral data to arrive at the various factors is described in the appendix of the handbook. If we know the concentration in meat and we know the concentration in plants, then we can make up a diet. We can carry that through the uptake and the half-life stages; then we can arrive at a concentration in the tissues. In many cases we run up against a situation where we just do not have any data. We do not know the concentration in the rat, we do not know the concentration in man, and we do not know the concentration in any portion of the environment, except maybe rock. In that particular case, then we make the worst-case assumption: that the concentration of that particular element in the tissue is derived from the ratio between the concentration of mercury in the soil and mercury in the kidney. In other words, the worst-concentration ratio between the soil and the tissue is the one we assign for all those elements about which we know absolutely nothing. We feel pretty confident that the real dosage will come out to be less than our estimate because we have overestimated the environment-to-body concentration ratio. When a particular element like that is singled out as being one of the major hazards, it is a warning that here is an area where you need to do some biological research to provide the data. Most of the radionuclides that turn out to be important on our lists, it turns out, are not these worst-case unknowns. We know quite a bit about the biology of most of them. In what Ng will present subsequently, you will see that by making these worst-case assumptions we have been able to eliminate nearly all the elements for which we have no biological data whatsoever. We have been able to eliminate them by showing that they will contribute very much less dose than the things we know more about. Therefore they are insignificant and really even more insignificant than we say they are because of our worst-case assumptions. So it does help to solve the problem by doing it this way. If you find an element like antimony sitting at the top of the list, that means that, if you want to change your dosage estimate, you must get the biological data. It points out a critical area for research.

FOSTER: How about the dose to the GI tract?

TAMPLIN: We mixed up the diet and just calculated the dose rate to the diet. We said that was the dose rate to the tissue because we just assumed the GI tract was a continuous tube. Whatever the diet was getting for a radiation dose, that was what we assumed was the dose rate to the GI tract when none of the radionuclide was being absorbed. In the case of milk, we had to allow a 3-day passage time; so we gave it a half-life of 3 days.

DUNSTER: That does not conform with your conservative approach to the rest of the calculations, does it? The absorption of liquids in the diet while passing through the gut results in a dose substantially higher than the dose rate to the diet.

TAMPLIN: We do not assume any liquid in the diet.

DUNSTER: Your diet, then, is on a dry-weight basis.

TAMPLIN: No, it is on the normal basis.

DUNSTER: But there is a factor of 5 or 10 of concentration on a mass basis into the feces.

TAMPLIN: My impression was that the feces was damp and a little more damp than the meat and the bread. And excluding the liquids I might take in on my diet, if I did not have soup for dinner, then the consistency I got out one end was like the consistency I put in the other. So on that kind of basis we did not assume a change in concentration.

DUNSTER: Having answered question 1 from your table (what is the worst situation that could develop?), you said that you have the information to answer question 2 (what is the most likely situation that will develop?). If that is so, can you give us some feeling for some typical nuclides about the factor between the questions 1 and 2?

TAMPLIN: In Table 1—if all the material equilibrated with the aquatic system, this was assumed to be the worst case; if one-tenth of it equilibrated with the aquatic system, this was considered to be an average case. It turned out in this particular exercise that did not make much difference. You could assume that all the material equilibrated, or only 10% of it, and you did not change your estimate very much. Now there is one additional worst case that I can make. Included in these calculations is the fact that it is the entire Gulf of Panama that is equilibrating with the radionuclides. That is a volume of some 10^{12} m^3. I could simply change the situation to where I just flood the crater, then I have the people living on the fish and everything that is growing in the crater. That will then change these dosage estimates. That would be the situation you might expect very close to the crater itself—very close to the canal. And as you began to move away from the canal, you would begin to reduce these estimates. But your worst case would be to just flood the canal and not mix it with the rest of the water. This would also be unrealistic.

DUNSTER: Let us go in the other direction—your calculations include a whole range of maximized assumptions. What sort of figure does that bring out for the best guess as opposed to the safest guess for say, antimony? A factor of 10, 100, or 1000 down?

TAMPLIN: The estimate given for antimony I would say is pretty good. The best and safest estimates are about the same (maybe a factor of 10 different). Some of the others will be different.

CRAWFORD (LRL): You assume no movement of water out of the Gulf of Panama?

TAMPLIN: Yes I do—that is where the aquatic half-life comes in. I used the observation that the Gulf of Panama during a 3-month period of the year has a persistent southerly to northerly wind that blows surface waters out to the Pacific, and there is intense upwelling. So, in making this calculation of the aquatic half-life (T_c), I assumed that the water in the Gulf of Panama exchanged once each year. In other words, that the half-life of the water in the Gulf of Panama was 1 year. There again it did not make much difference in the dosage estimates.

ESTIMATION OF THE MAXIMUM DOSE TO MAN FROM THE FALLOUT OF RADIONUCLIDES ON AGRICULTURAL LAND

YOOK C. NG
Bio-Medical Division, Lawrence Radiation Laboratory, University of California, Livermore, California

ABSTRACT

A method is described for estimating the maximum internal dose that could result when radionuclides are released to the atmosphere and deposited on agricultural land. By means of this analysis, one can identify the nuclides that could contribute most to the internal dose and determine the contribution of each nuclide to the total dose. The calculations required to estimate the maximum dose to the whole body are presented to illustrate the overall method. The results are shown to serve the basic aims of preshot radiation safety analysis and of guidance for postshot documentation. The usefulness of the analysis in providing guidance for device design is pointed out.

We have developed a practical state-of-the-art approach for predicting the dosage to man from each and all the radionuclides produced in the detonation of a nuclear device. This approach is presented in a series of reports.[1-6] Part I of this series presents the approach we use to estimate the fallout levels as a function of cloud travel time for periods up to 50 hr postdetonation. This paper, Part II of the series, shows how these fallout estimates can be combined with radionuclide production estimates and biological uptake relations in the terrestrial environment to arrive at estimates of burden and dosage for man. Part III shows how this predictive approach can supply guidelines for the design of nuclear devices for peaceful purposes. Part IV is a handbook that lists the input parameters required for the estimation of dosage. Part V presents our approach for predicting the dosage to man from aquatic foodstuffs. Part VI discusses the transport of nuclear debris by surface and groundwater.

In developing this approach, we could have asked ourselves three questions concerning the outcome of a nuclear detonation. It is essential that the reader recognize which of the three is the question we are trying to answer and why we feel that it is the most appropriate question to answer. The three questions are:
1. What is the worst situation that could develop?
2. What is the most likely situation that will develop?
3. What would be the situation if everything went off perfectly?

We choose to answer the first question and to direct our efforts toward predicting the worst case. However, in the process of answering the first question, we can also answer the second. Quite obviously the answer to the third question has no meaning with respect to public health and safety.

By worst case, we do not necessarily mean a possible but highly improbable case. In the case of nuclear device test, by worst case we mean that the dosage estimates should be made by assuming that the radioactive cloud intersects a heavy rainstorm and that all the activity is deposited by the rain. We suggest that only the worst case should be compared with prescribed tolerances in a preshot radiation safety analysis. We make this suggestion because it is only when we know the worst case that we can establish an adequate system of postshot monitoring to document the actual case and to ensure that appropriate countermeasures are instituted when and if needed.

Furthermore, we are attempting to be quite thorough in our analyses and are considering each and every radionuclide recorded on the chart of the nuclides. In this respect, our estimates may indicate that a particular radionuclide is a hazard for one of two reasons: (1) either it will be a hazard because of what we know about it or (2) it will be a hazard because of what we do not know about it. If a pertinent relation is not known concerning a particular radionuclide, we make worst-case estimates of the relation and hence maximize our estimates of hazard. Nevertheless, even though it is conservative, this approach still allows us to eliminate most of the radionuclides from consideration and to indicate those that are potentially the most hazardous. Obviously, it also allows us to estimate the upper limit of the potential burden and dosage; however, owing to the perversity of nature, the precise dosage can only be determined by postshot documentation in the affected areas.

Thus through our predictive approach, we want to be able to indicate what should be measured, where it should be measured, and with what precision it should be measured. There would appear to be no other way to assure that the dosimetry of future events is unambiguous and that the need for countermeasures is recognized in time so that they can be planned for and instituted when and if needed. In this respect the most appropriate countermeasures lie in device design. Our approach has been so planned that it can supply guidelines for the design of nuclear devices that might be used for such projects as the construction of a sea-level canal.

This predictive approach is meant to serve three purposes: (1) in preshot radiation-safety analysis, by determining whether or not a particular event can be conducted without exceeding existing tolerances; (2) in guidance for postshot documentation, by indicating what should be measured, where it should be measured, and with what precision it should be measured; and (3) in guidance for device design, by indicating the maximum amount of a radionuclide that can be produced and subsequently released to the environment without exceeding prescribed tolerances.

Although the examples that we cite deal with nuclear explosive devices, the approach applies equally well to other means of introducing radionuclides to the environment.

This paper presents a general method for the analysis of environmental contamination by radionuclides released to the atmosphere. By means of this analysis (1) the radionuclides that could contribute most to the internal dose in man can be identified, (2) the maximum internal dose to tissues and organs of man can be estimated, and (3) contributions of individual nuclides to this dose can be determined.

The biological exchangeable pool concept has been utilized for the analysis.[7] When this approach is used, the passage of a radionuclide through the biosphere is presumed to be governed by the same factors that govern the distribution of the related stable isotopes within the biological exchangeable pool. It must be assumed, of course, that the radionuclide is biologically no more available than the related stable isotopes within the environment.

The basic calculation required in our approach is an estimation of the unit-rad deposition for each radionuclide encountered; a complete description of the procedure has been published by Burton.[8] The unit-rad deposition, F_1, is the minimum deposition that could result in a 30-year internal dose of 1 rad. Estimated maximum doses are calculated from F_1 and from known or predicted values of deposition.

Two modes of entry into man are assumed: (1) direct deposition on forage leading into the forage-to-cow-to-milk pathway and (2) deposition on the terrain followed by equilibration in the biological exchangeable pool, for which the soil—root pathway is required for entry into plants.

We will illustrate the overall method by presenting the calculations required to estimate the maximum 30-year internal dose to the whole body and then will show how the results can be used to fulfill the basic objectives relating to preshot radiation-safety analysis, postshot documentation, and device design. Estimates of the maximum dose to the whole body are especially useful since the radiation protection guides for the general population are described in terms of doses to the whole body and to the gonads.[9] It is also worthwhile to estimate the maximum internal dose to other organs. Estimates of the maximum dose to the gonads and various somatic organs have been made, but they will not be considered here.

THE FORAGE-TO-COW-TO-MILK PATHWAY

When radioactive fallout is deposited on plants, the forage-to-cow-to-milk pathway can contribute relatively large quantities of radioactivity to the diet. This route can be significant for all radionuclides except those of very short half-life. For short- and intermediate-lived nuclides, it can be regarded as the worst case because relatively large contaminated areas can be grazed daily by the cow and because the resulting transfer of radioactivity to man via milk can be achieved in a period that is short relative to the effective lifetime of the radionuclide on forage.

The Unit-Rad Deposition

The forage-to-cow-to-milk model assumes an instantaneous steady state with respect to the secretion of activity in milk following deposition on forage. This assumption maximizes the dose estimate. The minimum deposition that could lead to a 30-year internal dose of 1 rad when a liter of milk is consumed daily[8] is given by

$$F_1 = \frac{(7.04 \times 10^{-8})}{(UAF) \, Qf \, T_P T_E} \frac{(1 - T_P/T_E)}{(1 - T_P/T_E - e^{-20.8/T_E})} \tag{1}$$

where F_1 = unit-rad deposition ($\mu Ci/m^2/rad$)
(UAF) = "utilized area factor," the effective area of pasture grazed daily by the cow (m^2/day)
Q = energy absorbed in the tissue per unit disintegration (Mev)
f = fraction of the quantity of isotope ingested daily by the cow that is deposited in man's tissue per gram
T_P = effective half-life on forage (years)
T_E = effective half-life in man's tissue (years); the effective half-life is a measure of the rate of loss of activity in the tissue as a result of radioactive decay and normal biological turnover; the effective half-life is equal to the product of the biological and radiological half-lives divided by the sum, i.e., $T_E = T_B T_R/(T_B + T_R)$

The relation

$$f = \frac{f_M f_B}{m} \qquad (2)$$

is used for the estimation of f. In Eq. 2 f_M is the fraction of the isotope ingested daily by the cow that is secreted in milk per liter, f_B is the fraction of the isotope ingested by man that is deposited in his tissue, and m is the mass of man's tissue.

Determination of Input Parameters

The radionuclides that are produced in underground nuclear explosions include activities induced in the terrestrial environment, activities induced in device materials, fission products, and tritium. Numerous radionuclides distributed over the entire chart of the nuclides would be released to the biosphere if nuclear explosives were used in the construction of a sea-level canal across Central America.[10] For reasons of public health and safety it is essential that no radionuclide be overlooked as a potential contributor to the internal dose and that the maximum credible dose never be underestimated. Thus, when the data required to estimate F_1 are not available, conservative worst-case estimates must be made.

We have estimated the unit-rad deposition of all the radionuclides listed on the Knolls Atomic Power Laboratory Chart of the Nuclides[11] that have half-lives of 12 hr or greater. The F_1 values were calculated for a number of tissues including bone, kidneys, liver, ovaries, spleen, testes, whole body, and GI tract. A set of rules was adopted for making conservative worst-case estimates of input parameters. These rules were followed whenever the input parameters were not directly obtainable from the ICRP tables* or from our own data file of the biological exchangeable pool.[7] It will be shown that, following this procedure, most radionuclides can be eliminated from consideration as potential hazards with great assurance.

The parameters of Eq. 1, which determine the unit-rad deposition via the forage-to-cow-to-milk pathway, include biological and non-biological terms. Values for the parameters are derived as follows.†

Values of UAF. A reasonable value can be assigned to UAF based on Koranda's[3] review of agricultural factors affecting the intake of

---

*The ICRP tables referred to throughout this report are included in Ref. 12.
†No attempt will be made in this report to list the input parameters used in the calculations. Input parameters and a comprehensive bibliography of the sources from which they were obtained appear in a continuously updated handbook.[4] The handbook is available upon request.

fallout by dairy cows. A median UAF value of 45 m^2/day was found for dairy cows in the United States.

Values of Q. Burton and Maxwell[14] have developed a procedure for calculating conservative Q values for all the radionuclides of interest; details of the calculations are being published.

Values of T_P. Reasonable and conservative values can be assigned to T_P, the effective half-life on forage, based on Thompson's review[15] of the half-residence time and effective half-life of fallout on pasture plants. The half-residence time was noted to be independent of isotope and to vary in most cases between 9 and 14 days. The effective half-life on forage expressed in days can thus be determined from T_R, the half-life for radioactive decay, using the simple expression

$$T_P = \frac{14\, T_R}{14 + T_R} \tag{3}$$

Values of T_E. The effective half-life in man's tissue, T_E, is determined by the biological half-life, T_B, which was assumed to be 1000 years if not known. That is, if T_B was not known, it was assumed essentially to be infinite and T_E was assumed to be equal to T_R, the half-life for radioactive decay.

Values of f. The fraction of the quantity ingested daily by the cow that is deposited in man's tissue per gram, f, is shown by Eq. 2 to be composed of three quantities: f_M, f_B, and m. If f_M, the fraction secreted per liter of milk, is not known from tracer studies, it can be estimated from the elemental composition of forage and milk. In the steady state a constant fraction of the stable isotope ingested daily by the cow is secreted per liter of milk. Equation 4 expresses this relation.

$$f_M = \frac{C_M}{C_P R_{cow}} \tag{4}$$

In Eq. 4 C_M is the stable-element concentration in milk per liter, C_P is the stable-element concentration in forage, and R_{cow} is the daily intake of forage. For a conservative estimation[13] of f_M, it can be assumed that a cow ingests 10 kg of forage daily, i.e., $R_{cow} = 10^4$ g. If data were unavailable for an estimate of f_M by Eq. 4, it was assumed that 5% of the isotope absorbed daily by the cow is secreted per liter of milk. The f_M is then equal to 0.05 times a factor representing gut absorption. The fraction absorbed was assumed to be the ICRP value of the "fraction from GI tract to blood."[12]

The ICRP tables list (as f_W) many of the values of f_B, the fraction of the ingested isotope deposited in tissue. If f_B was not listed in the ICRP tables, it was assumed to be the fraction absorbed times the fraction from blood to the tissue. The fraction absorbed was assumed to be the ICRP value of "f_1, fraction from GI tract to blood," and the fraction from blood to the tissue was estimated from the ICRP values listed for "f_2^1, fraction from blood to tissue." In this procedure the particular tissue was assumed to take up all the absorbed isotope not known to be taken up by other tissues. Certain elements, i.e., H, C, N, O, Na, K, Cl, and Br, were assumed to be distributed uniformly; f_B was assumed to be the ratio of organ mass to total body mass, and the biological half-life was assumed to be the biological half-life for the total body.

The values for m were taken from revised values for the mass of the organs of standard man.[16]

It is to be noted especially that the worst-case assumptions adopted for estimation of the input parameters resulted in estimates that are overconservative, sometimes by more than an order of magnitude. It will be shown later that less conservative but more reasonable values based on collateral data have been substituted where possible for those nuclides shown to be the most hazardous using the worst-case assumptions mentioned above. On the other hand, no attempt was made to derive better estimates for nuclides that were shown by the worst-case assumptions to contribute only insignificantly to the dosage.

Estimated Maximum Dose from a Given Deposition

The unit-rad depositions calculated for the radionuclides rank the nuclides in order of their potential contribution to the internal dose under conditions of equal deposition. Under these conditions the estimated maximum dose from a radionuclide will vary inversely with its unit-rad deposition. The estimated maximum dose from a given deposition is simply the quotient of the deposition expressed in microcuries and the unit-rad deposition.

The estimated maximum dose from radionuclides released to the atmosphere in nuclear cratering events can be predicted if the activities produced are known. The prediction is based on estimates of the maximum deposition which are made as described by Tamplin.[1]

Prediction of Estimated Maximum Dose

In this procedure we first determine the m^2-rad based on the total activity produced. The m^2-rad is the quotient of the activity produced in the detonation expressed in microcuries and the unit-rad deposition, F_1, which is expressed in $\mu Ci/m^2/rad$. Let Σ represent the m^2-rad and P represent the activity produced in microcuries. Then

$$\Sigma = \frac{P}{F_1} \tag{5}$$

Tamplin[1] has presented estimates of the maximum deposition on agricultural land following an underground nuclear explosion as a function of cloud travel time. The estimated maximum fractional contamination, EMC, is the maximum fraction of the activity produced that is deposited per square meter; it is expressed in units of m^{-2}. The product of Σ and EMC thus gives an estimate of the maximum dosage, EMD:

$$EMD = \Sigma \times EMC \tag{6}$$

The EMC values listed in Table 1 can be used to estimate the maximum deposition at 12 hr. The values listed in Table 1 will be used in the calculations in this paper.

Table 1

DEPOSITION OF NUCLIDES[1] PRODUCED IN NUCLEAR CRATERING EVENTS [ESTIMATED MAXIMUM FRACTIONAL CONTAMINATION (EMC) AT 12 HR]

Isotope	EMC, m^{-2}
^{89}Sr, ^{137}Cs	5×10^{-11}
^{90}Sr, ^{91}Y, ^{140}Ba	2.5×10^{-11}
All others	10^{-11}

The m^2-rad values were determined for nuclides produced by fission and by activation of the environment. The m^2-rad was calculated per kiloton of ^{235}U fission and per kiloton of ^{239}Pu fission for over 80 fission products. The highest fission yields listed by Weaver, Strom, and Killeen[17] were assumed. The m^2-rad of activation products produced in granite was calculated per mole of thermal neutrons and per mole of 14-Mev neutrons.[18] The nuclides considered include over 125 activation products produced by close to 180 neutron activation reactions. Activities induced in major rock types other than granite have been calculated, and the m^2-rad estimates of these are available.

Relative Importance of Individual Nuclides

Very conservative values have been assumed for biological parameters when experimental data were not readily available. It is essential to note that, when this approach is used to analyze situations involving radiation exposure to the public, most radionuclides can still be eliminated from consideration as potential internal hazards despite the worst-case assumptions. Table 2 lists some m^2-rad values for activation products in granite selected from the series of calculations. The unit-rad depositions from which the m^2-rad values were derived are also shown. The unit-rad depositions are approximately the same, dif-

Table 2

ESTIMATED MAXIMUM 30-YEAR DOSE VIA MILK TO THE WHOLE BODY OF THE CHILD FROM ACTIVATION PRODUCTS PRODUCED IN GRANITE (UNIT-RAD DEPOSITION AND M²-RAD PER MOLE OF 14-MEV NEUTRONS)

Radionuclide	F_1, $\mu Ci/m^2/rad$	Σ, m^2-rad/mole
^{24}Na	24	4.3×10^{11}
^{32}P	11	3.8×10^{9}
^{58}Co	33	1.2×10^{5}
^{59}Ni	14	8.4
^{123m}Sn	25	6.3×10^{1}
^{124}Sb	73	8.2×10^{3}
^{121m}Te	54	1.9×10^{-1}
^{129m}Te	87	1.5
^{186}Re	52	5.5×10^{4}
^{192}Ir	22	9.4×10^{4}
^{197}Hg	44	2.1×10^{4}
^{205}Pb	24	3.6×10^{-5}

fering by less than a factor of 10. Although the F_1 values are comparable, the m^2-rad values, and therefore the estimated maximum doses, differ over a range of 10^{16} units. Obviously, relative to that from ^{24}Na and ^{32}P, the dose from the other nuclides can be considered insignificant.

Thus it is clear that this approach allows us to focus attention on the few nuclides that are singled out as potential hazards. The number of nuclides found to be potentially hazardous may then be further reduced following a critical reevaluation of the assumed biological and physical parameters.

The m^2-rad values presented were calculated for the whole body of the child (mass, 10 kg). The m^2-rad values are arranged in decreasing order. Only the highest values are shown for the reasons discussed above.

The M²-Rad and Estimated Maximum Dose from Fission Products

As an example of the calculations for fission products, the m^2-rad values via the forage-to-cow-to-milk pathway per kiloton of ^{239}Pu fission are shown in Table 3. The total m^2-rad summed over all the nuclides is listed at the bottom. The m^2-rad values range from the 3×10^{10} maximum of ^{131}I to the 3×10^{-14} minimum of ^{144}Nd, an extreme range of 10^{24} units. Except in the case of ^{111}Ag, the input parameters of the nuclides at the top of the list are well known; so the m^2-rad values are largely reasonable.

The estimated maximum doses via milk from the ^{239}Pu fission products are also shown in Table 3. The estimated maximum doses

Table 3

PRINCIPAL CONTRIBUTIONS TO THE ESTIMATED MAXIMUM 30-YEAR DOSE TO THE CHILD'S WHOLE BODY BY FISSION PRODUCTS VIA THE FORAGE-TO-COW-TO-MILK PATHWAY (M^2-RAD AND ESTIMATED MAXIMUM DOSE IN MILLIRADS PER KILOTON OF ^{239}Pu FISSION)

Radionuclide	Half-life	Σ, m^2-rad/kt	EMC,* m^{-2}	EMD = EMC × Σ, mrad	Percent of total EMD
^{131}I	8.05 days	3.1×10^{10}	10^{-11}	310	25
^{136}Cs	13 days	2.6×10^{10}	10^{-11}	260	21
^{111}Ag	7.5 days	1.9×10^{10}	10^{-11}	190	15
^{133}I	21 hr	1.4×10^{10}	10^{-11}	140	11
^{99}Mo	66 hr	9.8×10^{9}	10^{-11}	98	7.9
^{90}Sr	28 years	2.1×10^{9}	2.5×10^{-11}	53	4.3
^{89}Sr	50.4 days	1.6×10^{9}	5×10^{-11}	80	6.5
^{137}Cs	30 years	1.3×10^{9}	5×10^{-11}	65	5.3
^{132}Te	78 hr	9.2×10^{8}	10^{-11}	9	0.7
^{112}Pd	21 hr	8.0×10^{8}	10^{-11}	8	0.6
^{140}Ba	12.8 days	4.4×10^{8}	2.5×10^{-11}	11	0.9
^{105}Rh	36 hr	3.5×10^{8}	10^{-11}	4	0.3
^{131m}Te	1.2 days	3.3×10^{8}	10^{-11}	3	0.3
^{129m}Te	33 days	2.7×10^{8}	10^{-11}	3	0.2
^{125}Sn	9.4 days	2.0×10^{8}	10^{-11}	2	0.2
^{130}I	12.5 hr	1.4×10^{8}	10^{-11}	1	0.1
Total		1.1×10^{11}		1200	

*From Table 1.

listed include only those that are at least 0.1% of the total. Isotopes of iodine, cesium, and strontium contribute over 70% of the total estimated maximum dose; ^{99}Mo, ^{140}Ba, and isotopes of tellurium contribute an additional 10%.

Estimated Maximum Dose from Fission Products in a Series of Detonations

The calculations just presented can serve to establish limiting fission yields that could be used in nuclear cratering events, such as those proposed for the construction of a canal across Central America using nuclear explosives.[10] For example, the estimated maximum dose from fission products in a single detonation would be

$$EMD = 1.2 \ (rad/kt) \times Y \ (kt)$$

where Y is the fission yield. For a series of detonations where the fission yields are comparable, the estimated maximum dose would be

$$EMD = 0.1 \times 1.2 \ (rad/kt) \times Y_T \ (kt)$$

where Y_T is the total fission yield. A third factor, less than unity, has been introduced into the calculation. We have arbitrarily assumed 0.1. We feel justified in using this factor for planning purposes since we are considering a series of detonations, only a very few of which could be expected to be worst cases at the same location.[1] Whether or not any particular fission yield would be acceptable in a given situation would have to be decided with due consideration of the radiation protection guidelines for the population at large.[9]

The M^2-Rad and Estimated Maximum Dose from Activation Products Produced in the Environment

The second source of radionuclides to be considered is neutron activation of the environment surrounding the device. Table 4 gives the

Table 4

PRINCIPAL CONTRIBUTIONS TO THE ESTIMATED MAXIMUM 30-YEAR DOSE TO THE CHILD'S WHOLE BODY BY ACTIVATION PRODUCTS PRODUCED IN GRANITE VIA THE FORAGE-TO-COW-TO-MILK PATHWAY (M^2-RAD PER MOLE OF 14-MEV NEUTRONS)

Radionuclide	Half-life	Σ, m^2-rad/mole
^{24}Na	15 hr	4.3×10^{10}
^{32}P	14.3 days	3.8×10^{9}
^{42}K	12.4 hr	3.8×10^{9}
^{86}Rb	18.7 days	3.8×10^{9}
^{84}Rb	33 days	2.8×10^{9}
^{134}Cs	2.1 years	8.8×10^{8}
^{22}Na	2.58 years	3.7×10^{8}
^{45}Ca	165 days	3.3×10^{8}
^{82}Br	35.3 hr	1.2×10^{8}
Total		5.9×10^{10}

m^2-rad values (forage-to-cow-to-milk pathway) for activation products produced in granite per mole of 14-Mev neutrons. By assuming 14-Mev neutrons rather than thermal neutrons, we can be more certain of not overlooking a significant nuclide. Thus a table of m^2-rad values per mole of thermal neutrons would not differ substantially from Table 4, except that ^{84}Rb and ^{22}Na would not appear. All the m^2-rad values listed are directly convertible to the EMD, using the conversion factor 10^{-11} m^{-2}. Isotopes of group I elements are noted to be especially prominent among those at the top of the list. The isotope ^{24}Na contributes most to the total estimated maximum dose, about 75%. As a consequence of its relatively short half-life, the quantity of ^{24}Na actually secreted in milk is less by more than an order of magnitude than the quantity estimated on the basis of an instantaneous steady state. Accordingly, we have reduced the m²-rad calculated for ^{24}Na by a factor of 10. The input parameters of the nuclides at the top of the list are well known or are reasonable values; hence their m²-rad values are also reasonable. The estimated maximum dose from ^{24}Na exceeds that from the next highest, ^{32}P, ^{42}K, and ^{86}Rb, by a factor of about 10.

Estimated Maximum Dose from Activation Products in a Single High-Yield Detonation

Consider the estimated maximum dose from ^{24}Na in light of the proposed construction of a canal using nuclear explosives. The neutron yield[19] per megaton of fusion is about 10^{27} neutrons. If $1/_{1000}$ of this number of neutrons were released to the environment following capture in the device and in the shielding materials, about 1 mole of neutrons per megaton of fusion would be released to the environment. The m²-rad per mole of neutrons would then be equivalent to the m²-rad per megaton of fusion.

Under the assumptions just described, the estimated maximum dose from the ^{24}Na released in a 1-Mt nuclear cratering event would be

$$\text{EMD} = 5.9 \times 10^{10} \text{ (m}^2\text{-rad)} \times 10^{-11} \text{ (m}^{-2}\text{)}$$
$$= 0.59 \text{ rad}$$

The estimated maximum dose from a 10-Mt detonation would be 43 rads. The EMD would be greater if the attenuation in the number of neutrons were less than 1000, as was assumed. The 30-year dose from ^{24}Na would be delivered in just a few days since ^{24}Na has a half-life of only 15 hr. Calculations similar to those previously shown for the fission products can readily be performed to estimate the maximum ^{24}Na dose from a series of detonations.

The calculation points to the urgent need to reduce to very low levels the neutrons released to the environment through adequate shielding or other measures. In the course of reducing ^{24}Na production, the production of other activities induced in the environment would be reduced as well. Practical problems relating to countermeasures, if they are ever needed, are simplified in the case of ^{24}Na by virtue of its short half-life.

THE SOIL—ROOT PATHWAY

The second mode of entry into man is the soil—root pathway. This pathway involving equilibration over the soil—root system can be significant only for the relatively long lived radionuclides, which have the potential to equilibrate within the biological exchangeable pool before their disappearance by radioactive decay.

The soil–root model relates to a food crop grown under conditions of normal agricultural practice. The basic assumptions are (1) that fallout depositing on the terrain is immediately distributed and retained within the plow layer and (2) that radionuclides equilibrate instantaneously within the biological exchangeable pool exclusive of man. The assumption that equilibration of radionuclides is instantaneous maximizes the internal dose estimate for a given deposition since man's diet would then have maximum specific activity,* which would be equal to that of food-chain constituents and of the environment.

The Unit-Rad Deposition

The minimum deposition on agricultural land that could lead to a 30-year internal dose of 1 rad is determined using the expression[8]

$$F_1 = \frac{3.71 \times 10^{-1} \rho d}{Q} \left(\frac{C_S}{C_B}\right) \frac{1}{[T_R (1 - e^{-20.8/T_R}) - T_E (1 - e^{-20.8/T_E})]} \quad (7)$$

where F_1 = unit-rad deposition ($\mu Ci/m^2/rad$)
ρ = density of the soil (g/cm^3)
d = depth of the plow layer (cm)
Q = energy absorbed in the tissue per unit disintegration (Mev)
T_R = half-life for radioactive decay (years)
T_E = effective half-life in man's tissue (years)
C_S = stable-element concentration in soil
C_B = stable-element concentration in the tissue

Determination of Input Parameters

The parameters of Eq. 7 that determine the unit-rad deposition via the soil–root pathway (equilibration in the biological exchangeable pool) include Q, ρ, d, C_S, and C_B. The Q term has the same value that was used to estimate the unit-rad deposition via the forage-to-cow-to milk pathway. A soil density of 2 g/cm^3 and a depth of 20 cm have been adopted.

Rules were adopted for conservative estimation of C_S, C_B, and the C_S/C_B ratio when they were not known. When concentration in soil was not known, it was estimated from data on abundance in the earth's

---

*The specific activity is the ratio of radioactive to total nuclides of the element. In most systems of interest, the radionuclides constitute a negligible fraction of the total, and the specific activity can be regarded as the ratio of radioactive to stable nuclides.

crust. When concentration in the tissues was not known, it was assumed to exceed the average soil concentration by a factor of 100, and the C_S/C_B ratio was assumed to be 0.01.

Unit-rad depositions via the soil−root pathway to the same tissues considered for the forage-to-cow-to-milk pathway were calculated for radionuclides of half-life greater than 30 days. The effective half-life term of Eq. 7 was assumed to be zero if it was not known, which serves to minimize F_1. The effective half-life also was set equal to zero in calculating F_1 values for the infant.[4] Since an infant experiences very rapid growth, he will come into equilibrium with his diet and environment (soil) much more rapidly than an adult. Setting $T_E = 0$ serves to account for this rapid equilibration. The m^2-rad values were then calculated on the basis of the total production values used previously.

Initial M² -Rad of Fission Products

Calculations for m^2-rad to the whole body via the soil−root pathway per kiloton of ^{239}Pu fission led to the ordering of nuclides shown in Table 5. The observed ranking of the nuclides, however, resulted

Table 5

RANKING OF THE ^{239}Pu FISSION PRODUCTS ACCORDING TO THE INITIALLY CALCULATED M²-RAD PER KILOTON TO THE WHOLE BODY
(SOIL− ROOT PATHWAY)

Rank	Nuclide	Rank	Nuclide
1	^{106}Ru	11	^{115m}Cd
2	^{144}Ce	12	^{151}Sm
3	^{147}Pm	13	^{113m}Cd
4	^{103}Ru	14	^{125m}Te
5	^{129m}Te	15	^{162}Gd
6	^{127m}Te	16	^{124}Sb
7	^{141}Ce	17	^{154}Eu
8	^{155}Eu	18	^{123m}Sn
9	^{91}Y	19	^{90}Sr
10	^{125}Sb	20	^{137}Cs

from the use of worst-case assumptions. Unit-rad depositions and m^2-rad values of all the nuclides above ^{115m}Cd in Table 6 were calculated assuming worst-case values for input parameters, usually that the C_B/C_S ratio was equal to 100.

Reevaluation of Input Parameters

Using ^{106}Ru as an example, we can illustrate how collateral data on the behavior of elements in the biological exchangeable pool can be used to make more reasonable estimates of the C_B/C_S ratio and, there-

Table 6

PRINCIPAL CONTRIBUTIONS TO THE ESTIMATED MAXIMUM 30-YEAR WHOLE-BODY DOSE BY FISSION PRODUCTS VIA THE SOIL-ROOT PATHWAY (M^2-RAD PER KILOTON OF ^{239}Pu FISSION)

Radionuclide	Half-life	Σ, m^2-rad/kt Adult	Infant
^{129m}Te	33 days	4.6×10^8	6.6×10^8
^{106}Ru	1 year	3.7×10^8	5.0×10^8
^{127m}Te	105 days	1.4×10^8	1.6×10^8
^{103}Ru	40 days	3.9×10^7	1.7×10^8
^{115m}Cd	43 days	1.7×10^7	9.5×10^7
^{113m}Cd	14 years	1.4×10^7	1.5×10^7
^{125}Sb	2.7 years	7.9×10^5	8.3×10^5
^{123m}Sn	125 days	4.9×10^5	1.3×10^6
^{125m}Te	58 days	4.0×10^5	5.0×10^5
^{90}Sr	28 years	3.7×10^5	1.7×10^6
^{137}Cs	30 years	3.6×10^5	3.7×10^5
^{144}Ce	285 days	2.6×10^5	7.6×10^5

fore, of the unit-rad deposition and m^2-rad. Known data on the distribution of ruthenium in the biological exchangeable pool are: (1) the plant-to-soil ratio[20,21] of ruthenium concentration, C_P/C_S, in leaves and stems of crop plants at or approaching maturity varied between 0.02 and 0.7 and (2) the concentration[22] of ruthenium in beef, C_{steer}, has been found to be about 10^{-9} g/g.

We must assume that uptake and distribution are basically similar in steer and man. In the steady state the daily intake of ruthenium, I_{steer}, is related to the total-body concentration by the equation[12]

$$f_1 I_{steer} = \frac{0.693}{T_B} (m_{steer} C_{steer}) \qquad (8)$$

where f_1 is the fraction from GI tract to blood and T_B is the biological half-life in the total body. Iwashima[23] has noted that the ICRP values of f_1 and T_B led to estimates of the ^{106}Ru burden in human muscle which were low by a factor of 10 to 100. We have therefore assumed a value for f_1 that is 10 times greater than the ICRP value. The value adapted for T_B is based on long-term measurements of ^{106}Ru retention in the rat[24] and dog[25] and also exceeds the ICRP value by about a factor of 10. Substitution of $f_1 = 0.3$, $T_B = 130$ days, and C_{steer} into Eq. 8 leads to the calculation of

$$I_{steer} = 8.9 \times 10^{-6} \text{ g/day}$$

as the daily intake of ruthenium in a 1000-lb ($\sim 5 \times 10^5$ g) steer.

The daily intake of ruthenium is equal to the daily intake of forage times the concentration in forage:

$$I_{steer} = R_{steer} C_P \tag{9}$$

If the daily intake of forage is 10 kg and the daily intake of ruthenium is 8.9×10^{-6} g, as calculated, the ruthenium concentration in forage would be

$$C_P = \frac{8.9 \times 10^{-6}}{10^4} = 8.9 \times 10^{-10} \text{ g/g}$$

The plant-to-soil ratio of the ruthenium concentration, C_P/C_S, in forage was noted to vary between 0.02 and 0.7; so the concentration in soil would be 1.4 to 50 times greater than that in forage. The ruthenium concentration in soil, C_S, thus would vary between 1.3×10^{-9} and 4.5×10^{-8} g/g. Since the analysis is more conservative as the C_{steer}/C_S ratio is increased, the minimum concentration in soil is selected. The tissue-to-soil ratio for ruthenium concentration in beef would be

$$\frac{C_{steer}}{C_S} = \frac{10^{-9}}{1.3 \times 10^{-9}} = 0.8$$

The C_{steer}/C_S ratio is rounded off conservatively to 1.

By a similar approach it can be shown that man will not concentrate ruthenium from his diet. Thus the final C_B/C_S ratio for the whole body of man is taken to be 1. With a C_B/C_S ratio of 1 rather than 10^2, the m^2-rad of ^{106}Ru can be reduced by two orders of magnitude.

Using basically similar approaches we can also reduce the m^2-rad value of all the other nuclides above ^{115m}Cd, and many of the nuclides below, in some cases by orders of magnitude. In many cases it can be shown that a C_B/C_S ratio of 100 could only be consistent with a daily intake of the element measured in grams, which would be orders of magnitude above the possible levels. In many cases a C_B/C_S ratio of 100 could be consistent only with a C_B greater by orders of magnitude than that reported for soft tissues and bone of animals and man. The revised values of the input parameters are found in Ref. 4, and their derivation is described in detail.

Revised M² -Rad of Fission Products

The revised listing of the principal m^2-rad contributions via soil from fission products is shown in Table 6. Only those m^2-rad values are shown which are higher than 0.1% of the highest.

It must be remembered that information is not always available to permit the downward revision of a worst-case m^2-rad value to insignificant levels. The m^2-rad values listed in Table 6 for the isotopes of Te, Ru, Sb, and Ce represent revised estimates. Data are unavailable on the distributions of these elements in soils and plants and in animal and human tissues to permit the calculation of less restrictive m^2-rad values. The radionuclides listed in Table 6 include ^{129m}Te, ^{127m}Te, ^{103}Ru, ^{115m}Cd, ^{123m}Sn, and ^{125m}Te, which have half-lives substantially less than 1 year. The specific activities of these nuclides in plants that grow to maturity and are consumed by man would be much less at the time of ingestion than at the time of deposition even if equilibrium were rapidly attained. The specific activities in foods derived from animals that feed on plants and in processed foods derived from plants would differ from that in the plants at the time of deposition by an even greater amount. The m^2-rad (via soil) values for these intermediate-lived nuclides are clearly overconservative. It may be desirable in certain cases to examine the kinetics of uptake of intermediate-lived nuclides in plants. For the present, however, we have chosen simply to treat the intermediate- and long-lived nuclides alike, and we obtain results that are at least consistent with the conservative aspects of the analysis. The m^2-rad of the metastable nuclides were calculated assuming that 100% of the nuclides produced would be in the metastable state, which is also in keeping with our conservative approach. In any event it is essential for public health and safety that these values be accepted until additional data become available and more reliable estimates can be made. It is clear from these examples that the analysis reveals areas in which experimental data are needed and indicates the nuclides for which postshot documentation is essential.

Initial M² -Rad of Activation Products Produced in the Environment

The m^2-rad values to the whole body via the soil—root pathway calculated per mole of 14-Mev neutrons in granite led to the ordering of nuclides shown in Table 7. The m^2-rad values for all the nuclides above ^{22}Na were calculated assuming a C_B/C_S ratio of 100. More reasonable estimates of C_B/C_S can be made to reduce the m^2-rad estimates to levels below that of ^{22}Na.

Revised M² -Rad of Activation Products

The revised listing of the principal m^2-rad contributions via soil from activation products produced in granite is shown in Table 8. Only those m^2-rad values are shown that are greater than 0.2% of the ^{22}Na value. The nuclides listed in Table 8 include ^{114m}In, ^{182}Ta, ^{185}W, ^{152}Eu, and ^{192}Ir, for which the m^2-rad values are conservative or worst-case values based on incomplete data. In addition, the half-lives of ^{114m}In, ^{182}Ta, ^{185}W, ^{35}S, ^{84}Rb, and ^{192}Ir are substantially less than 1 year. The

Table 7

RANKING OF THE ACTIVATION PRODUCTS PRODUCED IN GRANITE ACCORDING TO THE INITIALLY CALCULATED M²-RAD PER MOLE OF 14-MEV NEUTRONS TO THE WHOLE-BODY (SOIL–ROOT PATHWAY)

Rank	Nuclide	Rank	Nuclide
1	^{152}Eu	11	^{166m}Ho
2	^{46}Sc	12	^{175}Hf
3	^{154}Eu	13	^{169}Yb
4	^{182}Ta	14	^{114m}In
5	^{160}Tb	15	^{141}Ce
6	^{170}Tm	16	^{88}Y
7	^{22}Na	17	^{185}W
8	^{192}Ir	18	^{35}S
9	^{139}Ce	19	^{153}Gd
10	^{181}Hf	20	^{36}Cl

Table 8

PRINCIPAL CONTRIBUTIONS TO THE ESTIMATED MAXIMUM 30-YEAR WHOLE-BODY DOSE VIA THE SOIL–ROOT PATHWAY BY ACTIVATION PRODUCTS PRODUCED IN GRANITE (M²-RAD PER MOLE OF 14-MEV NEUTRONS)

Radionuclide	Half-life	Σ (m²-rad/kt) Adult	Σ (m²-rad/kt) Infant
^{22}Na	2.58 years	5.7×10^6	5.8×10^6
^{114m}In	50 days	3.1×10^5	6.2×10^5
^{182}Ta	115 days	2.8×10^5	8.3×10^5
^{185}W	74 days	1.6×10^5	1.9×10^5
^{35}S	86.7 days	1.6×10^5	3.1×10^5
^{36}Cl	3×10^5 years	1.4×10^5	1.4×10^5
^{84}Rb	33 days	7.2×10^4	2.5×10^5
^{60}Co	5.26 years	3.9×10^4	3.9×10^4
^{134}Cs	2.1 years	3.6×10^4	3.9×10^4
^{152}Eu	12.4 years	2.5×10^4	2.9×10^4
^{192}Ir	74 days	2.3×10^4	3.0×10^4
^{65}Zn	245 days	2.3×10^4	1.3×10^5
^{204}Tl	3.8 years	1.3×10^4	1.3×10^4

m²-rad values of these nuclides are to be accepted until more reliable estimates can be made, in the same manner described previously for the m²-rad values of the fission products listed in Table 6.

Comparison of the Estimated Maximum Dose via Milk and via Soil

The revised estimates of the m²-rad values via soil (Tables 6 and 8) are lower than the m²-rad values via milk (Tables 3 and 4) by two or more orders of magnitude. These results indicate that the total internal dose to the whole body via the forage-to-cow-to-milk pathway would greatly exceed that via the soil−root pathway. It must not be concluded from this, however, that the total dose to individual organs via milk would also exceed that via soil.

ESTIMATED MAXIMUM DOSE FROM ACTIVITIES INDUCED IN THE DEVICE

A third and equally important source of radioactivity is the non-fission activities produced in the device itself. These include both tritium and induced activities. The major nuclide produced in nuclear explosions, tritium, is considered in other reports of this series.[5,6]

The m^2-rad calculations based on production of activities induced in specific devices would, of course, require the use of classified data. Calculations based on the unit-rad depositions already determined would be straightforward and would show m^2-rad values and ordering of nuclides in sharp contrast to those shown previously for fission products and activation products from the environment.

One of the most important applications for this analysis is to establish guidelines with respect to device design. We have performed a comprehensive analysis of radionuclides that could be induced in devices.[3] For this analysis it is necessary to examine critically every radionuclide from its potential production in a device to its eventual burden in man. For the consideration of activation of device components, it was therefore necessary to consider, in addition to single neutron capture, multiple neutron captures and charged-particle reactions. Worst-case calculations for activation of single elements were made, and m^2-rad values were determined on the basis of these results. The m^2-rad values were then summed for each parent element, and the total m^2-rad attributable to the parent element per gram was determined. These results, when considered in light of design requirements, relate the estimated maximum dose to the grams of an element in a device and hence establish limits to the quantities of materials that can safely be used. We have shown how similar calculations can be used to establish the limiting fission yields and to determine the minimum requirements for neutron shielding. In much the same way, we are attempting to establish for device design the guidelines that are essential to the development of the optimum in biologically clean devices.

INTERPRETATION OF THE DOSE ESTIMATES

These estimates were calculated using biological parameters estimated for standard man. Estimates of maximum internal dose therefore apply to the population at large and may be compared with the radiation protection standards established for the general population. The estimates can also be applied to individuals in the general population if one accepts the suggestion of the Federal Radiation Council (FRC)[9] that the majority of individuals do not vary from the average by a factor greater than 3.

It may be argued that the analysis described in this paper leads to estimates that are overconservative and hence too restrictive. Such arguments become unacceptable, however, when due consideration is given to the public health and safety. Indeed, strong arguments can be presented in favor of a more conservative approach. Certainly, for providing guidance for the establishment of an adequate postshot monitoring program, a more conservative interpretation of the estimates is essential. Thus we would suggest that the analysis is sufficient for preshot radiation safety analysis if, and only if, the system of postshot documentation is adequate both to determine the actual levels of environmental contamination and to assure that countermeasures would be instituted when and if required.

The Forage-to-Cow-to-Milk Pathway

The input parameters in the forage-to-cow-to-milk model include values estimated for standard man. In actual cases the values may depart considerably because of individual variability. The input parameters for the cow may also differ from those selected. Thus in individual cases a cow may secrete a greater fraction in milk than the value used, and it may graze over more than 45 m^2 of pasture daily. In addition, the residence half-time on forage may exceed 14 days. Any one of these situations could lead to an underestimate of dose by a factor of 2 or more. Although the probability is low that these situations would be encountered concurrently, the possibility does exist.

The following suggested guidelines therefore appear to be both reasonable and consistent with the guidelines for surveillance and control as set forth by the FRC.[26] It is suggested that monitoring of milk sheds be carried out in areas where the predicted maximum dose is greater than $1/100$ of the acceptable levels and that monitoring of individual farms be carried out where the predicted maximum dose is greater than $1/10$ of the acceptable levels. It is further suggested that activities be determined for those isotopes for which the m^2-rad estimates are within the first three orders of magnitude.

The Soil–Root Pathway

The input parameters assumed in the soil–root model apply to standard man and normal agricultural practices. The analysis is conservative to the extent that it assumes instantaneous equilibration of the specific activities in man's food chains and in the local terrestrial environment from which he is assumed to derive his entire food supply. There are, however, special food chains, such as the lichen–caribou–Eskimo chain, for which the analysis might not be sufficiently conservative. It is therefore reasonable to suggest that the rules for surveillance and control that were applied to the forage-to-cow-to-milk model be also applied to the soil–root model.

APPENDIX

Additional material not included in the formal publication was presented orally. Since this material was the subject of much of the ensuing discussion, it is included in an appendix.

The fractional depositions that were measured subsequent to nuclear device testing at the Nevada Test Site have been analyzed by Tamplin in Ref. 1. Figure A1 shows the maximum fractional wet and dry depositions that can be expected as a function of cloud travel time.[1]

Much of the discussion is related to the example presented to illustrate the basis for our choice of estimating the maximum or worst-case dosage. On Dec. 28, 1966, the U. S. Atomic Energy Commission sent this press release to the wire services: "The U. S. detected another Chinese Communist nuclear test in the atmosphere at their test site

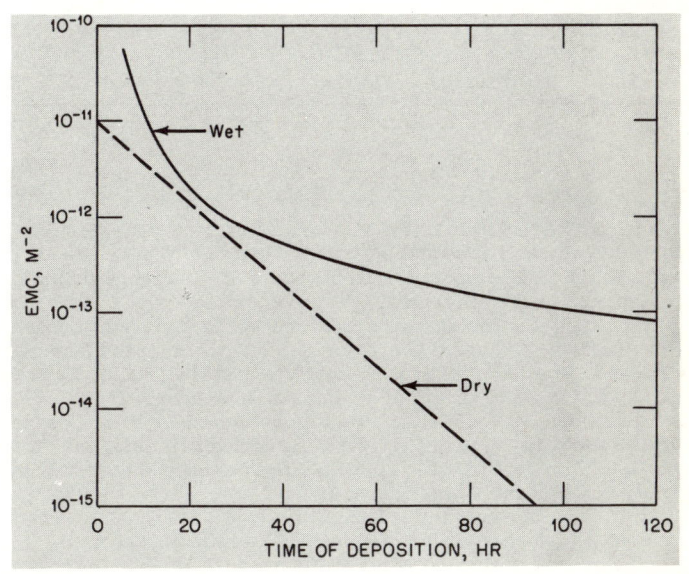

Fig. A1 — Maximum fractional wet and dry deposition vs. postdetonation time.[1]

near Lop Nor, on Dec. 28, 1966, Chinese time (December 27, U. S. time). The yield was a few hundred kilotons." The main contamination of Northern California from the event took place as dry deposition on Jan. 1 to 3, 1967 (5, 6, and 7 days postshot).

We assumed that 300 kt was within a factor of 2 of the reported yield of a few hundred kilotons. Using this assumption we estimated the maximum forage and milk concentrations that could be expected as a result of dry deposition some 6 days postshot. Table A1 shows the comparison of these estimates with the measured values.[27] A comparison of the values in the table strongly suggests that this represented a worst case of dry fallout. We would estimate that, if rain had occurred, these values would have increased by as much as a factor of 100. They would have exceeded the radiation protection guidelines for ^{131}I even though the test occurred 7000 miles away and 6 days before the contamination.

Table A1

DEPOSITION OF FALLOUT RADIONUCLIDES ON PASTURE GRASS AND TRANSFER TO COW'S MILK FOLLOWING THE CHINESE NUCLEAR TEST OF DEC. 28, 1966

	Forage, pCi/kg		Milk, pCi/kg	
Nuclide	Estimated	Measured*	Estimated	Measured*
^{131}I	1790	5000	1790	930
^{137}Cs	6	43	4	17
^{99}Mo	540	1050	67	20
^{140}Ba	2270	5740	68	71
^{132}Te	670	1510	34	7

*Reference 27.

REFERENCES

1. A. R. Tamplin, Prediction of the Maximum Dosage to Man from the Fallout of Nuclear Devices. I. Estimation of the Maximum Contamination of Agricultural Land, USAEC Report UCRL-50163(Pt. I), Lawrence Radiation Laboratory, University of California, Livermore, 1967.
2. Y. C. Ng and S. E. Thompson, Prediction of the Maximum Dosage to Man from the Fallout of Nuclear Devices. II. Estimation of the Maximum Dose from Internal Emitters, USAEC Report UCRL-50163(Pt. II), Lawrence Radiation Laboratory, University of California, Livermore, 1966.
3. C. A. Burton and M. W. Pratt, Prediction of the Maximum Dosage to Man from the Fallout of Nuclear Devices. III. Biological Guidelines for Device Design, USAEC Report UCRL-50163(Pt. III), Lawrence Radiation Laboratory, University of California, Livermore, 1967.
4. Y. C. Ng, C. A. Burton, S. E. Thompson, R. K. Tandy, H. K. Kretner, and M. W. Pratt, Prediction of the Maximum Dosage to Man from the Fallout of Nuclear Devices. IV. Handbook for Estimating the Maximum Internal Dose to Man from Radionuclides Released to the Biosphere, USAEC Report UCRL-50163(Pt. IV), Lawrence Radiation Laboratory, University of California, Livermore, 1968.

5. A. R. Tamplin, H. L. Fisher, and W. H. Chapman, Prediction of the Maximum Dosage to Man from the Fallout of Nuclear Devices. V. Estimation of the Maximum Dose from Internal Emitters in Aquatic Food Supply, USAEC Report UCRL-50163(Pt. V), Lawrence Radiation Laboratory, University of California, Livermore, 1968.
6. H. L. Fisher, Prediction of the Maximum Dosage to Man from the Fallout of Nuclear Devices. VI. Transport of Nuclear Debris by Surface and Groundwater, USAEC Report UCRL-50163(Pt. VI), Lawrence Radiation Laboratory, University of California, Livermore, in preparation.
7. Y. C. Ng, The Biological Exchangeable Pool, in Program Book for the Advisory Committee for Biology and Medicine of the U. S. Atomic Energy Commission, USAEC Report UCRL-14739, Part 2, pp. 19-32, Lawrence Radiation Laboratory, University of California, Livermore, 1966.
8. C. A. Burton, A Graphical Method for Calculating the Dose in Man from Individual Radionuclides in Fallout, USAEC Report UCRL-14922, Lawrence Radiation Laboratory, University of California, Livermore, 1966.
9. Federal Radiation Council, Background Material for the Development of Radiation Protection Standards, FRC Staff Report No. 1, Superintendent of Documents, U. S. Government Printing Office, Washington, 1960.
10. E. Graves, Nuclear Excavation of a Sea-Level Isthmian Canal, in Engineering with Nuclear Explosives, Proceedings of the Third Plowshare Symposium, University of California, Davis, April 21–23, 1964, USAEC Report TID-7695, pp. 321-334, Lawrence Radiation Laboratory, University of California, Livermore, 1964.
11. D. T. Goldman, *Chart of the Nuclides*, 8th ed., Knolls Atomic Power Laboratory, March 1965.
12. K. Z. Morgan (Chairman), Report of ICRP Committee II on Permissible Dose for Internal Radiation (1959), in *Radiation Protection. Recommendations of the International Commission on Radiological Protection*, ICRP Publication 2, Pergamon Press, Inc., 1960; or *Health Phys.*, 3: 1-380 (1960).
13. J. J. Koranda, Agricultural Factors Affecting the Daily Intake of Fresh Fallout by Dairy Cows, USAEC Report UCRL-12479, Lawrence Radiation Laboratory, University of California, Livermore, 1965.
14. C. A. Burton and J. H. Maxwell, The Available Disintegration Energy of All Radionuclides (for Use in Dosimetry Problems). I. Radionuclides with Half-Lives of 12 hr or Greater, USAEC Report UCRL-50164, Lawrence Radiation Laboratory, University of California, Livermore, 1966.
15. S. E. Thompson, Effective Half-Life of Fallout Radionuclides on Plants with Special Emphasis on Iodine-131, USAEC Report UCRL-12388, Lawrence Radiation Laboratory, University of California, Livermore, 1965.
16. W. S. Snyder, M. J. Cook, and I. H. Tipton, Revision of Standard Man, in Health Physics Division Annual Progress Report for Period Ending July 31, 1966, USAEC Report ORNL-4007(Pt. V), pp. 213-216, Oak Ridge National Laboratory, 1966.
17. L. E. Weaver, P. O. Strom, and P. A. Killeen, Estimated Total Chain and Independent Fission Processes, USAEC Report USNRDL-TR-633, U. S. Naval Radiological Defense Laboratory, 1963.
18. Y. C. Ng, Neutron Activation of the Terrestrial Environment as a Result of Underground Nuclear Explosions, USAEC Report UCRL-14249, Lawrence Radiation Laboratory, University of California, Livermore, June 22, 1965.
19. J. A. Miskel, Characteristics of Radioactivity Produced by Nuclear Explosives, in Engineering with Nuclear Explosives, Proceedings of the Third Plowshare Symposium, University of California, Davis, April 21–23, 1964, USAEC Report TID-7695, pp. 153-160, Lawrence Radiation Laboratory, University of California, Livermore, 1964.
20. W. B. Lane, J. D. Sartor, and C. F. Miller, Plant Uptake of Radioelements from Soil, USAEC File No. NP-13796, Stanford Research Institute, 1964.

21. J. D. Sartor, W. B. Lane, and J. J. Allen, Uptake of Radionuclides by Plants, USAEC File No. NP-16646, Stanford Research Institute, 1966.
22. R. C. Koch and J. Roesmer, Application of Activation Analysis to the Determination of Trace-Element Concentrations in Meat. *J. Food Sci.*, 27: 309-320 (1962).
23. K. Iwashima and N. Yamagata, Environmental Contamination with Radioruthenium, 1961-1965, *J. Radiat. Res.*, 7: 91-111 (1966).
24. J. E. Furchner, C. R. Richmond, and G. A. Trafton, Long-Term Retention of ^{106}Ru by Rats, USAEC Report LAMS-2526, Los Alamos Scientific Laboratory, 1961.
25. J. E. Furchner, C. R. Richmond, and G. A. Trafton, Metabolism of ^{106}Ru Chloride in Mammals: Progress Reports on Dogs, USAEC Report LAMS-2780, Los Alamos Scientific Laboratory, 1962.
26. Federal Radiation Council, Background Material for the Development of Radiation Protection Standards, FRC Staff Report No. 2, Superintendent of Documents, U. S. Government Printing Office, Washington, 1961.
27. G. D. Potter, D. R. McIntyre, and D. Pomeroy, Transport of Fallout Radionuclides in the Grass-to-Milk Food Chain Studied with a Germanium Lithium-Drifted Detector, *Health Phys.*, 16(3): 297-300(1969).

DISCUSSION

EVANS: In one of your figures you showed both wet and dry deposition on the ground. The two approached each other rather closely at a certain time. Could you say more about what that means?

NG: Figure A1 shows the estimated maximum contamination from wet and dry deposition as determined from analysis of fallout data collected subsequent to nuclear device testing at the Nevada Test Site. With few exceptions the wet depositions fell on or below the solid line. All the dry depositions fell on or below the dotted line. These are empirical data, and the two levels are about the same at about 24 hr.

EVANS: If you had a rainout at 20 hr, you would expect a bigger difference between dry and wet than appears on that curve.

TAMPLIN (LRL): In the case of rainout, you will get about a 30-fold increase in the wet depositions.*

NG: I wish to make a comment on a question that was previously asked of A. Tamplin. If we were at a loss to obtain an estimate for the concentration in organs, we assumed that the concentration in tissue was 100 times that in soil or rock.

EVANS: I think the safest curve is due to three factors. One is that the magnitude of the difference between wet and dry fallout would be increased by an increase in the size of the sample of rainout cases. The second is that the probability of being exposed to rainout increases as the cloud size grows; so you have a higher probability of rainout with increase in time. And probably the third factor is that the weather

---

*Author's note added in proof: The estimated maximum deposition by rainout would fall above the wet deposition curve of Fig. A1.

forecasters did a good job of ensuring that the probability of rainout was small on the first day or two after the shot was fired.

HAWLEY: Perhaps I should have asked this question of Tamplin. When you have a big cratering situation, such as a canal excavation, is there a chance that tearing up all that earth, which subsequently falls back and becomes available to the water by leaching, could change the amount of stable isotope in the water to such an extent that it would alter your calculations or possibly even change the ecological systems?

TAMPLIN: We purposely picked values that were either for estuarian or continental-shelf areas; so we picked areas where there were a lot of suspended materials. Also, we looked at the range of values depending upon what kind of geological surface was feeding the freshwater into the estuarian or shoreline area, and we tried to pick the higher values. The reason we suggest that all the radionuclides we have tabulated must be considered, even though the lowest one is contributing a factor of 1000 less than the top one on the list, is this question of biological availability. It may be that when you blow a canal you may find a large amount of the materials lower on the list entering the water and hence increasing the concentration of the stable element as you have suggested. There are experiments going on in the Bio-Medical Division that tend to suggest that is not going to be the case because these materials are not very soluble. This seems like a reasonable assumption for cratering projects, but, until you actually obtain postshot measurements, you must consider all the nuclides that are listed for the reason you suggested in your question.

CRAWFORD (LRL): The technique of taking worst cases for analysis is really a useful technique for identifying problem isotopes, which is what you are doing; but some of us are wondering what is the ratio of dose estimates between worst case and the expected case.

TAMPLIN: If you are going to do something, you had better be prepared for the worst case. You should have a monitoring program that will be distributed and able to respond in a timely way to the worst case. Everything may go perfectly, but these worst-case situations we present have happened in the past and probably will happen in the future, even with the Plowshare experiments or projects. The ratio between worst case and expected case is about a factor of 10 in the dry fallout and a factor of 50 in the wet fallout. In Table 3 the biology is well known for all the radionuclides shown. There were no worst-case assumptions associated with those data, except about rainout.

DUNSTER: Do you have children in this country 6 months old drinking fresh cow's milk (not dry milk) and nothing else?

TAMPLIN: Yes, all over. If Pendleton [Dr. Robert Pendleton, Radiobiology Department, University of Utah, Salt Lake City, Utah] were here he could name for you all the children in Utah that do.

DUNSTER: Although you can use these calculations for calculating the type of monitoring program you need for estimating worst-case situations, is not there also a very considerable danger that the calculations will also be used to prevent the test or project from happening at all?

TAMPLIN: That depends on which side of Panama you live on.

HOLLAND: I think it is essential to associate some concept of probability with these numbers. Obviously, if you talk about the expected case in the physical sense, this would be the average that would occur in a large number of trials. You are never going to have this kind of an experimental base. Associating a probability with something which has never before been done and which consists of a large number of parts (on many of which we have no statistical experience) is obviously impossible in any rigorous sense. If we could say when we give estimates like this whether we think this is a 1 percentile or a 0.1 or a 0.01, in terms of probability, the discussion would move to a more rational plane. We could argue about what is the probability of this being exceeded and examine the various factors that might or might not cause it to be exceeded, including an estimate of how many liters of milk a child drinks. We could then arrive at some sort of common terminology. I have a feeling the discussion is at cross purposes when only the term "worst case" is used, and then you try to define the relation between the worst case and the so-called expected case.

TAMPLIN: There were only four Chinese tests; so the chances are 1 in 4 that this will happen in the Chinese tests.

GOFMAN: I disagree with you heartily on your point of view and with those who always worry about these things being worst-case estimates and therefore not really related to reality. Actually it would be a very nice thing to talk about averages when you have had, for each kind of event, 100 or 1000 repetitions of the test. Now for the entire testing of nuclear devices there are not enough altogether to say anything about statistics. They were each done under different conditions, and so you cannot even talk about real statistics. What I am saying is, let us look at what has happened. Since we have so little experience, it is better to expect this kind of thing to happen again. Those who would like to go ahead with their program (and Dr. Dunster, I am fully in favor of going ahead with preparing for Plowshare) often say "But you are picking out the worst possible case. That is an atypical one. Wait until we have our typical shot." And then the very next shot is atypical again. So we still wait for the typical one. The Chinese come along. We made some estimates, and they were very close to the measurements. Well, it is said to be atypical — 7000 miles away and all that. These are realities; and we must stick close to reality rather than to averages we do not have from statistical distribution.

TAMPLIN: These are not actually worst cases; these are the maximum expectations based on a very small sample of experience.

GRAHN: You just said it is not the worst case. You are using the wrong language.

GOFMAN: Fine. I do not care about the language, whether "worst" or "maximum," but the issue that is being raised here is that we are making an unrealistic approach—that it is not going to happen very often in this way. I really do not want to debate whether we use the words "maximum expected" or "worst."

GRAHN: Yes, but Dunster's point was a very good one, namely, that, by a wrong choice of language, you are going to frighten people. If you are dealing with a really worst case, all right; but, if you are dealing with a situation you would normally expect, you should not call it "worst case."

TAMPLIN: I will give you a little history on the "worst case." The first time we presented this was to the Division of Biology and Medicine in Washington. At that time we did not use "worst case," we used estimated "maximum credible" case. They said you had better not say that because there may be a time when it will be even worse. So we changed it to "estimated maximum" and then we dropped that. It does not matter what word we choose, we will get into the same kind of semantic argument about it.

KNOX (LRL): I find it very intriguing that you have documented a case that approaches your worst-case estimate. Rather than argue about the language, I would like to ask some questions. I have listened to many talks about biology, notably Pendleton's; I enjoyed his talk very much. What he demonstrated was that you could get very great variability in local deposition due to differences in surface roughness and other factors. In one case a cloud could go over a field of grass and there would be no deposition on the grass. On the far side of the field there was a hay stack, on which the cloud was essentially swept out by attachment of fine particles in the process blowing around the hay stack. It is essential that one understands how the material was deposited. Was it deposited from dry deposition; was a hot spot involved, or some other alternative? Was it deposited by the mechanism of sweep out? The relevant place to look to solve some of these questions is to learn how the numbers really get so high. When you answer this question you are possibly closer to finding the solution to taking remedial measures. For instance, what do you do about the hay stack?

TAMPLIN: This was not a hay stack. It was pasture and widespread throughout California. There was 300 pCi per liter of milk found in northern California.

KNOX: How was it deposited, then?

TAMPLIN: It was deposited by dry deposition, by small particles impacting on the grass.

KNOX: That is not the question. Where did the forage come from that the cow ate?

TAMPLIN: Pasture — this cow was on pasture.

KNOX: How was it deposited?

TAMPLIN: God put it there. Or Mao put it there.

BRUNER: I am sorry I have not read the reference report UCRL-70301, but I am curious. Was our intelligence so good that you were able to identify the height of detonation, the materials used, etc., and arrive at the estimated value of 5000? Where did that information come from?

NG: The fission yields of the major fission products, ^{131}I for example, do not differ substantially among the various materials that could be used in a device. We estimated what the activity would be at the time of deposition and assumed the fractional dry deposition curve of Fig. A1. Then we used the relation that 45 m^2 of pasture yield 10 kg dry weight of grass. Using this relation and the fallout deposition, we arrived at the estimated concentration in forage.

BRUNER: What about the kilotonnage of the explosion?

NG: We assumed 300 kt since the AEC announced that it was a few hundred kiloton. It could have been 600 kt, which would have doubled the estimate.

COMAR: In one of your tables you made a comparison of ^{131}I and other nuclides on a whole-body basis. If that were calculated to the size of the thyroid gland in which the dose would be delivered, then it would come out that the dose to the thyroid gland would be something like 2000 times the dose of the other nuclides. I think that is rather a pertinent point.

NG: Yes. In actual practice, one would examine more closely any situation where a very high dose estimate is encountered. In the case of ^{131}I in a child's thyroid gland, one would certainly examine all the factors that determine the entry of iodine into his thyroid. One would more carefully consider the rate of increase of concentration of iodine in milk rather than assuming an instantaneous steady state. And one would also take into account the size of the thyroid gland in establishing the effective energy. For ^{131}I the dosage to the child's thyroid would be about 400 times the estimated maximum whole-body dose.

COMAR: For the initial type of survey work, you have to go through all the nuclides and take some given formula and crank them through, but I am hoping that the data we have on the metabolism of specific radionuclides will be quick to use, and that these can be looked at individually when the time comes to make some specific determination. Also, I would hope that some day there would be a very small test shot somewhere so that we can actually measure some concentrations on a tracer basis and see if that antimony really gets into the bones of animals and perhaps human beings.

SHORE (LRL): We have done that on Schooner, Cabriolet, and Buggy, but unfortunately we cannot present it here.

NG: These represent ongoing programs in the Bio-Medical Division.

GOFMAN: For each one of these things that come up as a potential worry, that is exactly what is done experimentally. First, we are trying to fill in the biological concentrations data with laboratory experiments so we will not have to use estimates like the worst ratio of tissue to soil values. Second, documentation in the field is now carried out on all the ongoing shots.

COMAR: I think it would be very satisfying if you obtain actual data that show that some of these relations do, indeed, exist.

NG: Many of our values for the fraction of the isotope ingested by the cow that is secreted in the milk per liter were based on Gil Potter's experimental programs. In other words, we make use of our own programs, as well as the worldwide literature to arrive at these estimates.

FOSTER: One of your tables shows that in the critical pathway via pasture to milk to the infant, ^{24}Na is one of the high limiting isotopes. It occurs to me that in order to have gotten that much from milk there must have been quite a bit on the pasture. Since ^{24}Na is a hard gamma emitter, what was the relative dose to the cow herd and the farmer who is tramping around in the pasture? Do you have a calculation made on that?

NG: I do not have a calculation based on the radiation dose to the herd. It should be noted that ^{24}Na is relatively short-lived, and, as far as our own estimates are concerned, they would be somewhat overconservative because of the assumption of instantaneous equilibration.*
We could use our Handbook to make an estimate of the dose to the herd.

HOLLAND: I would like to make one parting remark with regard to what John Gofman said. I do not want to imply that these calculations are unrealistic or overconservative. I am willing to accept the fact that these situations do happen in the real world and that maybe the worst case has been observed in some of them. What happens in the real world covers a wide range, and the various indices like dose or tissue concentration have some distribution of probabilities. We do not know what the distribution is, and we have no way of finding out what it is because we are not going to have a big enough experimental sample. But still, in trying to make judgments about the significance of levels within the range of possible levels, we will be influenced by both our estimates and the probability of their occurrence. Unless we can make some association of probability with magnitude, we will be groping

---

*Author's note added in proof: A correction for the assumption of instantaneous equilibration of ^{24}Na has been incorporated in the published text (pp. 105-106).

around in the fog forever. I do not know how we should arrive at estimates of probability that we can agree on and use as a basis for decisions. I think the discussion on that level would be a more rational one where one looks for evidence that would lead to assignment of one degree or another of probability to certain values that are estimated.

TAMPLIN: We only expect these estimates to represent part of a dialog. Since the early testing at the Nevada Test Site, the accuracy of meteorology has increased considerably. This has been partly because these tracers were injected into the atmosphere; and meteorologists suddenly had data on atmospheric dispersal to work with. The meteorologists in the Plowshare program are able to define conditions before they fire a shot that would make the possibility of running into a rainout situation very small. But I do think in a preshot analysis of the Plowshare program that the meteorologists in Plowshare should address themselves to the probability of a rainout. If they can show, which I think they can, that this is a risk we can afford to take, then they fire the shot. We have made these risk estimates, and they have fired shots. I assume this represented part of the dialog.

RADIOACTIVE POLLUTION OF THE ATMOSPHERE

JOSHUA Z. HOLLAND
Fallout Studies Branch, Division of Biology and Medicine, U. S. Atomic Energy Commission, Washington, D. C.

ABSTRACT

Presently existing nuclear technology can expand for several decades at a maximum pace determined by supply and demand, while keeping the radioactive air pollution within acceptable limits. Presently known methods for improving existing technology can extend that period a few additional decades. But after that, if the peaceful applications of nuclear energy are to continue to expand at a rate commensurate with human needs, new methods will be required for industrial waste-gas handling and for evaluating the acceptability of proposed new sources of pollution. There is no reason to doubt that the science and technology can grow at a sufficient rate to be available when needed.

For orientation purposes I will begin with some physical facts. The atmosphere weighs 10 tons per square meter of earth's surface. There are 500 million square kilometers of earth's surface. There are therefore 5×10^{18} kg of air. At sea level 1 m^3 air weighs $1\frac{1}{4}$ kg; so the atmosphere contains 4×10^{18} sea-level cubic meters.

One of the interesting potential pollutants resulting from nuclear fission is ^{85}Kr. Since ^{85}Kr is a noble gas, it tends to pass through filters and iodine traps during chemical processing of reactor fuel elements and thus escapes to the atmosphere. There it accumulates, having a half-life of 10 years. About 0.4 Ci of ^{85}Kr is produced by the nuclear reactor per year for each kilowatt of electric power it produces. If the nuclear-power-generation rate were constant and all the generated ^{85}Kr were released to the atmosphere during fuel reprocessing, the total atmospheric burden would approach an equilibrium value about 15 times the annual production rate, or about 6 Ci/kw(e).

The concentration below which nuclear-power-reactor operators are required to hold the ^{85}Kr concentration outside their controlled area is 3×10^{-7} Ci/m^3. A steady production rate of 200 billion nuclear electrical kilowatts would be required to bring the average concentration of ^{85}Kr up to this level. Because of the slow rate of atmospheric mixing upward into the stratosphere and horizontally from regions of heavy to light industrial concentration, the air in the more heavily populated latitude band would reach this concentration at a lower steady power level, perhaps 50 billion electrical kilowatts. For comparison, the present total electrical generating capacity in the United States is about 0.3 billion kilowatts.

However, as long as power levels are rising rapidly from year to year, the global ^{85}Kr accumulation will lag behind. Thus at the time a nuclear generation rate of 50 billion kilowatts is actually attained, average ^{85}Kr concentrations may be half the equilibrium level and well below the present permissible level. On the other hand, when large populations are exposed, a guide level one-third of that currently used might be applied.

Local concentrations downwind of reprocessing plants will, of course, be severalfold higher than latitude averages. Local levels depend on the rate of release rather than on the cumulative atmospheric inventory. Therefore they will not lag behind the power levels. So much for the quantitative orientation.

It has been estimated that by the turn of the century nuclear energy will supply about half of a total U. S. electric power capacity exceeding a billion kilowatts. An additional nuclear-power-generation capacity of similar or possibly greater magnitude will exist elsewhere in the world. The nuclear power will be economically competitive with that produced by the combustion of fossil fuels and will continue to keep the radiation exposures of the general public within present-day guides of the Federal Radiation Council. This can be accomplished even if only present-day practices are employed for gaseous- and particulate-waste disposal to the atmosphere.

The next billion worldwide nuclear kilowatts would begin to present problems, but these problems can be solved by using presently known methods for improving the removal and containment of radioactivity from the off-gas streams of fuel-reprocessing plants. Krypton-85, ^{131}I, ^{133}Xe, and tritium will need to be controlled carefully so that: (1) reprocessing plants do not require such large exclusion areas to maintain the radiation exposure of nearby populations below present-day guides that the number of suitable locations becomes very limited and transportation costs increasingly large and (2) the increase in average radiation exposure for the population as a whole does not exceed a small percentage of natural background exposure.

Possibly, when the volume of fuel-reprocessing business expands, the reduction of the site size permitted by improved off-gas treatment and the consequent increase in the number of usable sites will save more money in fuel-transportation expenses than the improved off-gas treatment will cost. If so, the improvements in effluent control at the source can be justified on economic grounds alone. This alternative would be strongly favored from the viewpoint of social benefit, even if it were not justifiable economically and even though it would not be required by present-day regulations. Furthermore, the nuclear electric power industry may not be the only significant source of manmade radioactivity in the atmosphere as we progress into the nuclear age.

Somewhere around the tenth billion kilowatts of worldwide nuclear electric power, it appears that source controls going beyond applications of presently known principles will become mandatory in order to stay within today's guides. This could come before the middle of the twenty-first century.

Let us be bullish and assume that before too many decades there will be nuclear desalting and agro-industrial complexes and nuclear earth-moving projects that will transform the arid wastelands of the earth to bountiful homelands for billions of people. Let us assume also that many large vehicles and scientific stations will be carrying out useful and entertaining missions in space with the aid of nuclear energy. We then can leap quickly to a number of conclusions about the nature of the radioactive air-pollution problems in the nuclear age.

The peaceful applications of nuclear energy will be carried out without creating an unacceptable air pollution problem *by definition.* That is, since conventional alternative means exist for doing nearly all the essential things, the extent to which nuclear means are employed will be limited by the levels of atmospheric radioactivity which the public finds acceptable. The definition of acceptable limits will have to be reasonably consistent among all nations. It is reassuring to observe that effective means of international communication already exist in this field.

The question as to how far below the acceptable limits the radioactivity concentrations can be maintained will be decided largely on economic grounds. Until well into the twenty-first century, it appears that the levels of individual radionuclides released by power reactors and reprocessing plants can be held well below present-day guides. Eventually the waste-handling technology may be fully occupied in keeping within the guides.

At first the guides will be applied to one or a few "critical" nuclides at a time, all others being clearly far less important. As controls are instituted on one nuclide after another when they are projected to be approaching the guides, the number of nuclides from the nuclear power industry whose atmospheric concentrations are close to their permissible limits will become larger and larger.

At the same time other sources of ^{85}Kr, ^{131}I, and tritium, such as peaceful nuclear explosives or nuclear rocket motors and also other radionuclides, such as ^{181}W and ^{54}Mn from peaceful nuclear explosions and ^{238}Pu from space nuclear power systems, will be increasing. Initially, the growth of each of these nuclear technologies may be limited by such other factors as supply and demand. Ultimately, however, each may tend to be limited by the economic penalties imposed by the requirement to operate within the permissible limits of environmental pollution.

It can be assumed that the effects, whatever they may be, would be more severe if a dozen or more different radionuclides, rather than one, were at their maximum permissible concentrations in the atmosphere. Therefore it will be necessary to establish guides for limiting the atmospheric concentrations of variable mixtures of numerous radionuclides. The composition of the mixture will change with time, and each component will have some segment of the world's economy, perhaps even the total economies of some nations, sensitively dependent on its prorated share of the maximum permissible concentration.

The biomedical problem is to find out how the effect of a low dose, of the same order of magnitude as the natural background dose, depends upon the way it is distributed among the organs and tissues of the body. The practical problem is that, even though the effects of doses of the magnitude of the maximum permissible radiation doses may continue to be in considerable doubt, the doses adopted for design and control purposes must be well defined and reasonably stable. Imagine that all possible combinations of organ and tissue doses can somehow be covered by a set of "permissible limits" or perhaps several sets for individuals and populations of various sizes. Under existing concepts of radiation protection, the summation of radiation exposure due to atmospheric pollution, together with all other pathways of exposure, would be judged against these limits. The atmospheric radionuclides, in turn, must be evaluated in terms of their exposure pathways, such as immersion, inhalation, deposition, and food-chains, to arrive at a measure of their contribution to the individual or population dose. The dose attributable to each atmospheric nuclide must again be resolved into the part attributable to each source of contamination to affect the nuclear technology in a rational manner. The effects of various assumed combinations probably will have to be explored at both the source end and the dose end of the calculation to arrive at a compatible set of radionuclide emission licenses.

This bookkeeping, plus the optimization problem, apparently is not an unreasonable job for a computer if it does not have to be done too many times at too many places. It does require complete input data on existing and proposed radioactive pollution sources, good mathematical models for predicting the doses via all possible pathways, and a comprehensive set of dose-distribution limits. The type of research and development that would be required for such a system is under way but perhaps at a somewhat leisurely pace.

After all, we do not know how long it will take to get the needed research results for the design of such a system since some of the pathways and mechanisms probably have not yet been identified. We also do not know when the system will be needed, although possibly it will be evolving during the coming decades as rapidly as the scientific base permits. Even now, with essentially the same scientific base and the same book of rules in the hands of both the official regulatory agencies and the applicants for licenses, each significant new scientific finding has an impact on the licensing process.

Quantitative models will certainly be needed for predicting atmospheric transport, dispersion, and deposition on all spatial scales as a function of the physical and chemical properties of the contaminant material, the location and height of release, the nature of surrounding buildings and terrain, the time of day, the season, and the weather. Even for present-day applications, the uncertainties are larger than we would like them to be. Such present applications include the determination of permissible reactor containment-building leakage rates, the determination of exclusion-area requirements for fuel-reprocessing plants, the evaluation of the consequences of potential accidents affecting isotope power units for the space program, and the estimation of the effects of long-range dispersion or precipitation on the number of acceptable days for nuclear cratering or nuclear rocket-engine tests. These programs are in their infancy, and each has the potential to grow within a few decades to a size such that incremental costs of hundreds of millions to billions of dollars may well be determined by the outcome of such meteorological calculations.

I think that the problem of radioactive pollution of the atmosphere *can* be kept under control. To do so will require worldwide acceptance of common standards and effective regulatory mechanisms. These mechanisms and their scientific base must grow to keep ahead of the industry and not be allowed to lag behind as has occurred most commonly in the history of other technologies. The problem will become more and more complicated with the proliferation of sources and will probably require an international accounting system as well as rapid international dissemination of the best available technological information. The problem of evaluating the biomedical implications of proposed new sources of radioactive air pollution will continue to strain our scientific capabilities, despite the best research efforts we will be able to put forth, for some time to come. Nevertheless, feasible control levels, assuring an acceptable margin of safety, can be agreed upon.

The incentive for exploiting the benefits of nuclear energy will be very powerful. The incentive for keeping the atmosphere safely breathable will also be very powerful. Of course, the people who feel these two incentives most keenly may not, in general, be the same. As scientists we must provide both groups with a complete and objective information base and on a timely basis. As scientists we must also keep in mind the following possibilities: (1) that the worldwide nuclear technologies may grow more slowly or more rapidly than we are now predicting and (2) that the biomedical research may turn up information that will result in a change upward or downward in the acceptable levels of radioactive pollution.

DISCUSSION

HARLEY: Do you have any thoughts on how this particular pie may be sliced into allowable additions in the environment say by the USSR and the United States?

HOLLAND: I see this as a subject of some sort of negotiation. I think it would be quite interesting.

HARLEY: Perhaps each country could be allowed so many rads per unit population.

HOLLAND: I am not going to try to predict how this would be done. From what Mr. Parker says, the NCRP is thinking this way. You can assume, since the same people are involved, that the ICRP is going to think this way. Some of the committees, boards, and panels who advise on these subjects are going to be preparing against this day. And if they do it in a very conservative way, they will assign to each individual project a very small piece of the pie. The question is if this can be done without some kind of a great negotiation process. But certainly there are always going to be two sides on every one of these decisions. The people who want so much to carry out a technological advance will tend to push limits as high as they can, either because of their convictions about the benefits that will result or because they assume somebody else is taking the responsibility for worrying about the hazards. The people on the other side are not too sure what the benefits are going to be from the new technology but are sure that they do not want any more radiation than they can help. Both sides are represented within the government, so even the government does not represent one side. It is a very highly developed problem in the reactor field. As other activities begin to go after other pieces of the pie, the situation for the reactors and fuel processing plants also becomes very complicated. I do not think anyone can answer the question now.

DUNSTER: You associated 3×10^{-7} $\mu Ci/cm^3$ with 500 mrads/year. Krypton is essentially a beta emitter. How do you think krypton is going to work in the calculations on the true genetic dose?

HOLLAND: I believe this is the level that is used for off-site individuals, and it corresponded to 500 mr/year. Whether or not you would go to a level $\frac{1}{3}$ of this for the general population I do not know. Possibly it is not correct to calculate in this way.

DUNSTER: But, with the gamma contribution of about 100 mr, there is some additional contribution from krypton in the body. If we have to start partitioning power programs, things of that sort, this is one of the factors that might be worth considering before we decide on site locations.

HOLLAND: I must admit I have not done this calculation myself. I do not know if the 500 mr/year is from betas or gammas.

DUNSTER: It is from betas.

HOLLAND: In that case the genetic dose would be as you say, a very small fraction.

CRAWFORD (LRL): Everything you have said applies to any environmental pollution problem, either fossil fuels or radioactivity. I guess I am referring to what I said earlier; the thing that bothers me sometimes is that we all end up thinking of only our own area. Nobody looks at the balances of one vs. the other.

HOLLAND: But I am not talking about any other pollutant. There are certain considerations that are involved in radioactive pollution which one must look at regardless of what may be going on elsewhere in the environment. I hope that the other people are just as careful as we are.

GOFMAN (LRL): Can you or the Division of Biology and Medicine answer this question? Has anyone done a calculation of the fraction of people in the world that are called radiation workers as a function of time from 1945 on? Have you any idea what the fraction of radiation workers is over total people as a function of time?

PARKER: No, I do not, but we concluded that within the foreseeable expansion of the fissionists this was not a factor. I think if the fraction of radiation workers did become significant, you would have to change this 5 rem/year. In any case, radiation workers do not actually get 5 rem, they only *can* get 5 rem/year. One has no business coming anywhere near that. The average in the United States is less than 0.2 rem/year.

PARKER: I am confused about the numbers you gave for the growth in the nuclear electricity industry.

HOLLAND: In the United States we now have 300,000 Mw of total electrical power. I predict that there will be about a million megawatts before the year 2000, of which $\frac{1}{2}$ will be nuclear. Then there will be $\frac{1}{2}$ million megawatts of nuclear power in the rest of the world. The world will have about a million nuclear megawatts of electricity by the year 2000. In not too many decades after that, we will have another million. By the middle of the century we will be up around 10 million nuclear electrical megawatts in the world. This is what it takes to bring the average concentration of ^{85}Kr in the entire atmosphere up to this guide level. But I say that at 2 million we shall have to be doing something about local contamination and the maximum permissible concentration.

PARKER: That is all going to be solved because by that time we will design and build reactors in which fuel does not ever have to be reprocessed. This will be fairly simple to develop. You do not ever release any of these radionuclides if you do not process the fuel.

HOLLAND: That would solve the problem.

PARKER: It will have to be the solution, I think.

REACTOR RELEASES OF RADIONUCLIDES*

R. L. JUNKINS
Pacific Northwest Laboratory, Battelle Memorial Institute, Richland, Washington

ABSTRACT

The releases of radionuclides from reactors and the environmental effects of these releases have been studied since the early 1940's. Controls based on the knowledge gained from these studies have been adequate to maintain the radiation exposure of the public well within acceptable limits. The significant pathways of exposure have been identified. Over the years improved methods of waste treatment and containment technology for reactors have evolved to the point where release of waste heat from power reactors now appears to be receiving more public attention than the release of radionuclides.

In this review of the releases of radionuclides from reactors, I will first discuss chronic releases as contrasted with accidental, or the potential for, accidental releases. I will discuss the past and present generations of production and power reactors and attempt to look into the foreseeable future.

Chronologically, it seems appropriate to begin with the production reactors. Our first production reactors were built along the Columbia River at the Hanford site in the early 1940's. A total of six reactors have been added to the original three, the most recent being the N Reactor, a dual-purpose plutonium-production–power-production unit. The five oldest reactors have now been shut down and placed in standby condition.

The first eight production reactors built at Hanford were designed with once-through cooling systems. Water is pumped from the Columbia River, treated, filtered, passed through the reactors as coolant, and

---

*This paper is based on work performed under U. S. Atomic Energy Commission Contract AT(45-1)-1830.

then returned to the river, after monitoring, by way of retention basins. For our discussion on releases of radionuclides, the cooling system is the most important design feature of these reactors.

As the treated water passes through the active zones of the reactors, it accumulates radionuclides from various sources, e.g., from the activation of stable elements in the water by nuclear reactions, from the activation of stable elements in reactor hardware which are then passed to the water as a result of corrosion, from the fission of natural uranium in the water forming fission products, and from the fission products from failed fuel elements. The combination of these sources results in a very large number of nuclides present or potentially present in the water in small but measureable amounts.

A few words of elaboration on each of these sources of radionuclides may be helpful. The activation of stable elements in the water is illustrated by the formation of ^{51}Cr from a neutron-capture reaction in stable chromium, which is present in the water as sodium dichromate, a corrosion inhibitor. Chromium-51 is the most abundant radionuclide in the Columbia River at the point of nearest downstream usage. Other elements present in the water in trace amounts undergo neutron reactions and result in measurable amounts of radionuclides, such as ^{24}Na, ^{76}As, ^{65}Zn, and ^{32}P. Although the water-treatment process is highly efficient, we must remember that neutron activation is one of the most sensitive analytical tools currently available; even trace amounts of elements in the water result in activation products.

The second source of radionuclides is the corrosion of reactor hardware components. Elements present in the hardware, including alloying agents and trace impurities, become activated, and some eventually reach the cooling water by way of corrosion. Cobalt-60 and radioisotopes of iron and manganese are typical examples. Some of the same nuclides that are formed by the activation of the cooling water may also enter the stream as a result of corrosion, for instance, ^{24}Na.

Columbia River water upstream from the Hanford Plant contains small amounts of natural uranium. Some of this uranium enters the reactors in the cooling water and undergoes fission. The small amount of the fission-product mixture and the relative abundance of the individual fission products verify the source of the uranium as a result of estimating the irradiation time. The natural uranium is also the principal source of ^{239}Np in the effluent water.

Fuel-cladding failure releases some fission products to the coolant. This source of radionuclides is not a routine occurrence because reactors are not operated with a known failed fuel element in the core. When a failure is detected, the reactor is shut down and the damaged fuel element is removed.

The production reactors at the Savannah River site were built in the early 1950's, about a decade after the first Hanford reactors. Three of the original five Savannah River reactors are still in operation. These reactors are cooled and moderated by heavy water with a heat-exchange system to light water. The recirculated coolant is the most important difference between the Savannah and Hanford reactors for the purpose of this discussion on the release of radionuclides from reactors. This recirculation provides a barrier between the radionuclides in the coolant and the environment.

The same sources of radionuclides and mechanisms of formation described for the Hanford reactors also obtain for the Savannah River reactors except the traces of natural uranium in the cooling water at Hanford. There are notable differences, however, in the radionuclides formed and in the amounts released. As a result of irradiation of the heavy-water moderator and coolant, tritium is formed. Some of the tritium eventually reaches the Savannah River. Downstream measurements show that tritium is the most abundant radionuclide released from the reactors to the river.

A portion of the heavy-water coolant is continuously routed through a cleanup system to maintain its purity. The system includes ion-exchange equipment, and the resin is a source of stable sulfur. Traces of the stable sulfur reach the active zone of the reactor, and some is converted to ^{35}S, the second most abundant radionuclide released to the river by these reactors. The same resin and mechanism is also the source of ^{32}P, which is occasionally detectable in aquatic life downstream. Corrosion of activated reactor components results in infrequently detectable amounts of ^{51}Cr, ^{65}Zn, and ^{60}Co in the river. Occasional fuel-cladding failures result in traces of fission products being detected in the river.

Experience at the Chalk River, Canada, reactors is quite similar to Savannah River with regard to chronic releases. Various test reactors operating during the 1940's and 1950's involved similar mechanisms of formation and release of radionuclides. The principal differences are in amounts and kinds of radionuclides. For example, ^{41}Ar formed in air-cooled test reactors was released. This radionuclide, a short-lived gamma emitter, was the most abundant radionuclide released from air-cooled units.

Before discussing the current generation of reactors, I will review a few of the environmental aspects of the releases from production reactors. Obviously it is of paramount importance to evaluate the impact of the releases on man and his environment. Evaluation programs have been conducted for many years at the production reactor sites, and the results have been widely reported. The dose to the public has been determined and kept well within relevant limits and regulations.

The releases of radionuclides from the reactors have provided many opportunities for interesting research, both in the field and in the laboratory. I will identify some of the typical programs and highlight some of the results; starting again with the oldest production-reactor site, Hanford, which is in the southeastern part of the State of Washington (Fig. 1). The site covers about 570 sq miles as shown in the figure. McNary Dam was built in the early 1950's, and its pool extends approximately to the laboratories' area. Priest Rapids Dam was built more recently just upstream from the site. It influences the river level

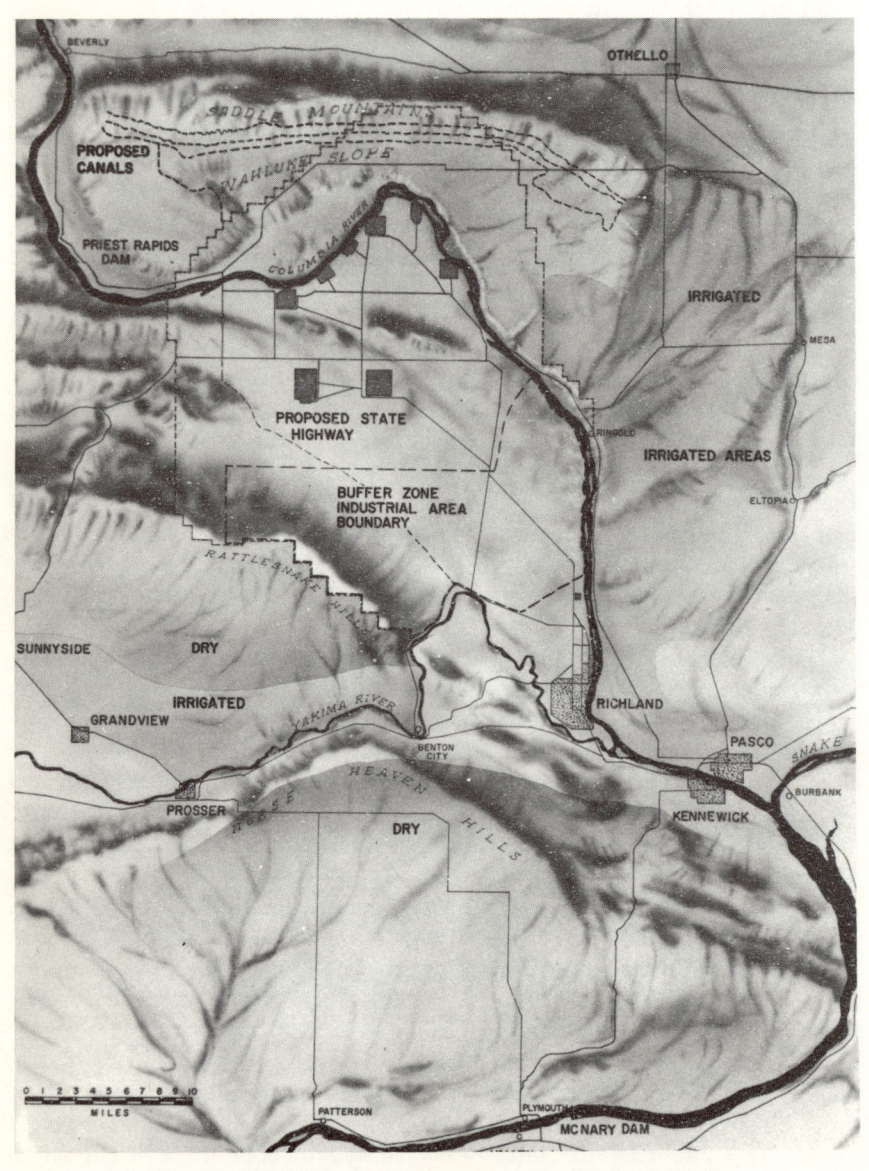

Fig. 1—*Oldest production reactor site, Hanford, Wash.*

markedly because of the fluctuating power generation and water-release rates.

Extensive environmental and life science surveillance and research programs have been carried out for many years. These programs have been and are currently sponsored by the U. S. Atomic Energy Commission.

Facilities for conducting biological studies on reactor effluent water are located in two of the reactor areas. Studies to determine the effect of the cooling water on various species of fish and other aquatic life have been conducted under controlled laboratory conditions for many years. This work is supplemented by analysis of samples of aquatic life from the river. The field studies also include an annual survey of the number of salmon nests in this stretch of the Columbia River. With regard to the radionuclides from reactor effluent water, the findings of interest include the tendency of organisms to accumulate ^{65}Zn and ^{32}P through the food web. The results have been widely reported and confirmed in other locations, e.g., Savannah River and Chalk River. The tendency of aquatic life to concentrate these nuclides varies, of course, with trophic level and feeding habits. The adult Chinook salmon, for example, does not feed after entering the river to spawn. The amount of ^{32}P and ^{65}Zn found in the adult salmon is extremely small compared to the amount found in other fish. Near the mouth of the Columbia River, a concentration of ^{65}Zn in shellfish is observed. The relatively short half-life of ^{32}P apparently limits the extent of its concentration in shellfish.

The Columbia River is a significant flyway for migratory waterfowl, and some ducks and geese nest there, particularly on the islands in the river. These birds show the same tendency to accumulate ^{32}P and ^{65}Zn, again accumulation depends primarily on feeding habits. Most of the ducks and geese are species that feed in surrounding fields rather than on the river. A small fraction of the ducks are the diving type and feed on river organisms. Of the waterfowl these ducks show the highest concentration of reactor-produced radionuclides. The surveillance program for waterfowl includes nest counts and population surveys. Nests are checked for numbers of eggs, and fertility is checked by success of the hatch.

The accumulation of 11 radionuclides in Columbia River sediments was studied intensively over a 3-year period. The nuclides in the sediment study were sufficiently long-lived to serve as useful tracers and were abundant enough to provide measurable amounts. They included ^{51}Cr, ^{65}Zn, ^{46}Sc, ^{54}Mn, ^{58}Co, ^{59}Fe, ^{60}Co, ^{95}Zr–^{95}Nb, ^{106}Ru, ^{124}Sb, and ^{140}Ba.

The study, covering 350 km in the lower river, showed that as much as 90% of the total activity of some of these nuclides was depleted by sedimentation. Much of this activity is deposited in the pool created by McNary Dam. The ratio of ^{65}Zn to ^{51}Cr was used as an index of age, and it was found that about 30% of the annual deposit moves downstream from the McNary pool as suspended solids during the spring freshet. Laboratory examination indicated that the nuclides are tightly bound by the sediments; they could not readily be replaced by contact with salt solutions. With the exception of ^{51}Cr, the nuclides remain in the same oxidation state they were in when they entered the river. Chromium is reduced in the river from the hexavalent to the trivalent state.

As shown in Fig. 1, there are about 5000 acres of land near the plant which are irrigated with Columbia River water taken downstream from the reactors. This land has been the object of several interesting studies on the effect of irrigation methods on uptake of radionuclides in farm products. Sampling has included all types of cultivated plant life, pasture, livestock, milk, and whole-body counting of members of some of the families living on these farms to identify the significant exposure pathways. Under more-controlled conditions, experimental plots of various crops are grown within the plant site and are irrigated with various concentrations of reactor effluent water.

The Tri-Cities now obtain their water supply from the Columbia River. Different water-treatment processes are used in each city, and information has been obtained on the efficiency of these systems for removal of various radionuclides. As implied earlier, the most important removal mechanism is the cleanup of suspended solids.

The foregoing is merely a sample of the kinds of research and surveillance programs associated with the release of radionuclides from reactors. Similar programs have been conducted at other production-reactor sites, e.g., Savannah River, Chalk River, and Windscale. I have chosen a few of the programs at Hanford because I think they are illustrative and because I am much more familiar with them. There are several objectives on which such programs are based: the protection of man and his environment, adding to the fundamental knowledge of the environmental and life sciences, and acquiring knowledge of the behavior of nuclides in the environment which would be useful in the event of a serious accident. Much has been learned on all these matters at the sites mentioned. The important pathways of exposure have been identified, and the dose to the public from the multiple sources has been well within the appropriate limits.

Over the years several trends have greatly influenced this work. The development of new equipment and techniques has vastly improved our ability to measure minute amounts of radionuclides in various media and to economically process large numbers of samples. J. Z. Holland in his paper (this volume) pointed out the influence of nuclides from other sources which complicate studies of reactor-produced nuclides. In effect, many of the nuclides involved in such studies are no longer unique. They may be present as a result of fallout, as effluent from chemical processing plants, or as effluent from reactors other than the one of interest. This is particularly true of the nuclides released to the atmosphere. In summary, these trends have provided improved opportunities and also have presented new challenges.

Turning now to the present generation of power reactors in operation and under construction, we find the same mechanisms for formation and the same potential for release to the environment. There are, however, several important differences. The technology of containment and the treatment of wastes have advanced greatly in the last two decades. It is now technically feasible to design and operate power reactors with waste streams containing concentrations of radionuclides exceedingly small compared to the production sites and much less than the limits set by regulations. Although it is not currently practical to remove the last picocurie from these waste streams, in general, experience shows that the releases from reactors are sufficiently small that the principal monitoring can be at the point of release. Comparatively little environmental monitoring is required, on the basis of the recommendations of the Federal Radiation Council.

There is much incentive to keep a power reactor operating a maximum fraction of the time. In the event of a fuel-element failure, it is desirable to continue operation until the next scheduled shutdown, provided this can be done safely and without damage to the reactor. The design of the system for decontaminating the reactor coolant is therefore based on the cleanup of such fuel debris, i.e., removal of fission products, corrosion products, and nuclides produced by activation reactions. These systems are highly efficient, but no engineering equipment is 100% efficient all the time. Current power reactors do not provide for the separation of the noble-gas fission products, xenon and krypton. In some power reactors it is feasible to store the noncondensable gases sufficiently long to allow all but ^{85}Kr to decay. Krypton-85 is discussed later. Where no long-term storage of noncondensable gases is provided, the short-lived isotopes of xenon and krypton are usually dominant in the release to the atmosphere. In general, most of the other radionuclides are accumulated in ion exchangers, as evaporator bottoms and the like for eventual disposal as solid radioactive wastes in approved locations remote from the reactor.

Various miscellaneous liquid-waste streams contain traces of radionuclides; condensate from waste evaporators, waste from the laundry of protective clothing, and waste from the decontamination of tools and equipment are typical examples. After monitoring has determined compliance with limits, these streams are normally combined and diluted with the much larger flow of turbine condenser cooling water before release to the environment as waste water.

Of the radionuclides released from present reactors, those with short half-lives — on the order of a year or less — approach an equilibrium amount in the environment depending on the rate of their release. They are generally of local interest because they are not widely distributed. There are, however, other radionuclides of longer life which are of special interest. In this category ^{3}H, ^{14}C, and ^{85}Kr rate special attention. Tritium and ^{85}Kr are fission products. All are difficult to contain and tend to be widely distributed in the environment. Tritium and ^{14}C are formed in nature as a result of cosmic radiation and also by nuclear reactions in reactors and in weapons testing. They are important in biological research studies, the age dating of materials, and the like. Krypton-85 has no comparable value in biological research to my knowledge. Since Holland has discussed the importance of ^{85}Kr as a function of growth of the nuclear power industry, I will merely emphasize that most of the ^{85}Kr formed in the reactors will be contained in the spent fuel shipped to fuel reprocessing centers. Its release to the environment, or potential for release, from fuel-reprocessing plants will therefore greatly exceed its release from reactors.

Next, consider the release of radionuclides as a result of reactor accidents — the experience to date and postulated accidents of greater severity than any which have occurred. The accident on which design is based is usually called the maximum credible accident. For present thermal-neutron reactors, both gas and water cooled, the maximum credible accident is believed to be a total loss of coolant. Of the few reactor accidents that have occurred, none has approached the degree of severity of total loss of coolant during operation. The experience gained at Windscale was the most informative regarding release of radionuclides. This was due, in part, to the nature of the accident — the overheating and oxidation of a portion of the metallic uranium fuel. However, a large measure of the credit for the knowledge gained must be attributed to the diligent efforts of the staff in gathering the maximum amount of data and in analyzing the impact on the environment. The path of release was through a stack to the atmosphere. The reactor had been shut down long enough before the accident to minimize the amount of short-lived radionuclides, particularly the noble gases. Under these conditions the ^{131}I released resulted in the largest exposure potential by way of the milk pathway, as expected. Much valuable information was obtained also on ^{137}Cs release and behavior. Except for the noble gases, these nuclides are among the more volatile of the fission products. Numerous excellent reports were prepared, and these were a major information source for the British Medical Research Council study that resulted in recommendations for permissible exposure of the population under emergency conditions. Their recommendations included ingestion rates for ^{131}I, ^{137}Cs, and ^{89}Sr and ^{90}Sr.

The releases from other reactor accidents, such as Chalk River and the SL-1 in Idaho, were such that not nearly as much information was obtained for evaluating the consequences of reactor accidents in terms of release of radionuclides to the environment.

The evaluation of postulated accidents today is included as a part of the safety analysis reports required in the application for a reactor construction permit and later for the operating license. Numerous potential accidents are considered, the most severe of which, for thermal-neutron reactors, is total loss of coolant during operation. The consequences of such an accident are currently evaluated in terms of estimated dose to thyroid and total body at the exclusion-zone boundary and the low-population-zone boundary as defined by the Reactor Siting Guide in the *Code of Federal Regulations*. Since the accident postulated presumes loss of coolant, the path of release is through the atmosphere.

There is a reasonable amount of experimental data which shows the fraction of the various fission products volatilized from molten fuel, the tendency of some fission products to deposit on relatively cooler surfaces in the containment, the removal by pressure-suppression and fog-spray systems, and removal by other mechanisms, such as filtration and absorption. There are several important research programs in progress to better define these parameters.

The containment systems and appurtenances are designed to withstand the pressure of the release of stored energy in the coolant and the radioactive decay energy of the irradiated fuel. However, the containment system is assumed to leak at some rate. Currently the state of the art indicates that about 0.1% per day of the contained volume is the lowest demonstrable leak rate.

Those who design reactors have done an excellent job of providing engineering safeguards to prevent an accident from occurring and, in the unlikely event of a severe accident, to mitigate the consequences. In practice, the reactor operator must convince the AEC Division of Reactor Licensing and the Advisory Committee on Reactor Safeguards that the facility will be operated within the long-term permissible release limits and that a severe accident is highly unlikely. Even in such an unlikely event, the estimated dose would be well within the reactor siting criteria: 300 rems to thyroid and 25 rems to total body at the relevant boundary distances.

Fast-neutron reactors introduce a new type of potential accident. Plutonium fuels and sodium coolant appear to be the materials of choice at this time. These materials and the configuration of the reactor result in a postulated core-compaction prompt-critical reaction terminated by explosive disruption of the core as the design-basis accident. The current containment designs consider the shock and pressure loading from such a reaction and the possible addition of energy as a result of a sodium fire. Under these circumstances a portion of the fuel is assumed to be vaporized, not merely molten as in the assumed loss-of-coolant accident for thermal-neutron reactors. Under postulated fuel-vaporization and sodium-oxidation conditions, new, challenging problems must be solved. Fission products and fuel materials that are only slightly volatile under molten-fuel conditions presumably would be released from the vaporized fuel almost quantitatively. Several studies have been completed and others are in progress to assist in the evaluation of the consequences of such accidents and to identify effective mechanisms for mitigating the consequences.

In conclusion, I think it is indicative of the success of the industry in controlling the release of radionuclides from reactors that the focus of attention has turned toward the release of heat. As you are probably aware, recent trends in reactor-licensing hearings have emphasized the problem of release of waste heat to water. Some of the states have recently passed legislation on disposal of waste heat to rivers. As a result, the nuclear industry appears to be turning toward cooling towers using the atmosphere as the heat sink. It is my opinion that this may not be the ultimate solution, particularly if urban siting of large power reactors becomes a reality. The additional atmospheric heat load may be less acceptable in metropolitan areas than the additional freshwater or saltwater heat load.

DISCUSSION

FLEMING (LRL): Can you give the total volume per day of water flow through all those reactors?

JUNKINS: No, I cannot. It is classified information.

KNOX (LRL): Are you able to say what the tritium levels are in the water supply of the city of Richland or the tritium levels in the downstream reservoirs?

JUNKINS: With respect to the concentration of radionuclides measured downstream from the plant, this is unclassified information. I do not recall the numerical data, but the essence of it is, in the case of tritium, that the tritium reaching the river environment is small compared to the total tritium that is in the river already. Some of the tritium reaching the Columbia River from Hanford facilities is released from the fuel-reprocessing plants and travels through the groundwater.

[Subsequent to the discussion the following information was obtained. On the basis of paired positive values only, the 1968 annual average tritium concentration in the Columbia River at Priest Rapids and Richland was 1720 and 1850 pCi/liter, respectively. If all data are included (using the values less than the detection limit as 1000 pCi/liter), the respective values are <1540 and 1740 pCi/liter. Priest Rapids is upstream from all Hanford facilities.]

KNOX: Have the people studying the river made any theoretical models of turbulent diffusion in the river?

JUNKINS: Yes. They have done a great deal of this work, and it has been reported. Computer programs have been developed that are based on the models. R. F. Foster has been involved in this work. Would you like to comment, Dr. Foster?

FOSTER: The dispersion of reactor effluent in the Columbia was studied by physical measurements made in the river before attempts were made to develop mathematical models. There are really three aspects to the problem. One aspect involves the full longitudinal and lateral dispersion with time and travel downriver over distances of tens of miles. Another aspect involves the dispersion pattern that occurs fairly close to the point of discharge—within a distance of tens to hundreds of yards. The third aspect involves the hydraulics right at the point of discharge of the outfall; this is one we are working on at the moment.

KNOX: Are these buoyant plumes, these outfalls? They must have some excess temperature and rise to the surface.

FOSTER: Only to a small extent. They do have an excess temperature; but the discharge pipe itself is aimed upward so that what might otherwise be considered heat buoyancy is largely the force associated with the velocity of the water as it leaves the discharge pipe.

PARTICIPANT: May I ask what is the source of ^{65}Zn in the effluent water?

JUNKINS: It is a neutron activation product that comes from the reactions with the hardware and the traces in the cooling water. The neutrons react with the stable zinc, and zinc is present, for example, in aluminum in the construction materials of the reactor.

UNITED KINGDOM STUDIES ON RADIOACTIVE MATERIALS RELEASED IN THE MARINE ENVIRONMENT

H. J. DUNSTER
Radiological Protection Division, United Kingdom Atomic Energy Authority, Harwell, Didcot, Berks., England

ABSTRACT

For a number of reasons, the United Kingdom has always been seriously interested in the discharge of wastes to the sea, and this paper summarizes the current policy for the disposal of radioactive wastes. As an example of this policy in practice, an account is given of the discharges of liquid waste from the fuel-reprocessing plant at Windscale to the Irish Sea. The development of discharge criteria is discussed, together with the current basis of control and the results of the monitoring program. The principal discharges from other sites of the United Kingdom Atomic Energy Authority are mentioned briefly.

The stringent control exercised by the Authority and by the relevant government departments achieves a high standard of safety so that there is no damage to the marine environment and no limitation on man's use of that environment. In short, the discharges to sea are effected without creating pollution.

Partly because of its geographical situation, high density of population, and extensive utilization of ground and river water, the United Kingdom has always been seriously interested in the discharge of wastes to the sea.

The three establishments of the UKAEA which have substantial provision for discharging radioactive waste to the sea are Windscale in the northwest of England, Dounreay in the extreme north of Scotland, and Winfrith in the south of England. Other establishments discharging some radioactive wastes to the sea include the nuclear power stations and the Authority's fuel production plant at Springfields in Lancashire.

WASTE-DISPOSAL POLICY

The underlying policy of the United Kingdom was first formulated in a government report, "The Control of Radioactive Wastes," published[1] in 1959. This policy can be summarized as follows:

(1) To ensure, irrespective of cost, that the radiation dose received by members of the public shall not exceed the dose limits recommended from time to time by the International Commission on Radiological Protection (ICRP).

(2) To ensure, irrespective of cost, that the whole population of the country shall not receive an average genetic dose of more than 1 rem/person in 30 years as a result of waste disposal.

(3) To reduce the actual doses as far below these limits as is reasonably practicable, having regard to cost, convenience, and the national importance of the subject.

The framework for the implementation of these policies was provided by the Radioactive Substances Act[2] of 1960, which requires *inter alia* that users of radioactive materials must be registered and permits discharges of radioactive waste (other than in defined trivial amounts) only in accordance with written authorizations from the relevant government departments. These authorizations are individually negotiated and limit the discharges to the amounts that are genuinely necessary. The amounts permitted are often many orders of magnitude lower than the limits that would be set by the capacity of the environment to accept the waste. During the negotiations various local authorities, such as district councils, river boards, water undertakings, and sea fisheries authorities, are consulted as necessary. Nevertheless, enforcement and inspection remain the responsibility of the relevant central government departments.

The authorizations for waste disposal issued to the Authority require appropriate samples to be taken and analyzed, both of the effluent itself and of the surrounding environment. The details of these programs are agreed upon through discussions between the appropriate officials of the Authority and the inspecting government departments. In addition, some independent measurements are made by the departments as a check on the accuracy and adequacy of the Authority's programs. In the case of the discharges from Windscale, where the resulting doses are a substantial fraction of the ICRP dose limits, the independent government monitoring program is a substantial one.

THE DISCHARGES FROM WINDSCALE

Windscale, on the Cumberland coast of northwest England, comprises the four Calder reactors (natural uranium, graphite moderated, gas cooled), one advanced gas-cooled reactor, the fuel-reprocessing plant dealing with all the natural and low-enrichment fuels from the United Kingdom power program and designed to handle 1500 metric tons of uranium a year, the plutonium plant dealing with the output from the reprocessing plant and handling a few metric tons of plutonium a year, a group of associated research and development laboratories, and the usual technical laboratories and services.

The main activity in the wastes to the sea comes from the reprocessing plant; mainly from the uranium and plutonium evaporation stages since the primary fission products are concentrated and stored. The main volume comes from ancillary plants, particularly from the fuel-element storage and handling ponds. A typical concentration in the discharged waste is 5×10^{-2} μCi/cm^3, with a volume of approximately 1.5×10^6 m^3 per year or about 1 million gallons per day.

The current authorization for the discharge of wastes from Windscale to the sea is summarized in Table 1. In addition to the limits on total activity and some individual nuclides, the control formula is an attempt to reflect the addition of doses to the gastrointestinal tract of the exposed population group. The numerator in each fraction is the number of curies discharged in a 3-month period. Table 2 shows the actual discharges[3] for 1967.

Table 1

DISCHARGE LIMITS FROM WINDSCALE TO SEA

Total β activity	75,000 Ci/quarter
^{106}Ru	15,000 Ci/quarter
^{90}Sr	7,500 Ci/quarter
Total α activity	450 Ci/quarter

$$\frac{^{106}\text{Ru}}{15,000} + \frac{^{144}\text{Ce}}{90,000} + \frac{\text{total }\beta\text{ activity}}{300,000} \text{ shall not exceed 1}$$

Table 2

AVERAGE 3-MONTH DISCHARGE OF LIQUID RADIOACTIVE WASTE INTO THE IRISH SEA FROM WINDSCALE, 1967

Activity	Average 3-month discharge, Ci	% of authorized limit
Total β	18,068	24.1
^{106}Ru	4,310	28.7
^{90}Sr	350	4.7
^{144}Ce	3,426	
Total α	239	53.1
	Controlling formula	37.6

The History of the Hazard Assessment

The progression from the original decision to discharge wastes to the sea to the present authorization issued in 1963 has been satisfyingly logical and scientific. Experimental work by the Atomic Energy Project and by the Ministry of Agriculture, Fisheries, and Food started in 1948. This work included hydrographic studies using fluorescein, drift poles and bottles, and current meters; adsorption studies on sand and mud; studies of fish movement, marketing, and consumption; studies of seaweed marketing and consumption; aquarium studies on uptakes; and measurements of the LD_{50} for fish. These programs clearly showed only four potentially critical pathways between discharge and man: the eating of seaweed or fish and the exposure to shore sand or fishing gear contaminated by bottom sediments. The first assessments made in the period from 1949 to 1952, and published[4] in 1955, indicated a safe rate of discharge of 3000 Ci/month. They included a deliberate safety factor of 10 because of the uncertainties in some of the data.

In 1952 a regular series of experimental discharges was started at a rate of between 1000 and 2000 Ci/month. Regular reviews of the environmental monitoring results confirmed the safety of the discharges and allowed a further estimate to be made of the safe limit. In 1956 the authorized limit was raised to 25,000 Ci/month, of which only 5000 Ci/month could be ^{106}Ru. Further discharges at rates up to 7000 Ci/month culminated in the issue of the current authorization in 1963. Thereafter the discharges have been regarded as purely operational. The results of the discharges and of surveys have been reviewed from time to time.[5-8] The commissioning of a new fuel-reprocessing plant in 1964, and careful attention to the treatment of some of the individual waste streams, has resulted in a steady or slightly reduced discharge rate over the last 5 years, in spite of an increase to about 5000 Mw in the output of nuclear power.

The Current Basis of Control

The basic standards applied to these discharges are those of the ICRP.[9] These basic dose limits are applied to the exposure of the critical group via the critical pathway.[10] The identification of the critical factors has been simple. The pathway is eating seaweed, and the group is made up of those who eat a great deal of seaweed. The difficulty has been in defining this group in quantitative terms.

The distribution of consumption among those who regularly eat the seaweed product, laver bread, is approximately log normal, with an average for the whole group (adults) of 16 g/day.[11] Of the whole group of about 26,000, 1500 have been included in the survey. The survey shows a small subgroup who eat more than would be expected from the log-normal distribution. If the sampling probability for this subgroup is the same as for the group as a whole, then the number in the subgroup is about 120. One of the ICRP requirements for a critical group is that it should be reasonably homogeneous.[10] The main group extends over a factor of more than 100 in consumption, but the subgroup has a much smaller spread of only about a factor of 2 from the median of 160 g/day. This figure is used to calculate the relevant derived working limit for seaweed. This calculation makes use of the ICRP maximum permissible daily intake of ^{106}Ru, and, since the critical group has been adequately defined, no further safety factor (such as $1/3$) need be applied.[10]

THE RESULTS OF THE MONITORING PROGRAMS

The Authority's program emphasizes the edible seaweed, *Porphyra umbilicalis*. Samples are taken at points over about 50 km of coast, with a monthly frequency for four points near the discharge pipeline and at a frequency of every 3 months from four points at greater distances. The combined average results for the four near-in points for 1967 are shown in Table 3 and compared with the derived working limits.

Table 3 shows that ^{106}Ru is the critical nuclide for this particular pathway. The monthly average results differ from the annual average by factors of up to about 2, or exceptionally 3, whereas occasional individual samples may be about an order of magnitude higher than the mean. In this context it is important to remember that the ICRP dose limits apply to annual doses, and consequently the derived working limits for seaweed also apply to annual averages. Therefore the variations due to nonuniform discharge rates and to varying weather conditions are of little real importance.

Table 3

AVERAGE CONCENTRATIONS OF NUCLIDES IN SAMPLES OF *PORPHYRA UMBILICALIS* (WINDSCALE 1967)

Nuclide	Mean activity, pCi/g	Derived working limit, pCi/g
^{106}Ru	87	300
^{95}Zr	6.9	2000
^{95}Nb	6.5	3000
^{144}Ce	3.2	300
^{90}Sr	0.10	10

The monitoring program of the Fisheries Radiobiological Laboratory of the Ministry of Agriculture, Fisheries, and Food is intended partly to confirm the safety of the discharges and partly to make quantitative estimates of the radiation dose to the critical group of seaweed eaters. The work is also concerned with making dose estimates for other noncritical groups and with making use of the discharges as a source of information for field research.

The sampling program for the edible seaweed extends over about 100 km of coast. This program, which is more detailed than that of the Authority, allows the mean activity to be calculated by weighting the results of each location by a factor proportional to the area's contribution to the total shipments of seaweed to the manufacturer of the final food product. In 1967 the average concentration of ^{106}Ru in samples of seaweed within about 5 km of the outfall was about 110 pCi/g (wet weight) compared with the derived working limit (DWL) of 300 pCi/g. The weighted average was 97 pCi/g for ^{106}Ru and 27 pCi/g for ^{95}Zr/^{95}Nb.

The Cumberland coast is not the only source of the edible seaweed eaten in the consumer area, but the dilution from other areas varies unpredictably and is not allowed for in setting the DWL. To make a more realistic appreciation of the true doses to consumers, the Fisheries Radiobiological Laboratory has measured the concentration of ^{106}Ru in the food product, laver bread, from each of the major manufacturers. The highest annual average figure in 1967 was 15 pCi/g, and the corresponding figure in the raw seaweed would have been about 30 pCi/g. This is substantially lower than the weighted average of 97 pCi/g for seaweed on the Cumberland coast in 1967. This difference can be attributed to dilution of seaweed from other sources.

The Laboratory also measures the activity of silt and the resulting gamma-radiation dose rate over silt banks. In 1967 the highest mean dose rate was about 130 µr/hr compared with a DWL of 1.5 mr/hr. The radiation is predominantly from ^{95}Zr and ^{95}Nb, in contrast to the importance of ^{106}Ru in seaweed. This indicates how a change in the composition of the effluent might change the critical nuclide, critical pathway, and critical group. It emphasizes the importance of a regular review of environmental monitoring programs and of the bases of limits of discharges of radioactive waste.

Fish, often thought of as an important pathway in the marine environment, are monitored by the Laboratory, but their activity has systematically been trivial. Table 4 shows the results of two age groups of plaice (*Pleuronectes platessa*) compared with the relevant DWL.

The work of the Fisheries Radiobiological Laboratory is summarized in annual reports of the monitoring results.[12-14]

Table 4

ACTIVITIES OF NUCLIDES IN PLAICE FLESH NEAR WINDSCALE, 1967

Nuclide	Mean activity in fish of various ages, pCi/g 0 to 1 year	1 to 2 years	DWL, pCi/g
^{106}Ru	1.4	1.9	1000
^{134}Cs	0.4	0.3	1000
^{137}Cs	0.8	0.7	2000
^{40}K	2.0	2.1	

DISCHARGES FROM OTHER SITES

Some of the principal discharges from other Authority sites are summarized in Table 5. These figures are all fairly typical of other years, except for the solid waste, which was unusually low in 1967. A more typical figure would be a few tens of thousands of curies. All these discharges have been the subject of studies similar in concept to those at Windscale though sometimes of a much simpler character. They have required a preoperational review of the environmental situation and a quantitative appraisal of the possible hazards. None of these programs has required any preoperational measurement of radioactivity because, in some cases, the degree of possible contamination of the environment was obviously trivial or, in others, because it was clear that the discharges would be large enough for the resulting activity to be readily detectable in the presence of background

Table 5

PRINCIPAL DISCHARGES OF RADIOACTIVE WASTE TO SEA FROM THE UK ATOMIC ENERGY AUTHORITY, 1967

Establishment and function	Quantity discharged, Ci	Receiving water
Windscale (fuel reprocessing)	70,000 (β) 1,000 (α)	Coastal waters of the Irish Sea
Dounreay (fuel reprocessing)	20,000 (β)	Pentland Firth
Springfields (fuel preparation)	600 (β)	Ribble Estuary
Chapelcross (nuclear power station)*	70 (β)	Solway Firth
All establishments (solid waste)	2,000	Atlantic Deeps

*Similar figures apply to the larger nuclear power stations of the Central Electricity Generating Board and the South of Scotland Electricity Board.

activity. Some of the programs of measurements associated with Windscale, particularly those in which samples have been taken at great distances from the plant, have been confused by the presence of radioactivity from other sources, but this confusion would not have been resolved by background surveys because these other sources of radioactivity were varying with time.

Both Winfrith and the Fisheries Radiobiological Laboratory have conducted measurements of radionuclides from fallout in seawater and marine materials and have obtained valuable information concerning the behavior of fallout materials in the marine environment. These studies are valuable in their own right but do not provide a justification for preoperational environmental monitoring. Perhaps the principal justification for preoperational environmental monitoring programs is that they provide training and a basis of experience for the monitoring and analytical teams. Unfortunately the majority of measurements made during operations will be specific to nuclides discharged in the effluent, and these may well not be present in sufficient quantities in the preoperational environment. The preoperational survey may then become a somewhat frustrating collection of negative results.

CONCLUSIONS

The discharge of radioactive waste to the sea from several establishments of the UKAEA produces measurable activity in the marine environment. However, because of the stringent control exercised both by the Authority and by the relevant government departments, the discharge rates are limited so that there is no damage to the marine environment and no limitation on man's use of the marine environment. The whole program represents an industry's successful disposal of waste without producing any problems of pollution.

REFERENCES

1. The Control of Radioactive Wastes, *Cmnd. 884*, Her Majesty's Stationery Office, London, 1960.
2. Radioactive Substances Act, 1960, Her Majesty's Stationery Office, London, 1960.
3. E. T. Wray (Ed.), Environmental Monitoring Associated with Discharges of Radioactive Waste During 1967 from UKAEA Establishments, *AHSB(RP)R86*, Her Majesty's Stationery Office, London, 1968.
4. H. J. Dunster, The Discharge of Radioactive Waste Products into the Irish Sea, Part 2, The Preliminary Estimate of the Safe Daily Discharge of Radioactive Effluent, in *Proceedings of the International Conference on the Peaceful Uses of Atomic Energy, Geneva, 1955*, Vol. 9, p. 712, United Nations, New York, 1956.

5. D. D. R. Fair and A. S. McLean, The Radioactive Survey of the Area Surrounding an Atomic Energy Factory, in *Proceedings of the International Conference on the Peaceful Uses of Atomic Energy, Geneva, 1955,* Vol. 13, p. 329, United Nations, New York, 1956.
6. H. J. Dunster, The Disposal of Radioactive Liquid Wastes into Coastal Waters, in *Proceedings of the Second United Nations International Conference on the Peaceful Uses of Atomic Energy, Geneva, 1958,* Vol. 18, p. 390, United Nations, New York, 1958.
7. H. J. Dunster, et al., Environmental Monitoring Associated with the Discharge of Low Activity Radioactive Waste from Windscale Works to the Irish Sea, *Health Phys.,* 10(5): 353 (1964).
8. H. Howells, Discharges of Low-Activity, Radioactive Effluent from the Windscale Works into the Irish Sea, in *Disposal of Radioactive Wastes into Seas, Oceans, and Surface Waters,* Symposium Proceedings, Vienna, 1966, p. 769, International Atomic Energy Agency, Vienna, 1966 (STI/PUB/126).
9. Recommendations of the International Commission on Radiological Protection (Adopted September 17, 1965), *ICRP Publication 9,* Pergamon Press Ltd., Oxford, 1966.
10. Principles of Environmental Monitoring Related to the Handling of Radioactive Materials: A Report by Committee 4 of ICRP, *ICRP Publication 7,* Pergamon Press Ltd., Oxford, 1966.
11. A. Preston and D. F. Jefferies, The ICRP Critical Group Concept in Relation to the Windscale Sea Discharges, *Health Phys.,* 16(1): 33-46 (1969).
12. N. T. Mitchell (Ed.), Radioactivity in Surface and Coastal Waters of the British Isles, *Technical Report FRL 1,* MAFF Fisheries Radiobiological Laboratory, Lowestoft, Suffolk, 1967.
13. N. T. Mitchell, Radioactivity in Surface and Coastal Waters of the British Isles, 1967, *Technical Report FRL 2,* MAFF Fisheries Radiobiological Laboratory, Lowestoft, Suffolk, 1968.
14. N. T. Mitchell, Radioactivity in Surface and Coastal Waters of the British Isles, 1968, *Technical Report FRL 5,* MAFF Fisheries Radiobiological Laboratory, Lowestoft, Suffolk, 1969.

DISCUSSION

PARTICIPANT: Would there be a change in your attitude if your releases were contaminating waters outside your own country?

DUNSTER: Let me answer this indirectly. We are not inhibited from reprocessing overseas reactor fuel at our chemical plant at Windscale. I think we would attempt to balance benefit on a worldwide scale against risk on a worldwide scale on the rather doubtful assumption that one can, in fact, balance these terms. We already get a fair number of questions from Ireland, of course. They are just on the other side of the Irish Sea, but so far supplying them with data has been sufficient to satisfy them. A certain amount of monitoring is also being done on Irish coastal seaweeds. Another situation which is exactly comparable is that of the Channel Islands, which are just across the water from the new French reprocessing plant at Le Havre. A monitoring program is being run by the Ministry for them, although the French discharges so far have not been large enough to make any significant difference. These are international problems and deserve an international outlook.

FOSTER: You mentioned earlier that you were perhaps just a little disappointed that the total quantities involved were greater in the United States. We certainly would not want you to leave the country thinking that there is anything second best here; and I would like to point out that your Windscale curies are fission-product curies, whereas ours are the much more innocuous neutron activation curies.

DUNSTER: I understand.

HATCH (LRL): Do you have any information about the exchange rates of offshore waters based on these experiments?

DUNSTER: Not that I can put into numerical terms. Generally speaking, we have done movement studies to a limited extent, and the process principally in operation here is one of turbulent diffusion. Much of the information that we have is from studies of salinity rather than radioactivity. There is very little bulk movement of water; in fact, the radioactivity moves about equally north and south, up and down the coast. There is a tidal cycle up and down, and the radioactivity tails off the ends of this cycle about equally in both directions. It goes around the Isle of Man and is swept out of the North Channel because there is a general flow up the Irish Sea, with a turnover of once about every 3 years. The rate of dispersion in the immediate vicinity of Windscale is predominantly determined by wind, which is variable.

HAWLEY: Dr. Dunster, I think you are one of the proponents of the theory that we have reached a point where we can now stop all this environmental monitoring and monitor only the sources. At the same time you are saying that changes in processes may shift critical pathways and so on. Are these two standpoints compatible?

DUNSTER: By the skin of their teeth. I think that when we start discharges that give as much as 10 to 20% of permissible doses, we probably cannot rely on monitoring at the source alone. With that reservation, it is probably better to establish a 5-year review program to see if the environment has changed, if the people have moved, and to see if they are still behaving the same way. It may be better to do that perhaps every 5 years than to do a program of radioactivity measurements. In much the same way, I am totally convinced that it is far better to do a preoperational study of what people do and eat and what the environment looks like than it is to measure preoperational levels of radioactivity. Some of you will recognize this as a long-standing hobbyhorse of mine. I have yet to see preoperational radioactivity measurements providing anything useful in the way of rational information for later use. If the levels in the environment are large enough to be of concern, you could not care less what was there before — especially when you are putting something into the environment that did not happen to be there before.

PARKER: This is a comment on the question arising from Dr. Foster's comment about the relative comfort we have with our activation curies vs. your fission curies. I think we ought to be quite sure we do not leave the impression that this is necessarily so. It would have been very different in our case if, for instance, we had happened to want galvanized iron cladding on our fuel elements; the ^{65}Zn would have been horrendous. The same thing could apply anytime to Plowshare.

DUNSTER: We have a case of a nuclear power station where the critical pathway is of ^{65}Zn into the estuary, into the oysters, and into man. The levels are low, but the pathway is quite clearly there. One of the interesting features is, if we were to apply to the discharges a concentration limit based on some practical drinking water concentration, such as the AEC control figure for ^{65}Zn, or the USSR figure, which is a little lower, these oysters would become totally inedible, just downright dangerous. Here is a case where the reconcentration factor into the oysters is so great and the volume of discharge is so great that a concentration limit errs seriously on the wrong side of safety. We have more or less discounted concentration controls for both liquid and gaseous waste in favor of controls based on activity per unit time, preferably curies per quarter for liquid wastes, and perhaps curies per week for gaseous wastes, where you have the swing-of-the-wind problem.

PARTICIPANT: Are your reactor licensing criteria in the United Kingdom based on defining this critical path?

DUNSTER: Yes. Individually, in fact. The most recent summary of this appeared in the IAEA symposium report on the disposal of waste to seas, oceans, and surface waters, where Alan Preston, who was responsible for several of the tables I used in my paper, gave a rundown of the preoperational surveys of the major power-station sites where the critical pathways were identified and evaluated by field work.

COMAR: Are the seaweed levels in a constant steady state with the discharges, or is there any cumulative effect?

DUNSTER: The principal nuclides in the seaweed are ^{106}Ru (300-day half-life), ^{144}Ce (about a year), and niobium (30 to 60 days), and so, speaking generally, there is no cumulative effect because of the relatively short half-lives. Being a production establishment we have a nonuniform discharge rate, and you can follow peaks of radioactivity. These decrease fairly noticeably. On occasions the peak levels have been substantially higher than the guide figures I gave of approximately 300 pCi/g, but the guide figures relate to annual averages. Perhaps I should add that we do not take into account the fact that not all the seaweed in South Wales comes from Cumberland. There is dilution by a factor of 3 to 5, depending on year-to-year supplies from other places, and variable from manufacturer to manufacturer. Therefore it is difficult to make use of it as a routine control measure; but it is a legitimate factor to put in when estimating actual doses to people.

PRESENCE AND PERSISTENCE OF RADIONUCLIDES; POSSIBLE COUNTERMEASURES AGAINST HARMFUL CONSEQUENCES OF RADIONUCLIDE CONTAMINATION

Certain radionuclides are extraordinarily persistent in the local surroundings of nuclear detonations. Others have been raised into the troposphere and the stratosphere from whence they gradually return to the earth. Both local and global radioecology are matters of concern, with the primary aims of monitoring the contamination of man's food supplies and of devising countermeasures to affect the transport pathways at various feasible stages. These topics are the subject of this session.

PERSISTENCE OF RADIONUCLIDES AT SITES OF NUCLEAR DETONATIONS

JOHN J. KORANDA and JOHN R. MARTIN
Bio-Medical Division, Lawrence Radiation Laboratory, University of California, Livermore, California

ABSTRACT

A brief history of nuclear detonation site studies is discussed with special emphasis on those of an ecological nature. The development of the Plowshare program and the execution of the SEDAN event stimulated detailed radioecological studies of long-lived radionuclides. The Bio-Medical Division, Lawrence Radiation Laboratory, began ecological studies of residual tritium in the SEDAN crater area in 1966. The distribution of tritium in the SEDAN ejecta field, climatic effects on this distribution, and inventory data are described in this research. The biological significance of residual tritium at SEDAN crater is evaluated in plant and animal studies. The organic fixation of tritium in herbaceous plants at SEDAN crater is effective in the trophic transfer of tritium to seed-eating mammals whose internal radiation dose from tritium is greater than that produced by external gamma sources.

Gamma-emitting radionuclide distribution and movement at SEDAN crater are also described. An integrated inventory of radionuclides in SEDAN ejecta indicates that tritium is the most abundant radionuclide on basis of $\mu Ci/sq$ ft. Recent cratering detonations have been studied and a surficial distribution of gamma radioactivity is apparent when the ejecta field is transected and the vertical and horizontal distribution of radionuclides is determined.

Why are we concerned with long-lived radioactivity at nuclear detonation sites? After all, most nuclear detonation sites in existence today are either in the controlled expanses of the Nevada Test Site or in the remote Pacific Proving Grounds. Early in the nuclear age, we might have offered such reasons as radiological safety considerations or the use of the detonation site for basic research projects. The detonation site may be considered a natural laboratory where realistic environmental parameters affect the persistence of radionuclides created in the detonation.

At this time, however, when there are at least two large nuclear engineering projects under consideration by the U. S. Atomic Energy Commission, and the detonation site has the potential of becoming a harbor[1] or an interoceanic canal, the study of the persistence of radionuclides at the nuclear detonation site becomes an extremely cogent subject pertinent to the peaceful uses of nuclear explosives. In addition, the detonation site can become a source region for radionuclide release into the surrounding environments, which probably would contain food organisms used either directly or indirectly by man.

One of the principal aims of our research is to define the distribution of radioactivity at the detonation site where earth has been moved to create a crater or a trench. Subsequent ecological studies are then directed toward the biological systems that come in contact with that radioactive substratum.

FISSION EXPLOSIVES

The first detonation site of the nuclear age was created in 1945 in Operation Trinity in New Mexico. The Trinity site became the subject of the first radioecological investigations as Warren, Bellamy, and others[2] studied the persistence of various kinds of radioactivity in the environment adjacent to the Trinity ground zero (GZ). Their approaches were similar to those we use today; however, in the 20-year interim, nuclear technology has produced more-sophisticated tools with which to study environmental radioactivity. It is now possible to quantitate simultaneously several gamma-emitting radionuclides in soil, plant, or animal samples by the use of solid-state gamma spectroscopy. Also, during this period liquid scintillation counting was developed to permit rapid, automatic assay of low-energy beta-emitters, such as tritium and ^{14}C.

Early studies of detonation sites, such as at the Trinity site and others at the Nevada Test Site, indicated that the radioactivity near GZ decreased with time more rapidly than the radiological half-life of the long-lived fission products, whose decay was reasonably well known. In an open system, such as a natural environment, other factors besides radiological decay affect the persistence of a given radionuclide, and such concepts as the environmental half-life were recognized. More significantly, during this period it was found that certain radioisotopes appeared in plants and animals which reinvaded detonation sites and that a potential problem area existed when radioactivity entered an organism by ecological and biological routes and delivered its radiation internally.

Later in the nuclear test period, we learned that the entire biosphere and its inhabitants, especially in the northern hemisphere, acquired a small but measurable burden of radioactivity by these ecological mechanisms. If you happened to be an Eskimo or a Laplander, you received a little more than your share because of the unique ecosystem in which you lived. The literature is replete with research concerned with the presence of the fallout radionuclides ^{137}Cs, ^{90}Sr, and ^{54}Mn in man's environment, man's food, and in man himself.[3-5]

Testing in the Pacific Proving Grounds took place in another unique environment — that of the coral atolls of the South Pacific. The substratum, biota, and the entire ecological system of the atoll are quite endemic. The knowledge obtained in the study of atoll detonation sites by Donaldson and his staff[6] during their years of research at Eniwetok and Bikini atolls could be applied to certain offshore or littoral radioecological problems currently being faced. Five years postshot on a Pacific atoll, the most abundant long-lived radionuclides in terrestrial organisms were ^{137}Cs and ^{90}Sr and in some cases ^{54}Mn. In marine organisms the activation products ^{65}Zn, ^{60}Co, and ^{54}Mn were still being concentrated from the water and bottom sediments. In the upper 2 in. of atoll soil, the following radionuclides were still detectable: ^{54}Mn, ^{65}Zn, ^{106}Ru, ^{144}Ce, ^{55}Fe, ^{125}Sb, ^{57}Co, ^{60}Co, and ^{137}Cs. These data do not differ significantly from those obtained in continental environments in North America and Europe, where the same radionuclides have been detected in environments receiving worldwide fallout.

However, in our own radioecological studies at Eniwetok atoll,[7] we found that tritium and ^{14}C occurred in locally enriched levels in the vicinity of old detonation sites. Water obtained from the bottom of Mike crater on Eniwetok atoll in 1964, 12 years postshot, indicated that a source of tritium was present in the crater-bottom materials, which was detectable in spite of frequent exchange of crater water with the open sea. Tritium content of rainwater and seawater at Eniwetok are shown in Table 1. Marine algae growing at the edge of Mike crater

Table 1

TRITIUM CONTENT OF RAINWATER AND SEAWATER AT ENIWETOK ATOLL

Sample	Location	Tritium units
Lagoon seawater	10 ft below surface near center of lagoon	≤60
Lagoon seawater	180 ft below surface at bottom of lagoon	≤60
Lagoon seawater	1 m from bottom of Mike crater	820 ± 40 840 ± 40
Pacific Ocean seawater	Marshall Islands, December 1963	7.9
Rainwater	Eniwetok Island, August 1964	≤50

were enriched in ^{14}C 10-fold over those growing in other parts of the atoll where no detonations had taken place.

THERMONUCLEAR EXPLOSIVES

It was during this period that the nuclear explosive assumed a completely different character because of the development of the thermonuclear device. Previously the radioecologist was confronted with something like 73 fission products with half-lives longer than 1 hr and also a few activation products. The thermonuclear explosive produces

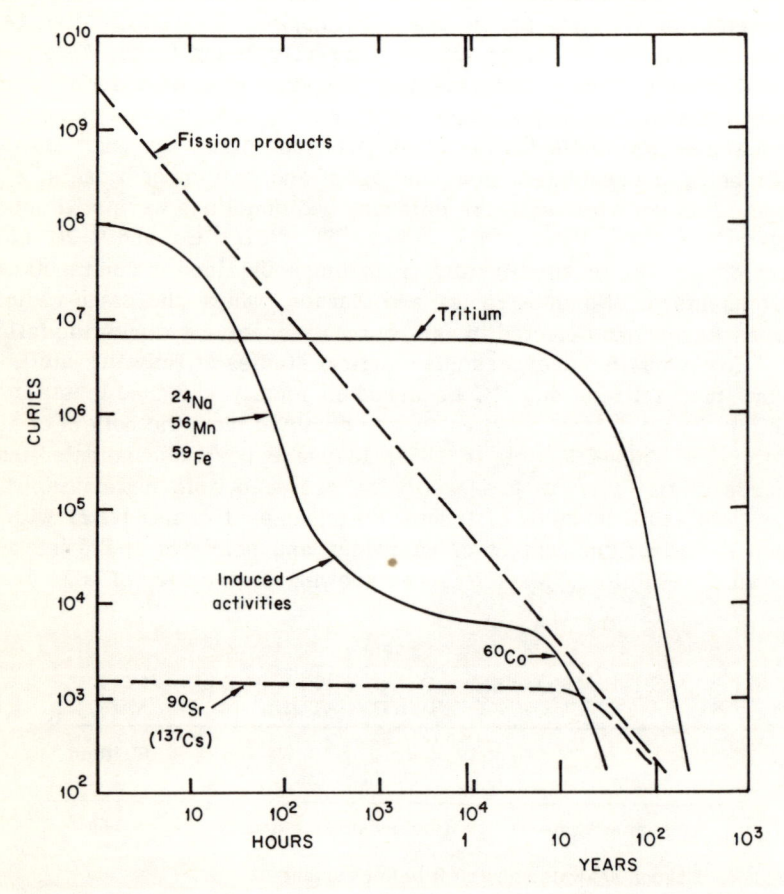

Fig. 1 — Tritium, ^{90}Sr, and other fission-product activities from a nominal 1-Mt fission–fusion (1 : 99) explosion in average crustal materials. (From F. W. Stead, Distribution in Groundwater of Radionuclides from Underground Nuclear Explosions, in Engineering with Nuclear Explosives, Proceedings of the Third Plowshare Symposium, USAEC Report TID-7695, University of California, Davis, 1964.)

a neutron flux of higher energy, activating more environmental materials, and also producing a new radioactive by-product in the form of residual tritium. A description of residual radioactivity half-life was made by Stead[8] for a 1-Mt explosion utilizing 1% fission (Fig. 1). When a thermonuclear explosive is used, the long-lived radioactivity consists primarily of tritium and activation products.

During the development and testing of the thermonuclear explosive, which took place at the Nevada Test Site as well as at the Pacific Proving Grounds, considerable attention was still focused on the volatile fission products which, if they left the detonation site in sufficient amounts, were potential public-health problems. The environmental behavior of ^{131}I and ^{90}Sr was studied in the close-in and intermediate-distance fallout fields.[9] Some research was conducted during this period on the biological availability of radionuclides in earth materials that were involved in one way or another with the nuclear detonation. Many detonations were conducted on towers or from low-altitude balloons, and the main effect on the ground surface was a fusion of the soil surface in which common soil constituents were activated.

THE SEDAN EVENT

In the late 1950's and early 1960's, the philosophy of the Plowshare Program was evolved with considerable imagination and farsightedness by scientists at the Lawrence Radiation Laboratory. In July 1962 an experiment utilizing a thermonuclear explosive to move earth was conducted in northern Yucca Flat at the Nevada Test Site. This was the Sedan event[10] in which a 100 kt explosive was detonated 320 ft below the surface of the desert in weakly consolidate alluvium. The resulting crater, shown in Fig. 2, was 1200 ft in diameter and 320 ft deep.

Approximately 5 million tons of ejecta were deposited on the landscape from the lip of Sedan crater to a distance of 5500 ft from GZ. In this mass of earth, not only fission and activation products were present but also residual tritium in the form of tritiated water. Because tungsten had been utilized in the explosive construction, several radioisotopes of tungsten were present in the nuclear debris and ejecta of the Sedan detonation. Project Sedan was a most significant event, however, because it provided the radioecologist with the first large-scale terrestrial detonation environment in which long-term ecological studies could be conducted.

The Sedan crater area and its contained radioactivity presented these unique features to the radioecologist: (1) it had been created by an explosive with a low yield of fission products relative to the total explosive energy; (2) tungsten radioisotopes were present, and their availability in nuclear crater ejecta was not definitely known; (3) biologically available residual tritium was present in the earth mass; and (4) a large radioactively "tagged" environment was created in which long-term ecological studies could be conducted.

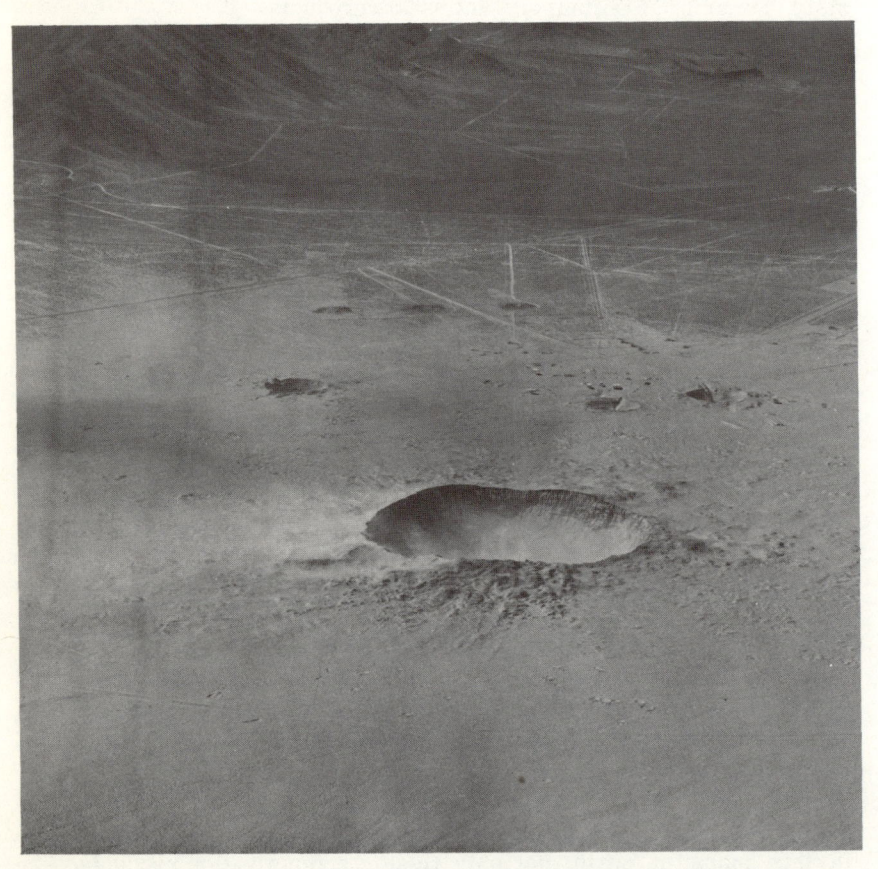

Fig. 2—*Aerial photograph of Sedan crater shortly after the detonation, July 1962.*

Early ecological studies at Sedan crater were focused on the behavior and biological availability of tungsten radioisotopes and on the uptake of ^{131}I and ^{90}Sr by animals in the fallout field. Basic studies concerned with the reestablishment of natural vegetation and animal populations on Sedan ejecta were also conducted. These studies were carried on mainly by the University of California at the Los Angeles Laboratory of Nuclear Medicine and Radiation Biology.[11,12]

TRITIUM FIELD STUDIES

In late 1964, studies progressed in the Bio-Medical Division of the Lawrence Radiation Laboratory at Livermore, and certain data became available in the Plowshare Division which indicated that tritium, perhaps one of the most significant radionuclides produced in the Sedan event, had been overlooked, at least from the standpoint of its ecological behavior. Tritium concentrations in the fallback in Sedan crater reported by Hansen[13] and discussed by Knox[14,15] indicated that this radionuclide indeed had been scavenged or retained in the ejecta mass rather efficiently. Their data are shown in Fig. 3. In early and mid-

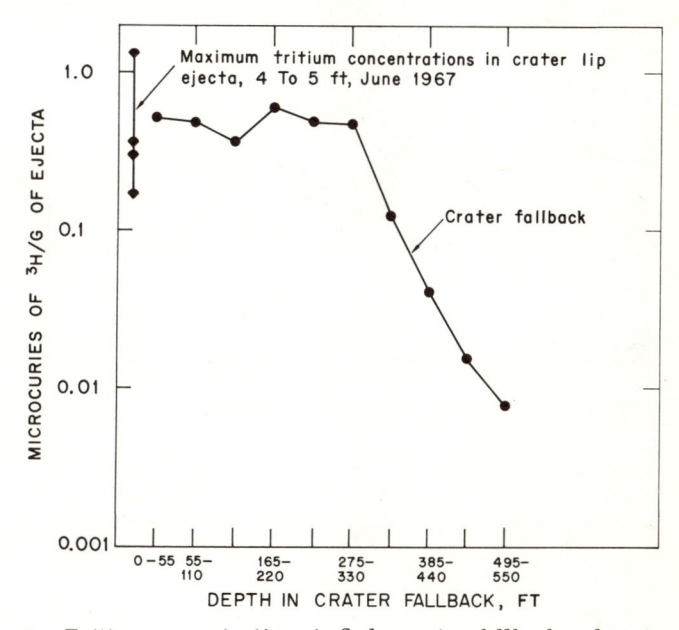

Fig. 3 — Tritium concentrations in Sedan crater fallback and crater lip.

1965, some preliminary measurements were made on tritium concentrations in Sedan crater-lip ejecta and at stations as far as 4000 ft from GZ by Bio-Medical Division scientists. In 1966, full-scale ecological studies on the persistence of residual tritium at Sedan crater were begun.[16] These studies have continued to the present time, being diminished in intensity only recently as other environmental research projects were initiated. Here are some of the salient results of our studies at the Sedan crater.

When you appear on the scene approximately 4 years postshot, you are faced with one serious problem in interpreting distributional patterns of radioactivity in earth materials moved by nuclear detonations. The distribution of radioactivity is either due to the original deposition of the ejecta, or else existing patterns are due to the integrated environmental effects since shot time. In Fig. 4 the tritium depth profiles for five crater-lip stations are shown. It is apparent

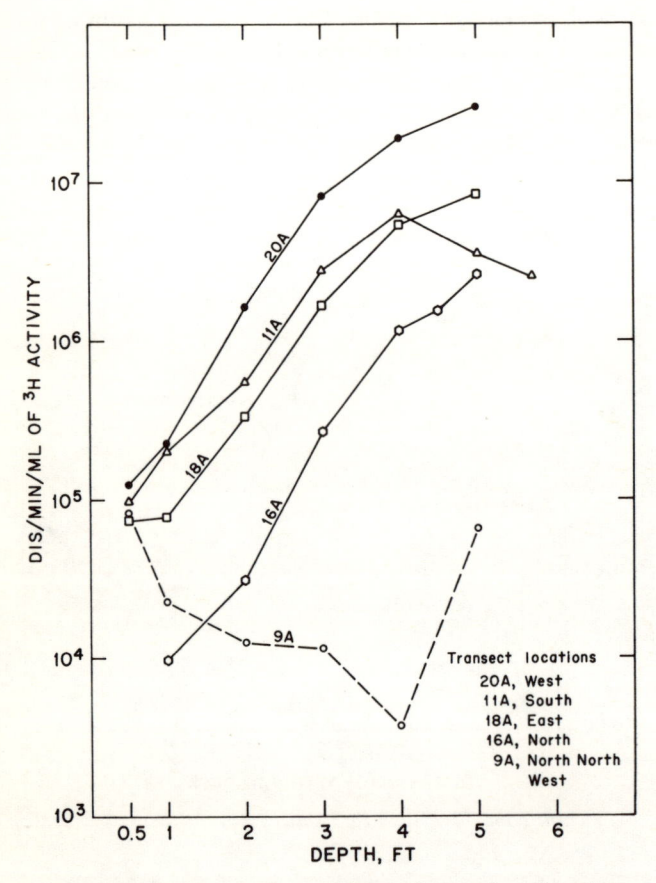

Fig. 4—*Tritium depth profiles at five crater-lip sites.*

that, except for the 9A area on the northwest lip of the crater, there is a consistent increase of tritium in soil water with depth in the ejecta. The concentration of tritium in interstitial water extracted from the fallback in the crater at the 187-ft depth (7.24 μCi/ml), which should be beyond the zone of environmental effects, is in the range of maximum tritium concentrations (2.2 to 9.5 μCi/ml) found at depths between 3 and 6 ft on the crater lip. The fallback data were obtained in 1964 by Hansen;[13] our crater-lip data were obtained in August 1966. It appears, therefore, that similar concentrations of tritium were retained in the fallback within the crater and in the crater lip and close-in ejecta.

A transect of the ejecta field along the east transect line (18A) was made in July 1967, and the data are shown in Fig. 5. From these data several observations can be made. There is a decreasing con-

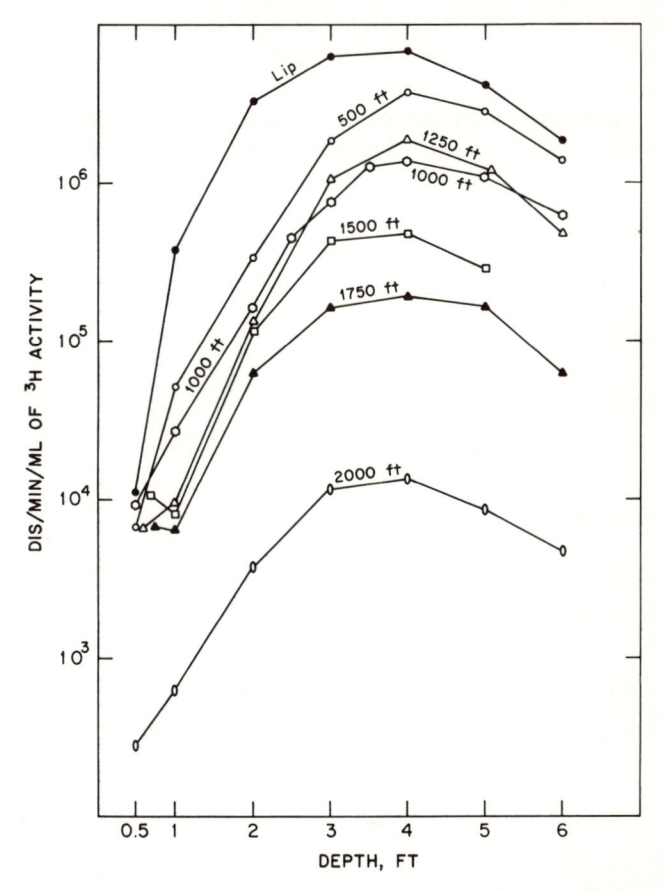

Fig. 5—*Tritium depth profiles along transect 18A of the Sedan ejecta field.*

centration of tritium with distance from the crater which may be related to the amount of ejecta and absorbed tritium deposited along a given azimuth from the crater. All the soil-water tritium profiles peak between 3 and 4 ft regardless of ejecta depth. Ejecta depth at the crater lip is 10.2 m or approximately 34 ft and decreases to approximately 1 ft at 2000 ft from the crater lip. Thus similar tritium profiles are present along a transect where ejecta depth is decreasing, indicating that the distributional patterns were all produced by the same process—rainfall leaching. The maximum concentrations of tritium at distances beyond 2000 ft from the crater are also found in the parent soil materials, beneath the ejecta or source layer, where they were eluted by winter rainfall. Although tritium responds to leaching and translocation within the ejecta profile, it is possible that other radionuclides, because of their physical–chemical nature in the ejecta materials, would exhibit another type of distribution.

A comparison of gross gamma radioactivity in the soil profile with tritium concentrations in the same samples is shown in Fig. 6. Gross gamma activity was used in this comparison merely to provide a tag for the ejecta layer. Gamma activity drops off steeply with depth at 1250 ft from the crater, and, at the depth where tritium maxima occur, it is barely above the gamma background for these earth materials.

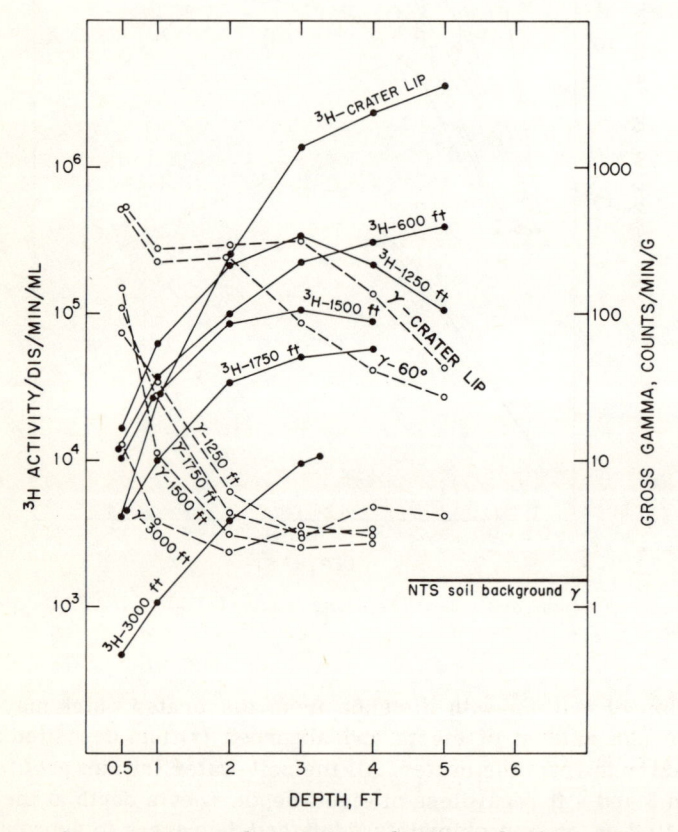

Fig. 6—*Gross gamma radioactivity and tritium depth profiles compared along a transect of the Sedan ejecta field.*

The tritium profiles shown in Fig. 5 have been produced by rainfall leaching; yet the maximum concentrations at the 3- to 5-ft depth are still very close to the tritium concentrations reported at depths exceeding 100 ft in the crater fallback. Apparently a slow-moving pulse of tritium has been produced in the Sedan ejecta and preshot soil beneath it, in which the maximum concentrations at or near the moving front have undergone little dilution from the driving force of the stable water column above it. Similar data have been reported by Zimmerman,[17] who applied tritium to the soil surface and followed this pulse in the soil profile as it moved downward after rainfall.

This phenomenon was actually simulated in the laboratory by setting up a large column of Sedan ejecta which was then leached with successive 1-in. rainfall water volumes applied to the top of the column. In Fig. 7 the column data are shown, and it is apparent that the first

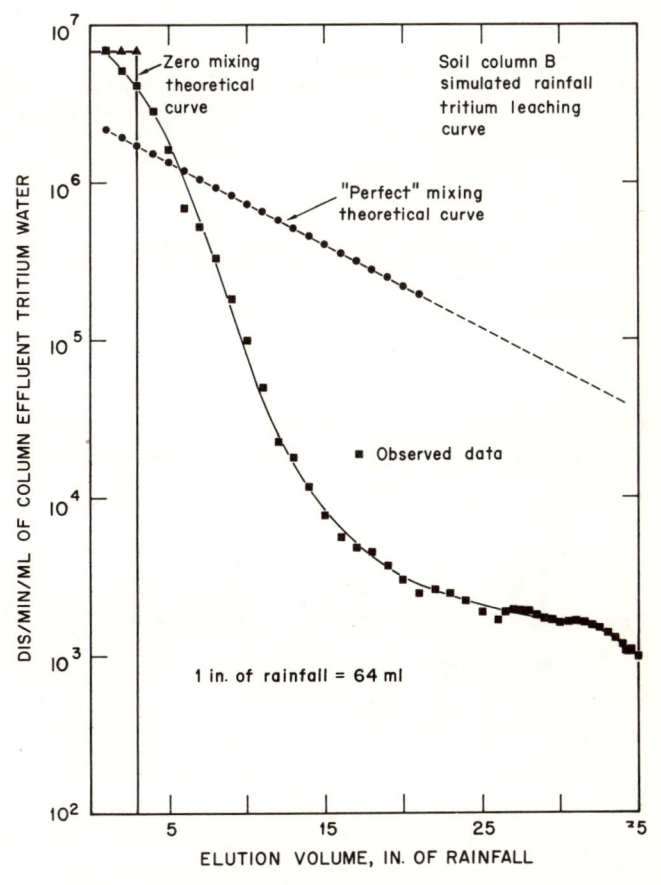

Fig. 7—Simulated rainfall leaching of Sedan ejecta.

pulse of water to be hydrostatically pushed from the column contained almost the same specific activity of tritium as the water extracted from the same soil sample by vacuum distillation. Vacuum-distillation data are represented by triangles at the top of the figure.

Soil-water movements are not simple in desert soils, and both upward and downward soil-water movements have affected the shape of these tritium profiles. Additional data indicate that the tritium maximum concentration occurs at a different depth in the summer and in the winter. The maxima are pushed down in the winter when the effective rainfall is received and move upward in the soil profile in the summer as soil water is depleted by evaporation from the top of the soil system.

The effect of an unusually large pulse of winter rainfall on the tritium depth profiles on the Sedan crater lip is shown in Fig. 8. Ap-

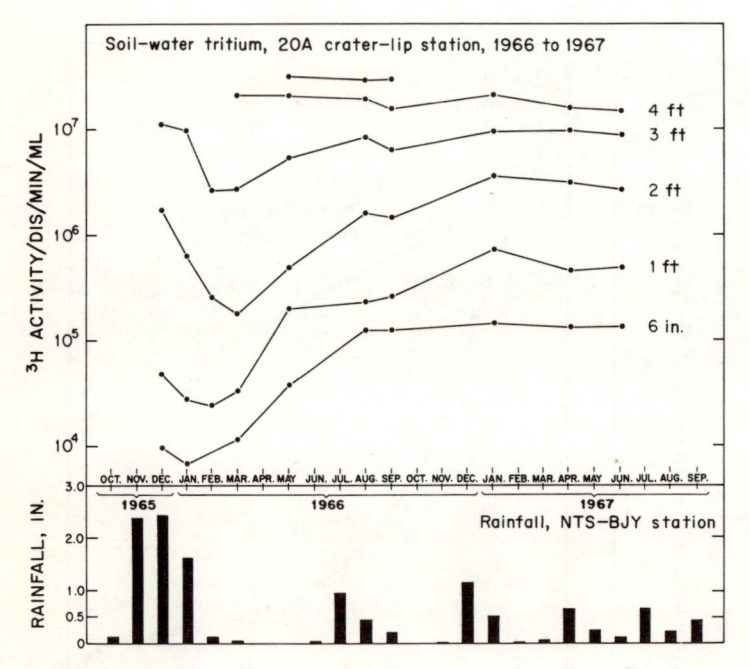

Fig. 8—*Seasonal variations in tritium concentration at a single crater-lip station.*

proximately 10 in. of rainfall was received in the winter of 1965 to 1966, and the dilution of soil-water tritium concentrations in the 6-in. to 3-ft stratum is obvious. During the period of high evaporation and soil-water use, mainly by herbaceous plants during the subsequent summer, the tritium concentrations in that depth zone returned to prerain values. The profile data obtained during the subsequent year,

1967 to 1968, show a gradual decline in the concentrations for this site, indicating that there is a loss from the zone being measured. One loss route would be via evapotranspiration and evaporation, but the most significant loss is very likely by the downward movement of tritiated water out of the sampling zone.

The soil-water tritium profile data were expressed on a disintegrations per minute per gram basis, and the concentration curve was integrated to obtain a surface value expressed in microcuries per square foot. A plot of these surface inventory values with time for a given site showed an exponential decrease from which the residence half-time of tritium at that location was determined. The inventory data for the 20A crater-lip site are shown in Fig. 9. The residence half-time for tritium at that site was 14 ± 2 months. An average of four crater-lip sites indicates a mean residence half-time for tritium in the Sedan crater lip of 17 ± 6 months.

The site inventory does not describe the irregularities that occur in ejecta distribution around the crater. By integrating the depth profile of tritium concentrations along a transect of the ejecta field, one

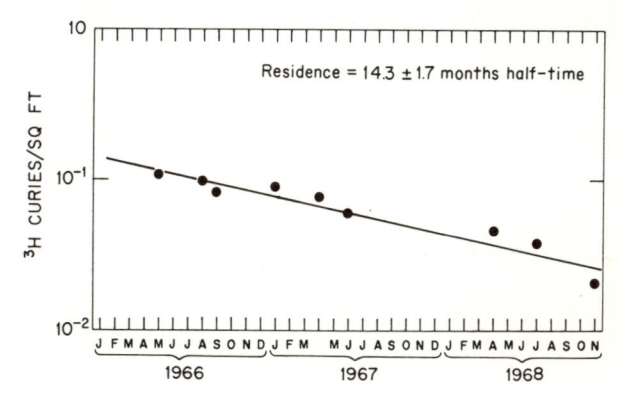

Fig. 9—*Tritium inventory and residence half-time data for a single crater-lip site (20A-L).*

can obtain an inventory of tritium in the ejecta field along a given azimuth. Two of these transect inventories are shown in Figs. 10 and 11. The shape of the transect-inventory curve is related to the deposition of ejecta along that azimuth. When the entire area of the ejecta field has been integrated by summing the inventories made on each wedge-shaped section of the ejecta field, a total inventory of tritium in the ejecta from the crater lip to 3000 ft from the crater is obtained.

This value determined in 1967 indicated that 8.4×10^4 Ci of tritium was present in the ejecta field. This value is between 5 and 6% of the estimated ejecta tritium inventory at shot time. This loss of ap-

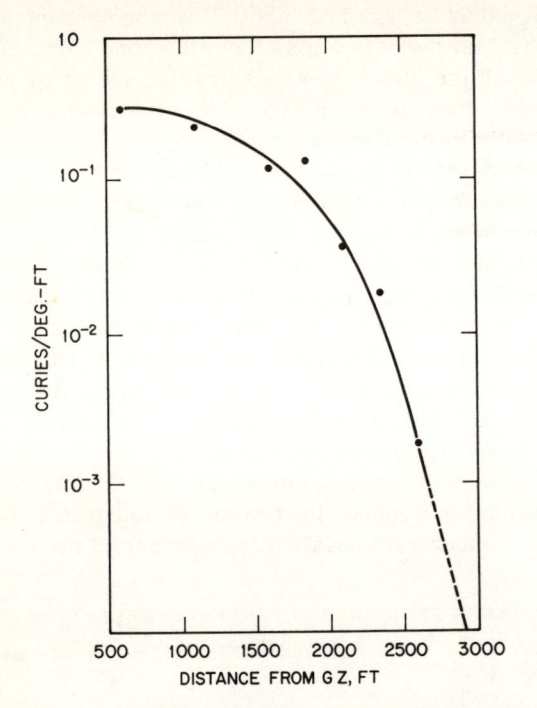

Fig. 10—Tritium inventory transects of the Sedan ejecta field, site 18A.

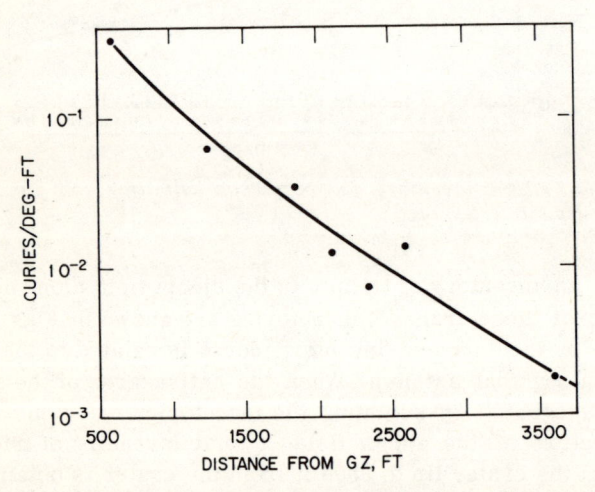

Fig. 11—Tritium inventory transects of the Sedan ejecta field, site 16A.

proximately 95% of the shot time estimated inventory of tritium corresponds to a residence half-time of 16 months, which is in good agreement with the site values obtained during a 3-year period.

It is encouraging that, in spite of a very low annual rainfall, the apparent residence time of tritium in the Sedan ejecta is rather short and that, under the influence of a higher rate of rainfall and a greater plant biomass, one could expect an even shorter residence time. Some of our current research has been concerned with tritium movement in the tropical rain forest, and some useful information will soon be forthcoming from those efforts.[21]

BIOLOGICAL STUDIES

Since our approach is primarily biological and ecological, we were concerned with the biological significance of the levels of tritium we had found in the ejecta substratum. The Sedan area was invaded by herbaceous plants within the next year after the detonation, and now at $6\frac{1}{2}$ years postshot, at least three perennial shrubs and almost a dozen species of herbaceous plants grow on the Sedan ejecta. One mammal abundantly occurring in the Sedan area is the kangaroo rat, *Dipodomys merriami*. Other mammals, such as ground squirrels, deer mice, and jackrabbits, also are found in the Sedan area. Flocks of horned lark are seen around the Sedan crater and apparently derive some of their food from plants growing on the Sedan ejecta because their bodies contain tritium.

Tritium concentrations in the tissue water of plants growing on Sedan ejecta are shown in Fig. 12. As with the soil profiles, a decrease in tritium concentration in plants with distance from the crater can be seen. As the plant grows and extends its root system deeper into the soil, it encounters higher concentrations of tritium in the soil water, as shown in Figs. 5 and 6. An increase in tissue-water tritium concentrations has been observed during the summer in most herbaceous plants. However, perennial woody plants, such as *Atriplex canescens*, have almost constant tissue-water tritium concentrations, as shown in Fig. 13. *Salsola kali* tritium concentrations approximate those in *Atriplex* at the end of their growing season or in midsummer to late summer. The presence of tritium in the tissue water of leaves and transpiring organs of plants suggested that transpirational water vapor, containing tritium, may increase the surface air levels of tritium.

Plant transpiration water-loss data are shown in Fig. 14. These data were obtained by taping a plastic bag over the plant branch and collecting the transpirational water from the bag after several hours of condensation had taken place. The rate of transpiration is accelerated by this method, but a sample of transpirational water is obtained. Gen-

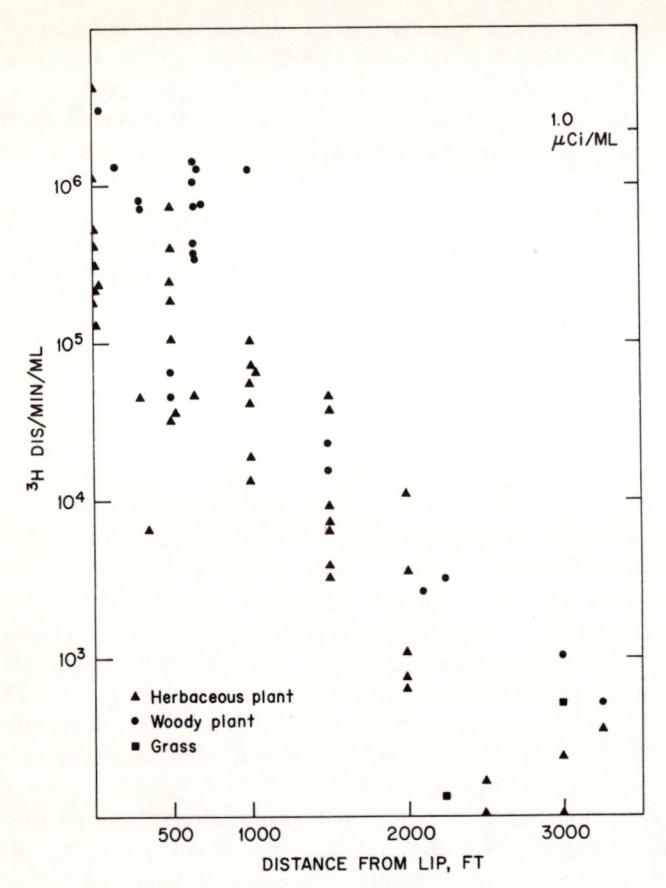

Fig. 12—*Tissue-water tritium concentrations in plants growing on Sedan ejecta, July 1968.*

erally, the transpirational water, collected by the plastic-bag method, has approximately the same tritium concentration as the tissue water. To obtain a more representative transpirational water sample, we have used a "cold finger" type condenser placed above the canopy of both the herbaceous and woody plants. The ground surface around the plant within the transpiration chamber is covered with a thick plastic sheet. Tritium concentrations in transpirational water vapor collected in this manner are shown in Fig. 15 and related to other measurements of tritium concentration in the same soil—plant system. These data suggest that transpirational water may contain a lower concentration of tritium than tissue water, perhaps because of the preferential transpiration of "lighter" water (HHO) or because of plant physiological factors concerned with the source of transpirational water and its

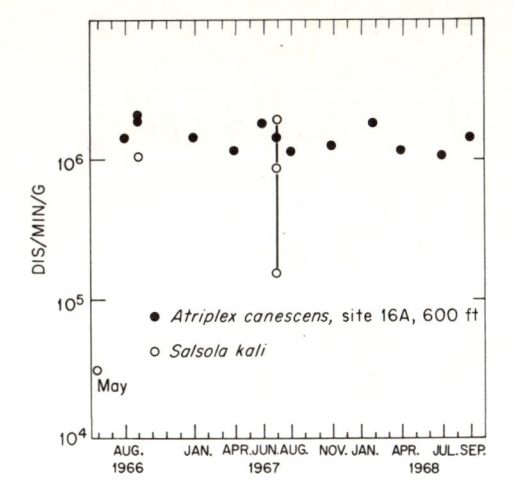

Fig. 13—Atriplex *(saltbush)* tissue-water tritium concentrations, 1966 to 1968.

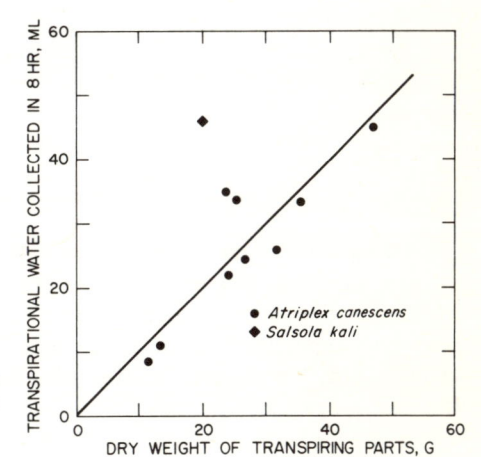

Fig. 14—*Plant transpirational losses of plants growing on Sedan ejecta, September 1968.*

relation to other water "pools" or compartments within the plant. These physiological and biochemical factors affecting tritium movement in such biological systems as trees are presently under study in the Bio-Medical Division.

Whatever the source, either plant transpiration or soil-surface evaporation, the surface air above the Sedan ejecta contains elevated concentrations of tritium. In August 1967, air concentrations of tritium were determined at two stations on the north side of the Sedan crater. These data ranged from 3.7×10^4 pCi/m^3 to 2.08×10^5 pCi/m^3 which were, respectively, 0.007 and 0.04 of the NCRP recommended MPC in air for occupational exposure.

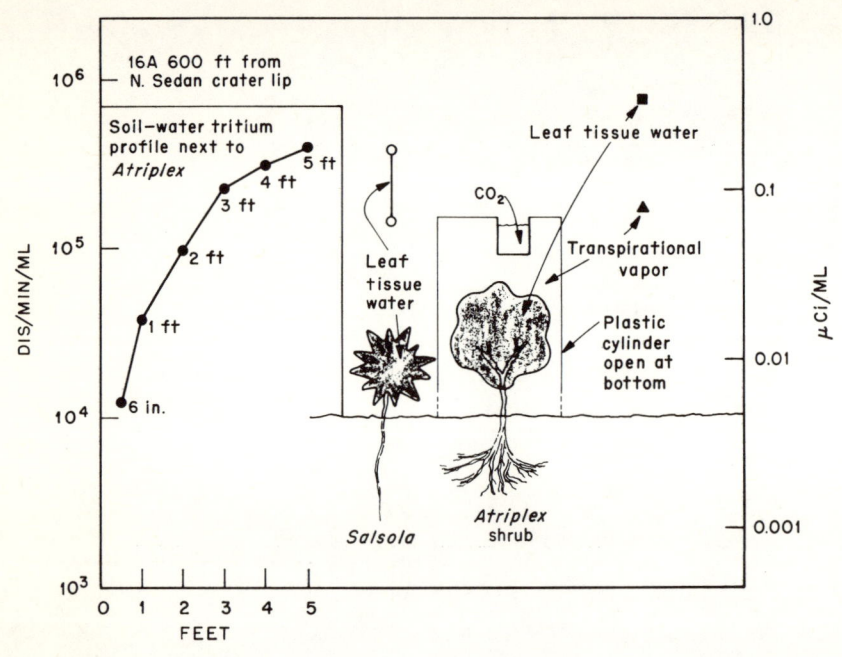

Fig. 15—Soil–plant transpiration study on Sedan crater ejecta, June 1967.

The plant-tissue water concentrations of tritium maintained throughout the growing season result in the fixation of tritium in the organic matter produced by the plants. If tissue-water and tissue-bound tritium data are expressed as disintegrations per minute of tritium per gram of hydrogen, the organic matter synthesized on Sedan ejecta has almost the same specific activity of tritium in the solid phase of the tissues as in the tissue water at maturity of the plant. These data are shown in Fig. 16.

This organically bound tritium is utilized by the resident mammals, mainly as seeds, but also to a limited extent as succulence. To determine the biological significance of this organically bound tritium, we have sampled and analyzed several kinds of animals living in the Sedan area. These have been mainly kangaroo rats; but insects, ground squirrels, lizards, and birds also have been analyzed for body-water tritium. In Fig. 17 the body-water tritium concentrations found in these animals during the past 3 years are shown. The maximum tritium concentrations in the body water of small mammals obtained in October 1965 delivered an annual internal dose of approximately 250 rads to the animal. This internal dose from tritium in the body water alone is approximately 10 times that received by the animal from the external

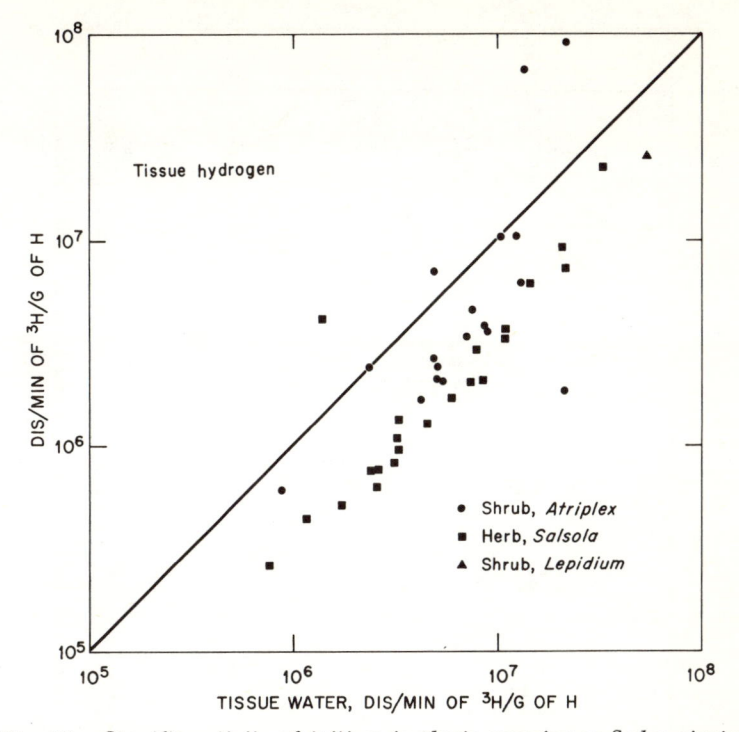

Fig. 16—*Specific activity of tritium in plants growing on Sedan ejecta.*

environmental radiation field. If the tissue-bound tritium concentrations are added to this value, the annual internal dose increases by about 30%.

The average values of each population sample of the kangaroo rat were plotted against time in Fig. 18, and the tritium half-time was determined to be 16 ± 3 months, which is in agreement with the residence half-time of tritium in the substratum.

It is possible that a portion of the body-water tritium burden measured in these animals had been obtained by the inspirational route, but soil-water tritium concentrations in the depth stratum in which burrows occur are one to three orders of magnitude lower than mammal body-water concentrations. The kangaroo rat drinks essentially no water but obtains all its body-water requirements from metabolic water produced in the digestion of its food.

Biological half-life studies have been performed on the Sedan kangaroo rats because of their unique chronic exposure to organically bound tritium. These studies were accomplished by bringing a large sample of animals from a given sector of the crater-lip area into the laboratory and maintaining them on food containing no tritium. The

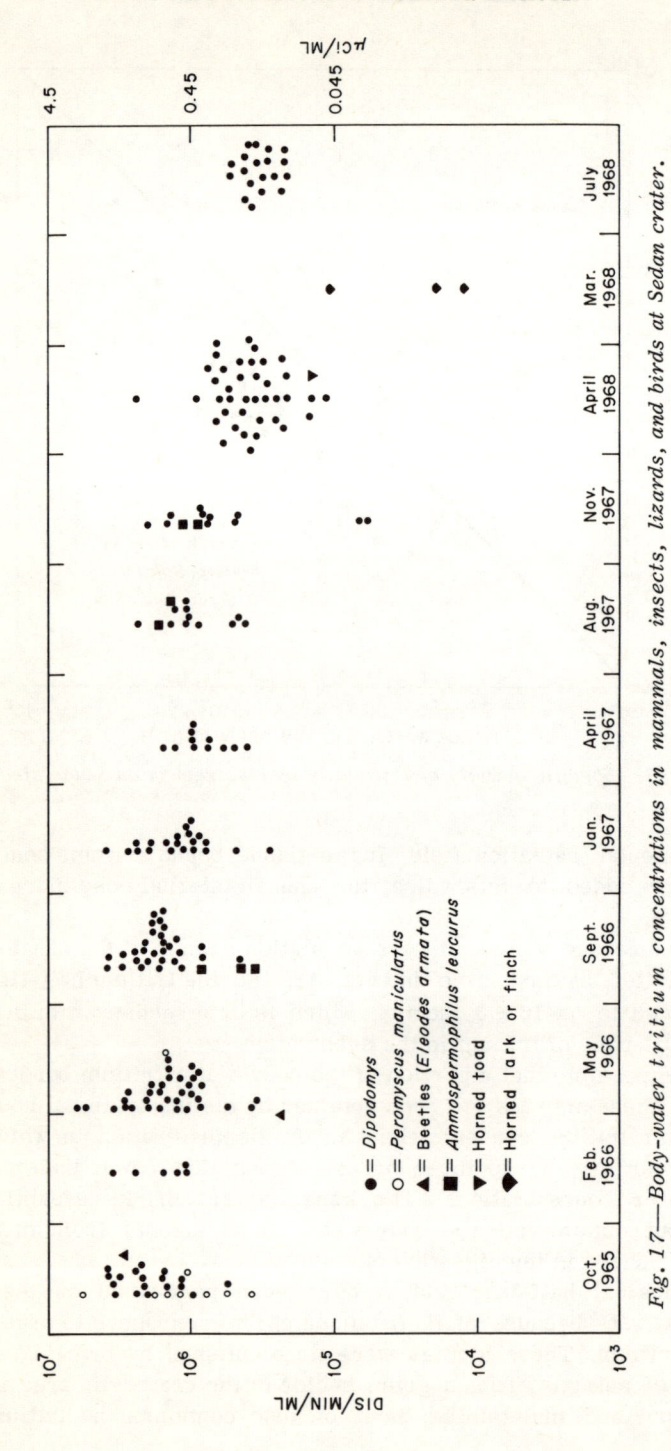

Fig. 17—Body-water tritium concentrations in mammals, insects, lizards, and birds at Sedan crater.

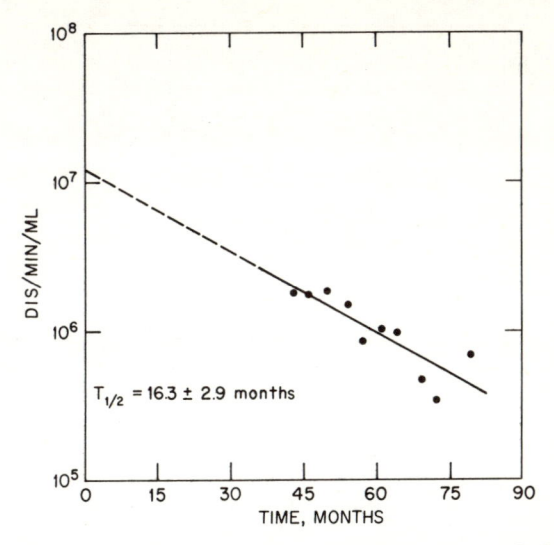

Fig. 18—Population half-time of tritium in Dipodomys *at Sedan crater.*

$T_{1/2} = 16.3 \pm 2.9$ months

body-water tritium concentrations decreased with a half-life of 15 to 17 days, which is in agreement with laboratory studies conducted with the same species of kangaroo rat. The tissue-bound tritium half-lives in various organs, however, were found to be considerably longer. The biological half-time of tritium in brain tissue was 45 ± 3 days.

Furthermore, the specific activity of tissue-bound tritium is greater at the time of capture than the specific activity of tritium in the body water. Tritium specific activity ratios between body-water and tissue-bound tritium in the brain during the period of a half-life study are shown in Fig. 19. The A_0 intercept value is 1.22, which means that kangaroo rats living in the Sedan area have 1.22 times the specific activity of tritium in the solid phase of their brain tissues as occurred in their body water. Ratios of 1.2 to 1.4 were found in other organs.

This phenomenon has not been observed in chronic exposures of experimental animals in the laboratory and gives further support to the assumption that these animals receive a unique chronic exposure to tritium via their food chain. Evans[18] reports ratios of 1.0 for body-water and tissue-bound tritium in deer receiving chronic exposure to tritium at the Savannah River installation.

GAMMA RADIOACTIVITY STUDIES

The gamma-emitting radionuclides determined in a 350-g sample of Sedan ejecta are shown in Fig. 20. These radionuclides are available

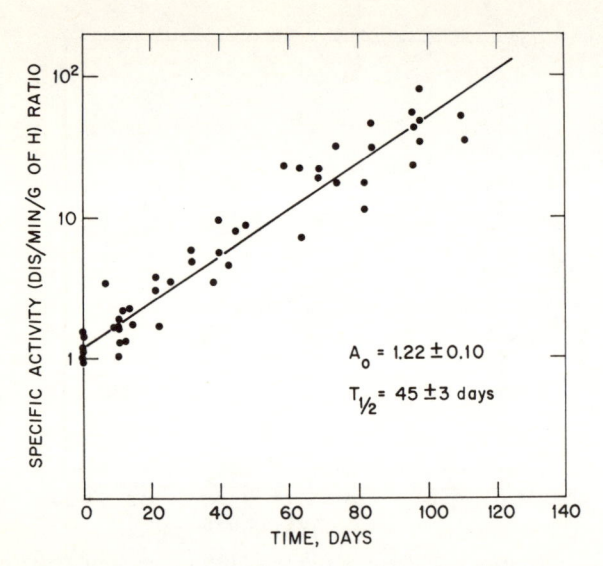

Fig. 19—Ratio of tissue-bound to body-water specific activity of tritium in brains of Dipodomys merriami *at Sedan crater.*

to plants growing on the Sedan ejecta. In Fig. 21 a plant gamma spectrum obtained with a 200-g sample of *Salsola kali* is shown. The plant gamma spectrum contains several gamma photo-peaks that were identified as ^{184m}Re, a radionuclide that is not evident in the Sedan ejecta. A radiochemical separation for rhenium was made on the plant tissue, and a pure spectrum of ^{184m}Re was obtained. We estimate that the plant would have to concentrate this radioisotope approximately 10 times for it to be evident in the plant and not in the ejecta. The uptake of rhenium by a plant is significant because rhenium is one of several elements that is accumulated in the thyroid gland, although it is not organically bound. The uptake of gamma-emitting radionuclides from Sedan ejecta was also studied by Romney and others[20] at the University of California at Los Angeles laboratories.

The rest of the prominent gamma radioactivity in the Sedan ejecta is a combination of long-lived fission products and certain activation radionuclides. These data agree with the residual radioactivity from a thermonuclear explosion as described by Stead[8] and shown in Fig. 1. Figure 22 shows the vertical distribution of these radionuclides and the integrated inventory per square foot of surface ejecta for each radionuclide, including three beta emitters, tritium, ^{90}Sr, and ^{147}Pm. All data are expressed as microcuries per square foot. It is obvious that tritium is the most abundant radionuclide in the ejecta at this time (2.39×10^4 μCi/sq ft), 5 years postshot, and this is true also for the biological systems that are present in the Sedan ecosystem. Tritium is

PERSISTENCE OF RADIONUCLIDES

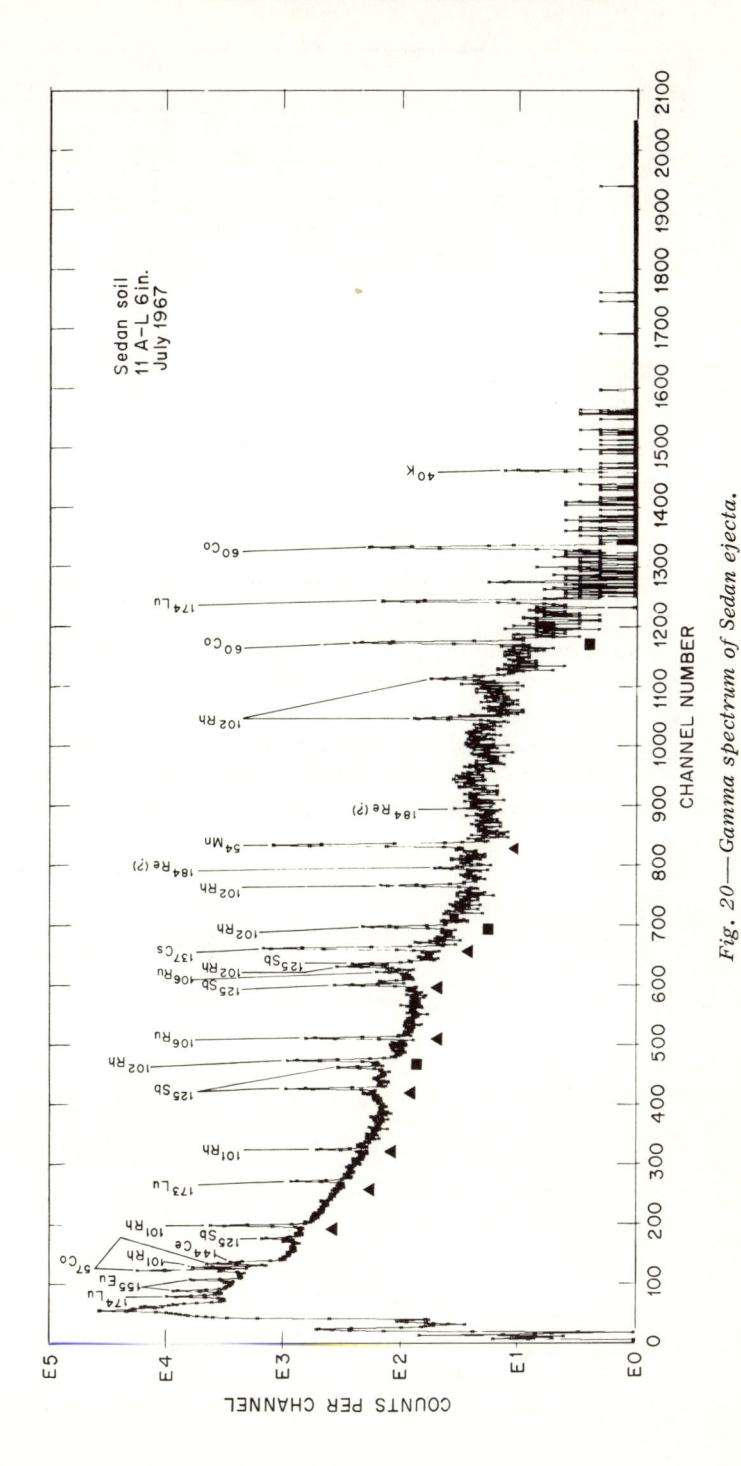

Fig. 20—Gamma spectrum of Sedan ejecta.

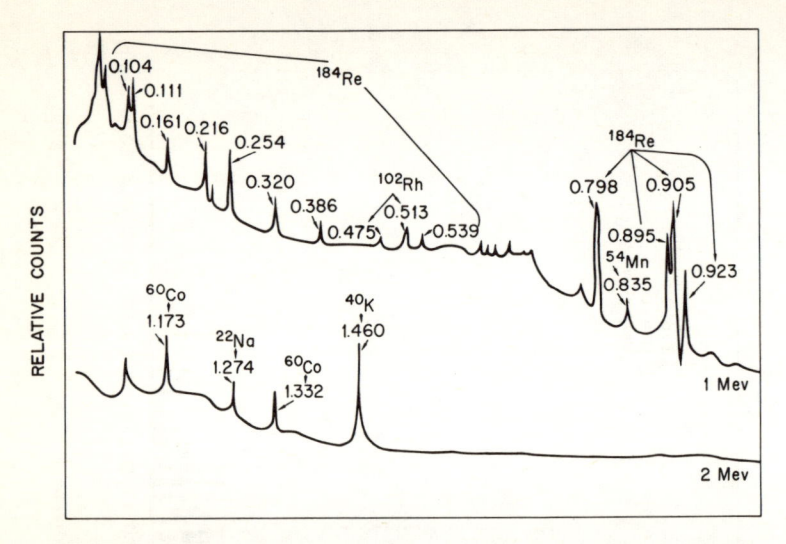

Fig. 21 — Gamma spectrum of Salsola kali *grown at Sedan crater.*

the most abundant radionuclide present in any biological sample, plant or animal, that we analyze from the Sedan area.

Most of the gamma radioactivity occurs in the upper 3 ft of the ejecta, as shown in Fig. 22. Apparently no large movement of any radionuclide has occurred that approximates that which has taken place for tritium. A slight leaching effect, however, has been seen for ^{137}Cs in Sedan ejecta.[22]

RECENT CRATERING EXPERIMENTS

Recently, three cratering detonations were conducted in hard-rock media at the Nevada Test Site. These cratering experiments provide an opportunity to study cratering phenomena in a different geological medium. Also, there is a significant difference in the climate of the higher elevations where these tests were conducted. In our attempt to sample the ejecta from a hard-rock cratering detonation we found that a new medium or substratum in a physical sense is created in this type of detonation. In a hard-rock detonation, bedrock is ground up to form the matrix of the ejecta, which also contains many large rock fragments. The interactions between this new medium and the radionuclides injected into it or condensed on it constitute another new phase of ecological research on nuclear crater sites.

The Cabriolet crater was created early in 1968, and in August 1968 it was possible to sample a large cross section of the ejecta field when the Nuclear Cratering Group of the Lawrence Radiation Labora-

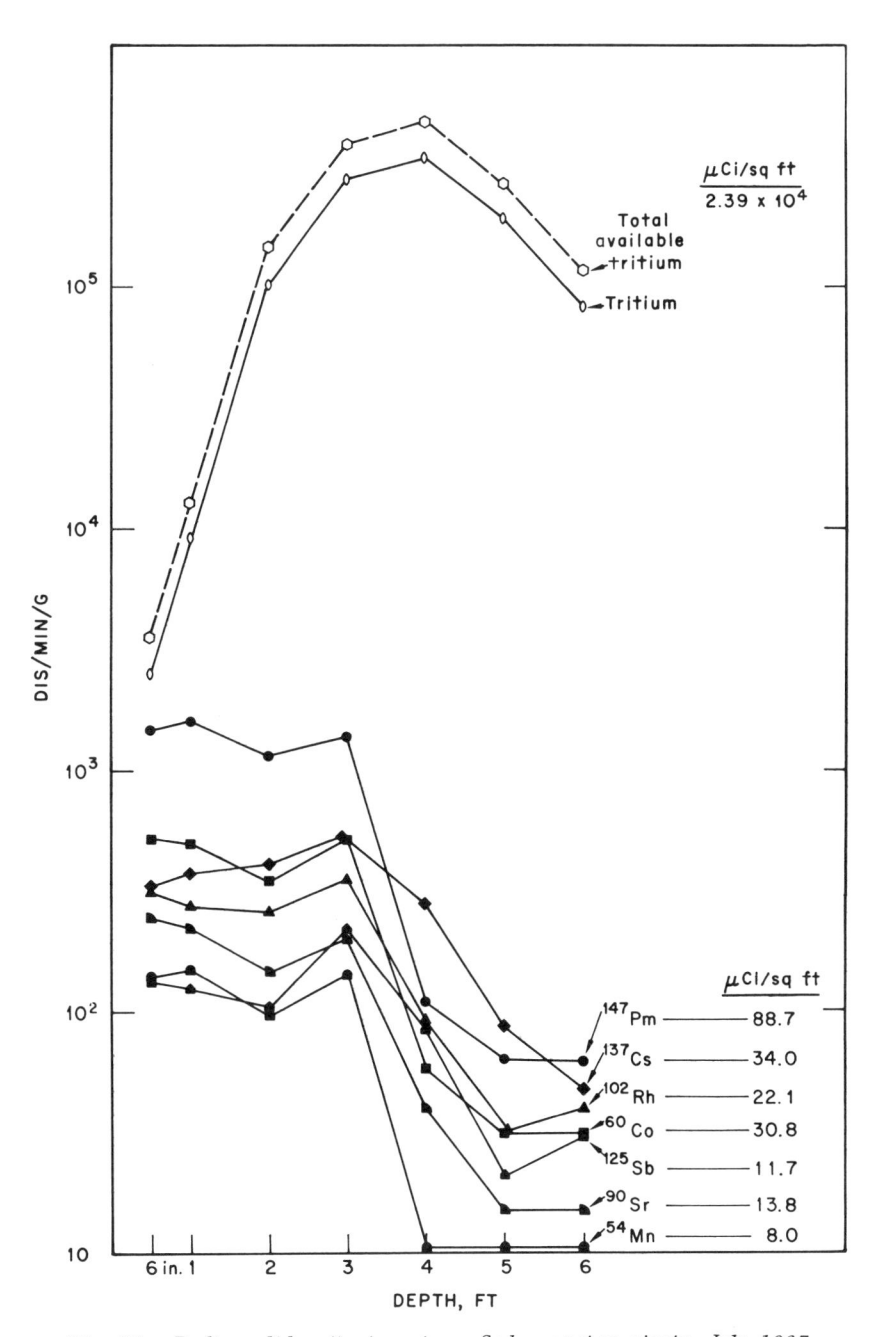

Fig. 22—Radionuclide site inventory, Sedan crater ejecta, July 1967.

tory excavated a trench in the ejecta up to the crater lip. The ejecta profile was revealed in a wide trench shown in Fig. 23. Samples of ejecta were obtained from the wall of this trench and analyzed for gamma-emitting radionuclides by solid-state detector gamma spectroscopy. The distribution of two radionuclides, ^{144}Ce and ^{95}Zr, is

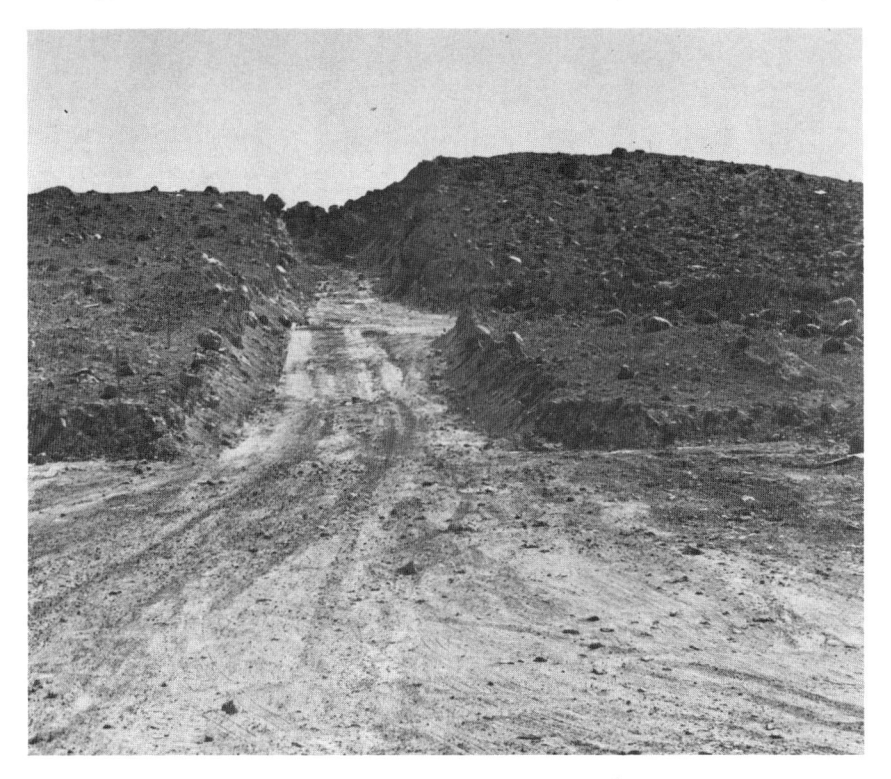

Fig. 23—Photo of Cabriolet trench.

shown in Fig. 24 for three stations along the trench, at 20, 55, and 85 ft from the crater lip.

We observed that these two fission products are not injected uniformly into the ejecta mass and that their concentration decreases by a factor of two for every 2 ft of depth. The distribution of other radionuclides generally follows that which is shown for ^{144}Ce and ^{95}Zr. Several feet of ejecta that overlies the parent materials does not have quantitatable concentrations of most radionuclides.

Our current explanation for the distribution of radionuclides found in nuclear crater ejecta is as follows. Apparently, radionuclides that condense at high temperatures have already done so before the mound of earth lifted by the detonation vents, and these radionuclides are then surface deposited on the bulk ejecta. The bulk ejecta is thrust upward

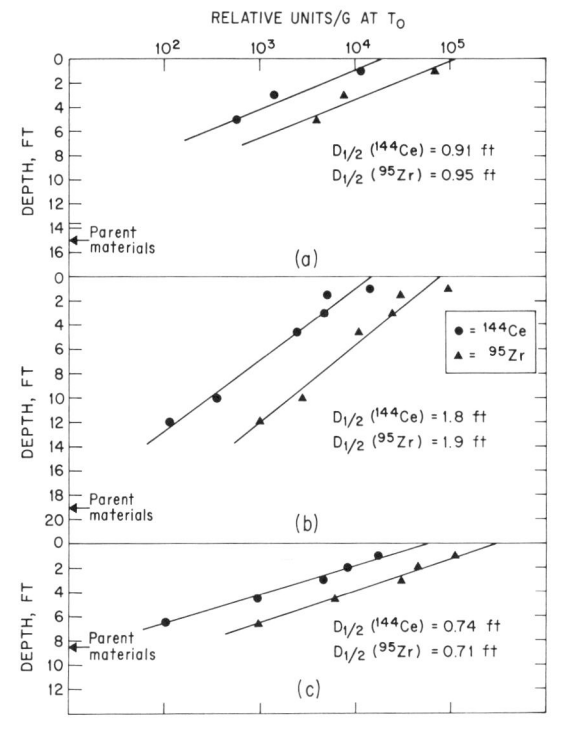

Fig. 24—*Radionuclide concentrations in Cabriolet ejecta at three distances from the crater: (a) 20 ft from crater lip; (b) 55 ft from crater lip; and (c) 85 ft from crater lip.*

and outward and inverted by the force of the explosion. The inside layer of the mound is deposited without much mixing on the surface of the close-in bulk ejecta. Volatile radionuclides permeate the overburden or mound more efficiently, and a deeper distribution of these radionuclides is to be expected. The hinging of the ejecta overburden was so regular at the Sedan crater lip that the stratigraphy of the alluvial strata was repeated above the hinge point, in reverse sequence to that below.

Certain radionuclides because of their physical–chemical behavior during cratering phenomena will therefore be distributed in a surficial manner whereas others of a volatile nature may be injected throughout the ejecta mass. The surficial distribution of many of the gamma-emitting radionuclides, especially fission products, will affect the postshot radiation field and possibly the time of reentry for conventional construction phases in an earth engineering project. This distribution of residual radioactivity around a nuclear crater also may be opportune in that radioactivity levels can be reduced significantly by removing the surface layer of ejecta.

REFERENCES

1. H. C. Rodean, University of California, Lawrence Radiation Laboratory, unpublished data, 1969.
2. Stafford L. Warren et al., The 1948 Radiological and Biological Survey of Areas in New Mexico Affected by the First Atomic Bomb Detonation, USAEC Report UCLA-32, University of California, Los Angeles, 1949.
3. W. C. Hanson, Fallout Radionuclides in Northern Alaskan Ecosystems, *Arch. Environ. Health*, 17: 639-648 (1968).
4. K. Liden and M. Gustafson, Relationships and Seasonal Variation of ^{137}Cs in Lichens, Reindeer, and Man In Northern Sweden, 1961-1965, in *Radioecological Concentration Processes*, International Symposium, Stockholm, Sweden, April 1966, Pergamon Press Ltd., Oxford, England, 1967.
5. P. Gustafson and James E. Miller, The Significance of ^{137}Cs in Man and His Diet, in Fallout Program, Quarterly Summary Report, September 1-December 1, 1967, USAEC Report HASL-184, 1968.
6. L. R. Donaldson, A. H. Seymour, and V. R. Donaldson, Radiological Analysis of Biological Samples Collected at Eniwetok, May 16, 1948, USAEC Report UWFL-18, University of Washington, 1949.
7. J. J. Koranda, Preliminary Studies of the Persistence of Tritium and ^{14}C in The Pacific Proving Grounds, *Health Phys.*, 11: 1445-1457 (1965).
8. F. W. Stead, Distribution in Groundwater of Radionuclides from Underground Nuclear Explosions, in Engineering with Nuclear Explosives, Proceedings of the Third Plowshare Symposium, USAEC Report TID-7695, University of California, Davis, April 1964.
9. W. E. Martin, Interception and Retention of Fallout by Desert Shrubs, *Health Phys.*, 11: 1341-1354 (1965).
10. M. D. Nordyke and M. M. Williamson, The Sedan Event, USAEC Report PNE-242F, Lawrence Radiation Laboratory and U. S. Army Corps of Engineers, 1965.
11. J. C. Beatley, Effects of Radioactive and Nonradioactive Dust upon *Larrea diraricata* Cav., Nevada Test Site, *Health Phys.*, 11: 1621-1625 (1965).
12. W. E. Martin, Early Food-Chain Kinetics of Radionuclides Following Close-In Fallout from a Single Nuclear Detonation, in Radioactive Fallout from Nuclear Weapons Tests, Germantown, Md., November 3-6, 1964, A. W. Klement, Jr., Ed., AEC Symposium Series, No. 5 (CONF-765), 1965.
13. S. M. Hansen, Preliminary Report of Results from Sedan Postshot Field Investigations Conducted During May and June 1964, USAEC Report UCID-4746, University of California, Lawrence Radiation Laboratory, 1964. (Classified)
14. J. B. Knox, Water Quality in Flooded Craters Produced by Nuclear Excavation, USAEC Report UCID-4741, University of California, Lawrence Radiation Laboratory, 1964.
15. J. B. Knox, H. A. Tewes, and T. V. Crawford, Production and Distribution of Tritium in Nuclear Cratering Events, USAEC Report UCRL-50297, University of California, Lawrence Radiation Laboratory, 1967. (Classified)
16. J. J. Koranda, Residual Tritium at Sedan Crater, in 2nd Radioecology Symposium on Radioecology, 1967, Ann Arbor, Mich., USAEC Report CONF-670503-6, 1967.
17. U. Zimmerman, K. O. Münnich, and W. Roether, Downward Movement of Soil Moisture Traced by Means of Hydrogen Isotopes, in *Isotope Techniques in the Hydrologic Cycle*, Geographical Monograph Series No. 11, American Geographical Union, National Academy of Science, National Research Council, Washington, 1967.
18. A. G. Evans, New Dose Estimates from Chronic Tritium Exposures, *Health Phys.*, 16: 57-63 (1969).

19. F. T. Hatch, J. A. Mazrimas, G. G. Greenway, J. J. Koranda, and J. L. Moore, Studies on Liver DNA in Tritiated Kangaroo Rats Living at Sedan Crater, USAEC Report UCRL-50461, University of California, Lawrence Radiation Laboratory, 1968.
20. E. M. Romney, A. J. Steen, R. A. Wood, and W. A. Rhoads, Concentration of Radionuclides by Plants Grown on Ejecta from the Sedan Thermonuclear Cratering Detonation, in *Radioecological Concentration Processes*, International Symposium, Stockholm, Sweden, April 1966, Pergamon Press Ltd., Oxford, England, 1967.
21. J. R. Kline, J. R. Martin, Carl Jordan, and J. J. Koranda, Measurement of Water Behavior in Tropical Trees Using Tritiated Water, in Radiation and Isotopes Technology in Latin American Development, American Nuclear Society Topical Meeting, San Juan, Puerto Rico, May 4–6, 1969.
22. J. J. Koranda, J. R. Martin, and R. W. Wikkerink, Leaching of Radionuclides at Sedan Crater, USAEC Report UCRL-70630, University of California, Lawrence Radiation Laboratory, 1968.

DISCUSSION

KNOX (LRL): We in Plowshare are very grateful to John Koranda for his work, and we have found it very helpful because he has described the distribution of radioactivity in the ejecta as a function of depth. With this information we can obviously improve our dose-rate calculations at the crater lip and in the crater. He also brought up the concept of migration of the pulse of radioactivity down through the ejecta and soil.

PARKER: You showed two curves in which the ordinates were in curies per degree-foot. Could you explain what that statement means?

KORANDA: These are values that came by integrating a depth profile, bringing it up to the surface value, and then also integrating for the area embraced by a 1° arc. The area progressively increases as you go out from the crater.

MASON: Our data picks up where Koranda's stops. The Public Health Service has a farm located $2\frac{1}{2}$ miles from the crater, and we have data to support what Koranda is saying. We have made one additional observation. We have a sprinkler irrigation system, and we think the tritium observed comes from the plants he has mentioned. There is a redeposition on the surface at the farm, and there is a significantly higher level in the irrigated area than outside. Our interpretation is that we are getting continuous deposition into this irrigated area. This results in a cycling of tritium where there is rainfall or an irrigation system. So there is a potential of maintaining tritium in this ecosystem longer than would be indicated by the theory of its going through the soil as a pulse.

KORANDA: This may take place in the tropics, especially. We have observed this in some Puerto Rican studies now in progress.

RADIONUCLIDES IN FOOD

JOHN H. HARLEY
Health and Safety Laboratory, U. S. Atomic Energy Commission,
New York, New York

ABSTRACT

The significance of measurements of low levels of radionuclides in foods for locating critical items in the diet for a particular nuclide and for studies on the mechanisms of entry of the radionuclides into the food chain is pointed out. Composite samples of food purchased in New York, Chicago, and San Francisco were analyzed for ^{137}Cs, ^{226}Ra, ^{90}Sr, and U. Tables are presented to show relative contributions of the various diet components to ^{137}Cs intake in Chicago, and ^{226}Ra, ^{90}Sr, and U in New York and San Francisco. A comparison of ^{137}Cs and ^{90}Sr intakes by the United States and the USSR showed that the Soviet intake of ^{90}Sr was twice and the ^{137}Cs intake, three times that in the United States.

The subject of radioactivity in foods is very broad; therefore I will limit myself largely to data obtained in our own laboratory. These data are much easier for me to find, and they are already in familiar form. This does not mean that there are not other institutions making diet studies throughout the United States; the California Health Department, for instance, maintains a very good program.

There are a number of reasons why we are interested in measuring the present low levels of radionuclides in foods. Certain groups make these measurements as a practice exercise with the intention of being prepared for a major nuclear disaster. Other groups find that the measurements produce data which have a certain scientific interest in their own right, even though the hazard from eating the particular foods is negligible. Regardless of the basic direction of the work, there is a need for setting up a program of sampling and analysis that has continuity.

The food measurements of the Health and Safety Laboratory started as a surveillance program but have been adaptable to the need for scientific information on the radionuclide content of the diet. This information is of interest to such groups as the U. N. Scientific Committee on the Effects of Atomic Radiation and the Federal Radiation Council when they are assessing the significance of dietary intake, when they are attempting to locate the critical items in the diet for a particular nuclide, or when the data are being used to study the mechanisms of entry of the radionuclides into the food chain.

The basic information required in our studies is the composition of the diet and the radionuclide content of the diet components. Our approach has been to set up a standard food-purchasing plan, based on Department of Agriculture statistics, and to buy foods in supermarkets in the large urban areas of New York, Chicago, and San Francisco. The total of 43 purchased food items are grouped into 19 categories, and these composite samples are analyzed. This system approximates the intake of the comparable urban population and thus gives us some predictive capability for estimating body burdens.

The program was, of course, originally designed for ^{90}Sr weapons test fallout. Analyses have also been made for ^{137}Cs, ^{226}Ra, and natural U. Work is in progress on the dietary intake of natural Th, ^{228}Ra, stable Pb, ^{210}Pb, and ^{210}Po.

Figure 1 shows the ^{90}Sr intake per day during our period of observation. The three cities have shown a consistent pattern in their

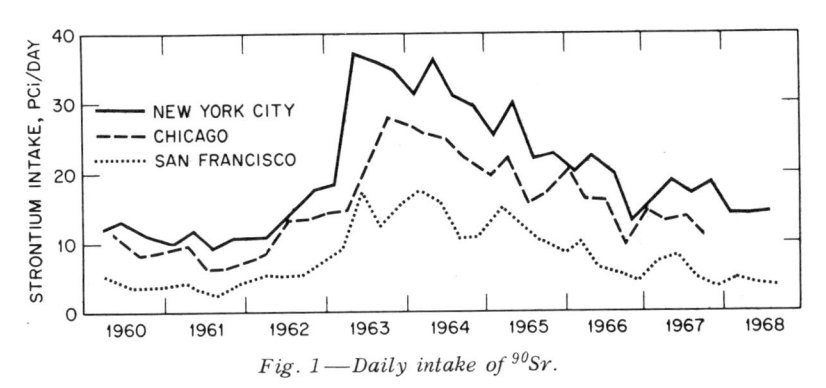

Fig. 1—Daily intake of ^{90}Sr.

relative values; hence we have finally dropped Chicago as a sampling site in the interest of economy.

The data for both New York and San Francisco show that the half-life for the disappearance of ^{90}Sr from the total diet is of the order of 3½ to 4 years. This rate of disappearance might be quite different for certain individual foods.

Typical data for a recent sampling are given in Table 1. In the table are shown the relative contributions of the various diet com-

Table 1
STRONTIUM-90 IN DIET*

Diet category	Intake, kg/year	Calcium, g/year	% of total intake	New York City (8/68) ^{90}Sr, pCi/kg	^{90}Sr, pCi/year	% of total intake	San Francisco (9/68) ^{90}Sr, pCi/kg	^{90}Sr, pCi/year	% of yearly intake
Dairy products	200	216.0	58	10.4	2080	38	1.7	340	23
Fresh vegetables	48	18.7		12.2	586		4.4	211	
Canned vegetables	22	4.4		9.3	205		1.9	42	
Root vegetables	10	3.8		4.9	49		4.5	45	
Potatoes	38	3.8		9.5	361		1.5	57	
Dried beans	3	2.1	9	3.6	11	22	5.4	16	26
Fresh fruit	59	9.4		18.2	1074		1.4	83	
Canned fruit	11	0.6		2.4	26		1.7	19	
Canned fruit juices	28	2.5	3	3.3	92	22	1.1	31	9
Bakery products	44	53.7		5.4	238		4.7	207	
Flour	34	6.5		6.9	235		3.4	116	
Whole grain products	11	10.3		8.5	94		6.3	69	
Macaroni	3	0.6		4.7	14		2.7	8	
Rice	3	1.1	20	2.3	7	11	9.7	29	29
Meat	79	12.6		10.0	79		0.7	55	
Poultry	20	6.0		2.4	48		1.1	22	
Eggs	15	8.7	8	3.4	51	3	1.5	23	7
Fresh fish	8	7.6		0.5	4		0.0	0	
Shellfish	1	1.6	2	1.4	1		0.3	0	0
Water	400	2–10		0.5	200	4	(0.2)†	80	6
Yearly intake (rounded)					5450			1450	

*Based on data given in E. P. Hardy, Jr., and J. Rivera (Eds.), Fallout Program, Quarterly Summary Report, September 1–December 1, 1968, USAEC Report HASL-204, January 1969.
†( ) = estimated.

ponents to ^{90}Sr intake. Some of these are obviously minor contributors for this nuclide, but analyses are still run for continuity, and the samples also are being used for other nuclides.

The same diet categories have been analyzed at Argonne National Laboratory for their ^{137}Cs content. Table 2 shows a recent sampling for ^{137}Cs and includes the potassium content of the various diet components. Note that the ^{137}Cs contribution of meat and fish is marked, whereas vegetables are less important than for ^{90}Sr.

At the Health and Safety Laboratory, we have also run our diet samples for ^{226}Ra and natural uranium. These do not require analyses over a period of years since the levels should be reasonably constant with the possible exception of seasonal changes. Table 3 indicates the dietary contributions to ^{226}Ra intake. Milk is not a major contributor of ^{226}Ra in comparison to fallout radionuclides. The uranium data in Table 4 are very similar, with even a wider distribution of contributors.

Table 2
CESIUM-137 IN CHICAGO DIET (ARGONNE DATA)*

		Potassium			^{137}Cs (10/68)	
Diet category	Intake, kg/year	G/kg	G/year	% of total intake	PCi/kg	PCi/year	% of total intake
Dairy products	200	1.4	280		18	3,600	
				21			29
Fresh vegetables	48	2.3	110		2	100	
Canned vegetables	22	1.3	29		9	200	
Root vegetables	10	2.9	29		7	70	
Potatoes	38	4.5	171		17	650	
Dried beans	3	13.9	42		5	10	
				29			8
Fresh fruit	59	1.9	112		4	240	
Canned fruit	11	1.2	13		18	200	
Canned fruit juices	28	1.9	53		26	730	
				13			10
Bakery products	44	1.2	53		21	920	
Flour	34	1.0	34		33	1,120	
Whole grain products	11	3.5	38		30	330	
Macaroni	3	1.8	5		19	60	
Rice	3	N.d.†			N.d.†		
				10			20
Meat	79	3.3	261		26	2,060	
Poultry	20	2.7	54		15	300	
Eggs	15	1.5	22		7	100	
				25			20
Fresh fish	8	3.4‡	27		194‡	1,550	
Shellfish	1	N.d.†			N.d.†		
				2			13
Water	400	N.d.†			(0.05)§	20	
Yearly intake (rounded)			1330			12,300	

*Based on data given in E. P. Hardy, Jr., and J. Rivera (Eds.), Fallout Program Quarterly Summary Report, September 1, 1968, USAEC Report HASL-204, January 1969, and P. F. Gustafson and J. E. Miller, Significance of Cs-137 in Man and His Diet, *Health Phys.*, 16:167-183 (February 1969).
†Not determined.
‡Based on 90% ocean, 10% freshwater fish.
§( ) estimated.

It is always interesting to see what is happening in other countries, and in recent years there has been a great deal of fallout information coming from the USSR. Naturally, they do not use the same groupings of diet components that we do, but it is of interest to compare the two dietary regimes by trying to regroup our values to fit their pattern. This has been done on a weight basis in Table 5. The agreement on total intake is remarkable, and the differences between countries for certain food groups can be quite instructive.

Tables 6 and 7 compare the U. S. and USSR intakes of ^{90}Sr and ^{137}Cs for 1966. The Soviet intake of ^{90}Sr is almost twice that in the United States, with over half coming from bread. This reflects their use of dark bread that includes ^{90}Sr from surface contamination of the wheat and rye.

The estimate of calcium intake from the USSR is about 0.6 to 0.8 g/day compared to our 1 g/day. This means that the dietary level in terms of strontium units (picocuries of ^{90}Sr per gram of calcium)

Table 3

RADIUM-226 IN DIET (1966)*

Diet category	Intake, kg/year	New York City ^{226}Ra, pCi/kg	^{226}Ra, pCi/year	% of total intake	San Francisco ^{226}Ra, pCi/kg	^{226}Ra, pCi/year	% of total intake
Dairy products	200	0.25	50		0.10	20	
				8			7
Fresh vegetables	48	0.50	24		0.48	23	
Canned vegetables	22	0.65	14		0.35	8	
Root vegetables	10	1.4	14		1.2	12	
Potatoes	38	2.8	108		0.14	5	
Dried beans	3	1.1	3		0.72	2	
				28			18
Fresh fruit	59	0.43	25		0.25	15	
Canned fruit	11	0.17	2		0.70	8	
Canned fruit juices	28	0.42	12		0.33	9	
				7			11
Bakery products	44	2.8	123		1.2	53	
Flour	34	1.9	66		1.4	48	
Whole grain products	11	2.2	24		2.1	23	
Macaroni	3	2.1	6		2.6	8	
Rice	3	0.76	2		0.24	1	
				38			47
Meat	79	0.01	1		0.01	1	
Poultry	20	0.76	15		0.43	9	
Eggs	15	6.1	92		2.0	30	
				18			14
Fresh fish	8	0.67	5		0.40	3	
Shellfish	1	0.80	1		1.9	2	
				1			2
Water	400	0.006	2		0.008	3	
				<1			1
Yearly intake (rounded)			590			280	

*Based on data given in N. A. Hallden, I. M. Fisenne, and J. H. Harley, Ra-226 in Human Diet and Bone, *Science,* 140: 74-75 (1963), and I. M. Fisenne, Health and Safety Laboratory, unpublished data.

Table 4

NATURAL URANIUM IN DIET*

	Intake, kg/year	New York City U, μg/kg	New York City U, μg/year	% of total intake	San Francisco U, μg/kg	San Francisco U, μg/year	% of total intake
Diet category							
Dairy products	200	0.07	14		0.3	60	
				3			13
Fresh vegetables	48	0.6	30		1.0	48	
Canned vegetables	22	0.2	4		0.2	4	
Root vegetables	10	0.7	7		0.7	7	
Potatoes	38	2.5	95		2.2	84	
Dried beans	3	1.5	4		3.8	11	
				30			35
Fresh fruit	59	1.2	71		0.6	35	
Canned fruit	11	0.2	2		0.2	2	
Canned fruit juices	28	0.1	3		0.2	6	
				16			10
Bakery products	44	1.8	80		1.6	71	
Flour	34	0.5	17		0.2	7	
Whole grain products	11	1.5	16		1.5	16	
Macaroni	3	0.4	1		0.6	2	
Rice	3	1.9	6		1.4	4	
				26			22
Meat	79	1.1	87		0.6	47	
Poultry	20	0.2	4		0.3	6	
Eggs	15	0.2	3		0.2	3	
				20			12
Fresh fish	8	0.4	3		0.6	5	
Shellfish	1	9.5	10		31	31	
				3			8
Water	400	0.03	12		N.d.†		
				2			
Yearly intake (rounded)			470			449	

*Based on data given in G. A. Welford and R. Baird, Uranium Levels in Human Diet and Biological Materials, *Health Phys.*, 13: 1321-1324 (1967).
†Not determined.

is about 19 for the United States and 54 for the Soviet Union. On the other hand, the levels of ^{90}Sr in bone tend to run slightly higher here than in the Soviet Union. This may have a number of causes, a favored one being a difference in the relative availability of ^{90}Sr from milk and cereals.

The cesium data show the USSR intake to be three times that in the United States. Again, bread is the big contributor, with meat second. As with ^{90}Sr, the body burdens are less than expected. At Argonne the reported body burden for 1966 averaged about 11,000 pCi with the diet shown, whereas the USSR data showed 8500 pCi with a much higher intake. This difference is being investigated.

The Russians have also maintained a strong interest in natural radioactivity and have recently presented data on their estimates of ^{210}Po intake (Table 8). Here the major contribution is from vegetables, with over 10% from water. Comparable data are not yet available from this country, but we will run some of our diet samples for ^{210}Po.

Table 5
COMPARISON OF U. S. AND SOVIET DIETS

U. S. category	Intake, kg/year	Total of group, kg/year	Soviet category	Intake, kg/year
Dairy products	200	200	Milk	110
Bakery products	44			
Flour	34			
Whole grain	11	89	Bread	220
Meat	79			
Poultry	20			
Eggs	15	114	Meat	60
Macaroni	3			
Rice	3	6	Cereals	20
Fresh fish	8			
Shellfish	1	9	Fish	4
Fresh vegetables	48			
Canned vegetables	22			
Root vegetables	10			
Potatoes	38			
Dried beans	3			
Fresh fruit	59			
Canned fruit	11			
Fruit juice	28	219	Potatoes and vegetables	220
Total		637		634
Water		400		440

Table 6
DIETARY ^{90}Sr IN THE UNITED STATES AND USSR, 1966

	U. S. diet (New York City)				USSR diet (country)*			
Diet category	Intake, kg/year	^{90}Sr, pCi/kg	^{90}Sr, pCi/year	% of total intake	Intake, kg/year	^{90}Sr, pCi/kg	^{90}Sr, pCi/year	% of total intake
Milk	200	13.4	2,970	42	110	14	1,540	12
Bread	89	17.4	1,580	22	220	33	7,250	55
Meat	114	2.8	320	4	60	10	600	5
Cereals	6	6.3	40	1	20	18	360	3
Fish	9	1.8	20		4	30	120	1
Potatoes and vegetables	219	8.3	1,800	25	220	12	2,640	20
Water	400	1.1	440	6	440	1.1	480	4
Yearly intake			7,170				12,990	

*Based on data given in E. V. Petukhova and V. A. Knizhnikov, Dietary Intake of Sr-90 and Cs-137, Publication A/AC.82/G/L.1245, United Nations Scientific Committee, Sales Section, New York, N. Y.

Table 7
DIETARY CESIUM-137 IN THE UNITED STATES AND USSR, 1966

Diet category	U. S. diet (Chicago, July)				USSR diet (country)*			
	Intake, kg/year	^{137}Cs, pCi/kg	^{137}Cs, pCi/year	% of total intake	Intake, kg/year	^{137}Cs, pCi/kg	^{137}Cs, pCi/year	% of total intake
Milk	200	22	4,400	25	110	56	6,160	12
Bread	89	46	4,100	23	220	111	24,420	46
Meat	114	44	5,000	28	60	188	11,280	22
Cereals	6	54	300	2	20	100	2,000	4
Fish	9	150	1,400	8	4	340	1,360	3
Potatoes and vegetables	219	12	2,600	14	220	32	7,040	13
Yearly intake			17,800				52,300	

*Based on data given in E. V. Petukhova and V. A. Knizhnikov, Dietary Intake of Sr-90 and Cs-137, Publication A/AC.82/G/L.1245, United Nations Scientific Committee, Sales Section, New York, N. Y.

Table 8
POLONIUM-210 IN USSR DIET*

Diet category	Intake, kg/year	^{210}Po, pCi/kg	^{210}Po, pCi/year	% of total intake
Milk	110	0.2	22	7
Bread	220	0.45	99	30
Meat	60	0.5	30	9
Cereals	20	0.1	2	1
Fish	4	0.4	2	
Potatoes and vegetables	220	0.6	132	40
Water	440	0.1	44	13
Yearly intake			331	

*Based on data given in A. P. Yermolayeva-Makovskaya, L. A. Pertsov, and D. K. Popov, Po-210 in the Human Body and the Environment, Publication A/AC.82/G/L.1260, 1969, United Nations Scientific Committee, Sales Section, New York, N. Y.

Table 9
ANNUAL INTAKE OF THE NUCLIDES AND ESTIMATED BODY BURDENS

Nuclide	Body burden	Annual intake	Burden corresponds to an intake for
^{90}Sr, New York	3,700 pCi*	5,450 pCi	8 months
^{137}Cs, Chicago	4,000 pCi†	12,300 pCi	4 months
^{226}Ra, New York	36 pCi	590 pCi	3 weeks
U, New York	54 μg‡	470 μg	6 weeks
^{210}Po, USSR	735 pCi	330 pCi	2 years

*This is the body content calculated from the diet using a discrimination factor of 0.25 going from diet to bone. It agrees with HASL measurements of childrens' bones (0–2 years) of 3.4 pCi/g Ca in 1968.
†This value is the same for corresponding intakes during the rise in dietary contamination (1962) and the fall in contamination (1968).
‡Skeleton only.

There is not a great deal of information available on the dietary intake of ^{210}Pb, the parent of ^{210}Po. Russian data on the same samples used for polonium show an intake of about 1500 pCi/year. The most striking comparison is with the intake estimate from Japan, which is 6200 pCi/year. The difference is accounted for by the Japanese estimate that about 70% of their polonium intake comes from seafood (see National Institute of Radiological Sciences, Annual Report on Radiological Sciences, 1967, Report NIRS-7, October 1968).

Considerable data on five different elements are shown in the tables, and it might be fruitful to attempt to compare these. Table 9 lists the annual intake of the nuclides and the estimated body burdens for the same time and location by the same investigators. About all that can be done with these two columns of figures is to show that the body burden corresponds to the intake over a certain period. These values are given in the final column.

These values in themselves do not have any marked scientific interest, and I have specifically stayed away from further inroads into the problem of radionuclides in man. However, the information on radionuclides in the diet is basic to the study of man, and this basic information can be most useful if it is part of an orderly, continuing plan of sampling and analysis.

DISCUSSION

HOLLAND: Would you comment on the dynamics required by the difference between milk and, for example, grains or cereals, with respect to radium and strontium. It seems to me it should come down to the secretion in milk. There may be some discrimination in the secretion of milk which is very markedly different for radium than it is for strontium.

HARLEY: This is true. I had intended to leave all this for Dr. Comar to comment on. For example, ^{90}Sr intake by the Russians is largely from cereals. The immediate thing that comes to mind is the relative availability, whether or not nuclides in cereals and grains may be much less available for any one of a number of reasons, such as combinations with phytates. Therefore, although their intake is higher, their uptake is about the same as ours.

HOLLAND: You were talking about retention in the body being different for radionuclides in the different food groups. But I am talking about differences between radium and strontium within single types of food, such as milk in one instance and cereal in another. It is the difference between radium and strontium rather than the difference between milk and cereal that I am interested in. Presumably you have the nuclides getting into the grain, grass, and so on, which the cow eats.

Then we have measurements of what goes into the milk. It turns out she puts a very much smaller fraction of radium into the milk than she does of strontium.

HARLEY: This goes back to what a number of us in UNSCEAR worked on for over a year. One concept was that as you went from one alkaline earth to another you kept having this factor of $1/4$ discrimination. The animal discrimination factor is roughly 4 with ^{90}Sr; with barium, 16 seems to fit better; and the factor is 64 with radium. As data improved, the numerical evidence for the concept disappeared. But the cow is discriminating against radium even more strongly than against strontium, the same as we do when we consume it again.

COMAR: I think one of the issues is the problem of surface contamination. The strontium data to date represent primarily surface contamination, and this is why the grains are so high. I would project that the Russian values will become much lower and grain less important when the wheat starts getting all its radionuclides via the soil pathways rather than from the surface. Differences such as these noted in the past have usually led to two types of explanation. One is that there is a physiological difference in the way people in other countries handle the radionuclides, i.e., have different discrimination factors. The other is that there are uncertainties in the analytical comparisons. And every time in the past that we have been able to resolve these differences, and we have in a number of instances, it has always turned out that physiologically there is a reasonable constancy but that the analytical comparisons have been faulty. In other words, one has to do the job properly. One must have actual diet samples and bones from people who have been on these diets. Usually what happens is that one gets diet samples from a given area and many fewer bone samples from specific locations. Then the relations are of limited validity. If I had to make a guess, I would suggest that is what happened in this case.

HARLEY: When I selected their figures, I used the Moscow area where they have the greatest amount of bone data. It is my impression that their system should be comparable with ours. In other words, they are getting bones from people they think lived in the same area where the diet data came from.

COMAR: Well, you remember that we had this sort of experience with the nursing mothers on which S. A. Lough worked with us. We thought we were on safe ground because we were taking food samples from the Boston area and then milk from nursing mothers at the Boston Lying-In Hospital, but the results made absolutely no sense at all until we took actual mothers and put them on various specific diets.

PARTICIPANT: Your data for calcium, cadmium, and uranium, all three, show that the mass of these elements per kilogram of vegetables eaten is very much smaller in canned vegetables than in fresh vegetables. Is there an explanation for that?

HARLEY: I should have thought initially that perhaps the canned vegetables were processed more or something like this. I think it holds up, but I do not see any good reason for it. It has been consistent in other parts of the study.

LOUGH: With regard to the Russian seafood intake, as I recall, you said the Russian intake is very high compared to ours and the body burden is relatively low, especially with regard to this intake. This cannot be explained along the lines that Dr. Comar was talking about with respect to collection of bones from the same area; so what can it hang on except analytical deviation?

HARLEY: There seems to be an agreement in other fields with regard to these analyses.

LOUGH: You have not actually exchanged samples, have you?

HARLEY: No, we have not. However, for example, the agreement with the measurements made on the Lapps, as opposed to the measurements made on the Eskimos by various U. S. groups, is very good. The data on Lapps are also compared with the Scandinavians, of course.

LOUGH: What is the half-residence time of cesium in humans in Scandinavia? Was it not low compared to Los Alamos figures?

HARLEY: According to the favorite Los Alamos figure, yes.

LOUGH: Have the Russians reported a half-residence time of cesium in their population?

HARLEY: I do not remember seeing this in the normal population; again, they did it for the Lapps and got comparable values.

COMAR: Would it make any difference if you put it on a Cs/K ratio basis?

HARLEY: This is the basis it was on, and I used the standard value of body potassium for both types. Maybe this could be in error, but it is unlikely it could be a factor of 3.

PARKER: May I first compliment you on an excellent summary and ask for a detail that you clearly did not have time to include. The activity of dried or canned food relates to the source of origin, and the consumption at any point can depend on rather incidental changes in wholesaling practice. If you bought Dr. Dunster's seaweed you would have high ruthenium, but, if you bought it in the West Coast markets, it comes from Japan and presumably is going to be low in ruthenium, etc. Do you actually find traceable changes that are referable to specific contamination items?

HARLEY: We aimed our study at trying to approximate the actual intake because we were interested in the people and the bones we could obtain from them. We tried to approximate their intake and were not concerned about the specific sources of the foods. We kept trying to randomize this. When our men shop for samples, they buy six cans of tomatoes of different brands. They go to two supermarkets to get more variety. We also try to randomize the sources. We have not really done much looking for data on food sources that would do what you mentioned, unfortunately.

GRENDON: Let me return to the point Dr. Holland raised. You do not have to resort to other people's data. You can take Table 1 and Table 2, for example, and compare the dairy products and the meat. Now here you have an animal and milk. If you look at the effect of the strontium where you have a relation in the two cases as percent of total intake, you have 38% (in New York City) vs. 3% for strontium, but in the radium case you find 8% vs. 18%. This substantiates the point of Dr. Holland that evidently there is more discrimination against radium in the production of milk in the cattle.

HARLEY: I am not sure you can treat these figures in exactly that way. But it does not seem impossible, does it Cyril, that the discrimination might occur in the secretion step?

COMAR: It is very hard to make this comparison, though. One has to take into account that dairy animals are probably fed a little differently than beef animals (e.g., different calcium supplements); so it makes the interpretations very difficult.

HARLEY: This sounds like a question for the Cornell Farm, rather than one to extract from survey data.

NELSON: In a similar sense, Table 1 sheds light on Dr. Parker's question regarding the origin of canned fruit. If you check canned fruit vs. fresh fruit and San Francisco vs. New York, you will see very clearly that New York purchases most, not quite all, of this canned fruit from California.

DOBSON (LRL): In your study of the Russian data, did you see any trends geographically analogous to the difference between San Francisco and New York?

HARLEY: The Russians reported their data on the basis of the republics, of which there are about 20. They had a very narrow range of data comparatively. Their range was about a factor of 2, whereas in the United States we run maybe a factor of 3. It was not an unreasonable range for an annual average. The differences seemed to be greater between north and south than between east and west. I had a little difficulty with this because there were certain places, like Uzbekistan, that I could not locate accurately on my maps.

STATUS OF REMEDIAL MEASURES AGAINST ENVIRONMENTAL RADIOCONTAMINATION

C. L. COMAR AND J. C. THOMPSON, Jr.
Department of Physical Biology, Cornell University, Ithaca, New York

ABSTRACT

The general principles of remedial measures are reviewed, and the critical factors are examined (important radionuclides, foods, and population groups). Since ^{131}I is considered as the most critical radionuclide under normal operating or accidental situations, the primary remedial measures for this radionuclide have been developed extensively. Models are shown which estimate total intake commitment from ^{131}I measurements in milk on any given day after the start of contamination. Methods to reduce this commitment are then discussed (stop drinking milk, remove cattle from pasture) along with the relative effectiveness of such measures. Other remedial measures relating to ^{90}Sr and ^{137}Cs are reviewed, particularly the effects of dietary additives (phosphate gels, alginates, Prussian Blue) and modifications of human dietary patterns. The general philosophy is discussed in regard to the likelihood of conditions that would require implementation of remedial measures. It is pointed out that the situation most likely to require remedial measures, namely, ^{131}I contamination, can be coped with; the circumstances that cannot be handled technologically, significant long-term ^{90}Sr contamination, fortunately seem unlikely to occur.

It is only reasonable and prudent that man having created radiocontamination of the environment should give some thought to mitigating the consequences by remedial or countermeasures. The data and concepts to date for the most part have been based on the effects of testing nuclear weapons and the potential of nuclear warfare, whereas it is hoped that any practical future concern will stem from the peacetime applications of nuclear energy. Many of the concepts already developed for fallout contamination are applicable to problems of developing technology. Since the overall developments in regard to remedial measures have been reviewed adequately in the literature,[1-3] this discussion is restricted to certain aspects of feasible large-scale measures.

GENERAL PRINCIPLES

Requirements

As clearly set forth in a report of the National Advisory Committee on Radiation to the Surgeon General,[2] a remedial measure to be useful from a public-health standpoint must fulfill certain requirements.

Effectiveness: It must substantially reduce population exposures below those which would prevail if the remedial measure were not used. This requirement has several implications. Reduction of contamination of the food supply will only be effective to the extent that food is the primary source of the radiation exposure. Reduction factors of about 2 in a single step of the food chain are not particularly useful; factors of about 10 or more may be required. However, consideration should be given to the fact that a series of small reduction factors in sequential steps of the food chain would be multiplicative and could produce a significant end effect.

Safety: The health risks associated with its use must be considerably less than those of the contamination at the action level. At low levels of contamination, the radiation risks are so small that they are most difficult to evaluate; this means that at such levels almost any remedial action would have greater risks. Thus the action levels for remedial action are usually much higher than those recommended for normal operating conditions in peacetime, which are controllable.

Practicality: The logistics of application should be worked out in advance; the cost must be reasonable in terms of degree of benefit to be obtained; and legal problems should be resolved.

Implementation: The responsibility and authority for its application must be well identified. Experience has shown that individual action has usually done more harm than good. Under our system state authorities have jurisdiction, with advice and help from the Public Health Service.

Other Considerations: Again, in terms of degree of benefit, the impact of the action on the public, industry, agriculture, and the government must be taken into account.

Importance of Distribution Pattern

The type of remedial action that might need to be undertaken depends largely on the size of the area that is involved, the crops affected, and the fraction of the population for which protection is deemed desirable. The terms "local" and "widespread" are used to denote the two limiting conditions of environmental deposition. Local deposition may occur from tropospheric fallout perhaps deposited under unusual meteorological conditions or from release to the atmosphere at ground level or to waters as from an industrial operation. Widespread deposition may result from the relatively uniform deposition of radioactive materials originally injected into the troposphere or stratosphere, a situation generally identified with nuclear explosions in the atmosphere.

Local situations could often be dealt with by introduction of uncontaminated food from clean areas or by restriction of consumption of local food products and water. Widespread situations, especially if continued in time, would require more difficult measures.

REMEDIAL MEASURES

General

In general terms the proposals for remedial measures have included: (1) bodily removal of contamination from the ground surface, (2) reduction of entry of radioactive materials into plants and animals, (3) decontamination of foodstuffs, and (4) dietary modifications or administration to man of substances that lessen the accumulation of individual nuclides in his tissue.

To deal specifically with the problem of environmental contamination, one must limit consideration to so-called "critical" factors: the nuclides responsible for the major radiation dose to be received by the population, the foods of major importance, and the population group that is most sensitive. Following the evaluation of many considerations, it appears that ^{131}I is the critical nuclide resulting from normal operation or accidental events in nuclear installations and during early periods after nuclear detonations. That is, unless ^{131}I reaches levels that require immediate remedial measures, it usually will not be necessary to consider other radionuclides. This may appear to be an oversimplification but can be explained in terms of the fission yield, the efficiency of transfer to the population, and the production of radiation dose. For example, in mixed fission products[4] at 24 hr after fission, the amount of ^{131}I present is about 4 times that of ^{89}Sr, about 600 times that of ^{90}Sr, and about 800 times that of ^{137}Cs. When the efficiency of transfer through the food chain and the production of radiation dose to the critical organ are taken into account, it appears that per unit of deposit the total exposure dose from ^{131}I will be about 2000 times that from ^{89}Sr, about 20,000 times that from ^{137}Cs, and about 2000 times the annual dose from ^{90}Sr. Under conditions where volatility is important, the relative exposure from ^{131}I would be further enhanced.

Other nuclides could become more important under unique or special conditions (radioactive effluents being discharged into fresh or seawater), but these situations are usually more localized and easier to control. An interesting example discussed by Dunster in this symposium is the existence of a critical exposure group in which the members consume a bread made from seaweed that contains ^{106}Ru discharged into the sea from the Windscale plant.[5] The radiation exposure of this group will govern the discharge permitted from the plant. Presumably, if on balance, it would be in the national interest to increase the discharge level, then the appropriate remedial measure would be to obtain raw materials from uncontaminated areas or eliminate the manufacture and consumption of the product. Since this condition affects a limited area and population, such steps could be taken when required. Thus the major research efforts have been concentrated on the broader problems concerned with ^{131}I and ^{90}Sr, remedial measures where more extensive planning is needed.

Remedial Measures Against ^{131}I

Important Factors. There are three main factors that govern the actions that can be taken against ^{131}I contamination. (1) Short half-life (8 days). (2) The fact that milk is normally the main source (although surface contamination from fresh fruits and vegetables can be important). (3) The fact that infants are the population group at greatest risk.

Primary Remedial Measures. A most important development in recent years has been an approach based on modeling of experimental data from dairy cows primarily undertaken by Lengemann and colleagues.[6-11] It is now possible to estimate the total intake commitment from measurement of ^{131}I in the milk on any given and known day after the start of contamination. This gives an approach to resolution of important aspects in regard to remedial measures, namely, the matter of surveillance, the determination of conditions under which action is to be initiated, and the time relations. The principles are briefly as follows: Figure 1 shows an experimentally determined curve and actual points that indicate the percent of ^{131}I per liter of milk as a function of time after contamination. Figure 2 shows the calculation of so-called "F factors" that represent the ratio of the total area under the curve to the level on any given day. The important factor is that, although the absolute heights of the curves may vary, the shapes of the curves are such as to give constant F values. Thus from the ^{131}I level in milk, one can calculate the total ^{131}I intake commitment.

There are two obvious and important countermeasures that can be invoked to reduce the intake of ^{131}I by the population: (1) stop drinking contaminated milk and (2) move cattle from pasture to uncontaminated feed.

As shown in Fig. 3, if man stops consuming contaminated milk on a given day, then the reduction of his intake commitment can be calcu-

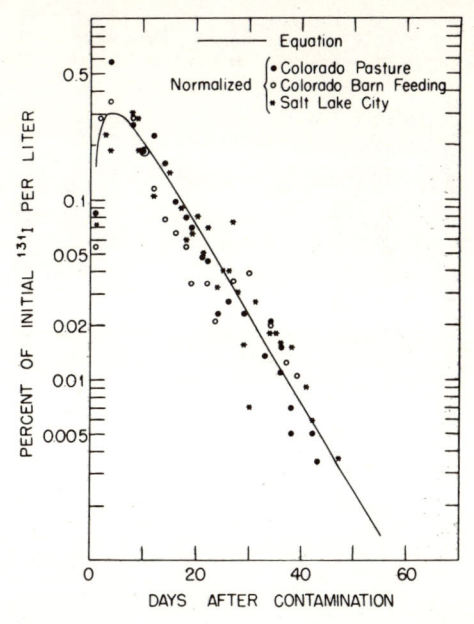

Fig. 1—Experimentally derived curve showing relation between ^{131}I levels in milk (percent per liter) and time after contamination.

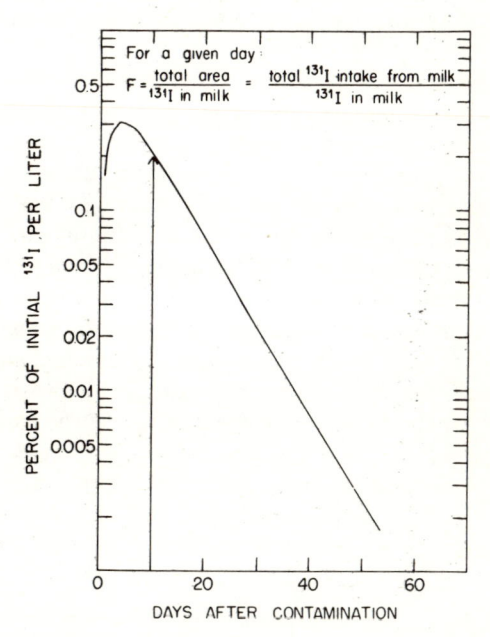

Fig. 2—Illustration of F value calculations used to determine ^{131}I intake commitments.

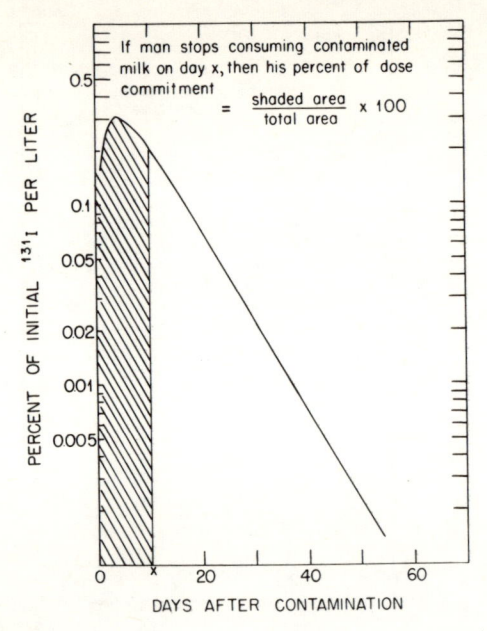

Fig. 3—Calculation of ^{131}I intake commitment when consumption of contaminated milk is stopped.

lated by the ratio of the appropriate areas under the curve. The same procedure can be used if animals are removed from contaminated pasture, as shown in Fig. 4. The net results are presented in Fig. 5, which allows us to make some important generalizations about the one factor that is important in governing the extent of reduced intake that can be attained—time. At early times (2 days), stopping milk consumption is about twice as effective as shifting cows; thereafter the difference becomes progressively smaller. In any event, action must be taken within about 4 days if the effectiveness[7,11,12] is to be of the order of 90%. These procedures may involve various logistic problems of fresh-milk replacement by stored or processed milk and feed replacement by stored rations which cannot usefully be discussed here. However, some interesting studies on the storage of fresh milk have recently been done by the U. S. Department of Agriculture as an outgrowth of the iodine problem.[13] It was found that, with modifications of the pasteurization procedure, summer milk could be stored under refrigeration for as long as 20 weeks and winter milk for as long as 6 weeks. Such storage could be an effective remedial measure for ^{131}I. In addition, these findings may have some implications in regard to general milk distribution.

Other methods of reducing ^{131}I effects on large populations, such as administration of high levels of stable iodine or other chemicals to

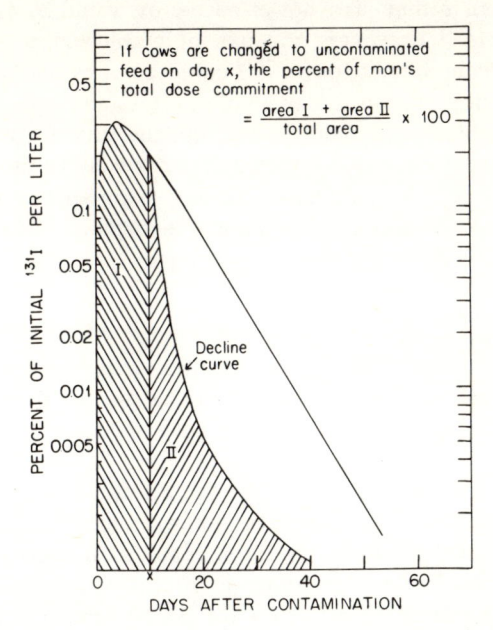

Fig. 4 — Calculation of ^{131}I intake commitment when cows are removed from contaminated feed.

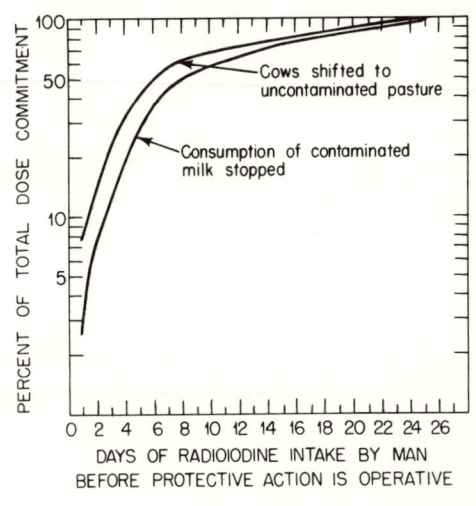

Fig. 5 — Comparison of ^{131}I intake commitments when consumption of contaminated milk is stopped and when cows are shifted to uncontaminated pasture.

cattle or to man either are not effective or would be difficult to apply on a large scale.[14] However, the use of stable iodine to block thyroid accumulation from inhalation of ^{131}I could be very useful under certain conditions, particularly in the event of reactor accidents.[15,16] The blocking dose to the human is about 30 mg, but the time for complete blocking is decreased to about $\frac{1}{2}$ hr if a 100 mg dose is used; after such a single dose, the uptake returns to normal after about 8 days. Repeated doses can be used to maintain blocking — schedules have been proposed of 35 mg/12 hr to 250 mg/48 hr.

Remedial Measures Against ^{90}Sr

Important Factors: The main factors that have to be taken into account in regard to ^{90}Sr are: (1) Long half-life (28 years). (2) Relations to calcium. (3) Contamination of both plant and animal sources of food.

The early measures required for ^{131}I as regards milk supply would also tend to reduce ^{89}Sr exposure since at early times surface contamination and milk would be the main vectors. In contrast to ^{131}I, there would be time available after an event during which plans could be implemented for minimizing exposure to ^{90}Sr occurring via contamination of all foods. A number of remedial measures have been proposed and are in various stages of research.[2]

Decontamination of Soil: The removal of massively contaminated vegetation might be effective, but the benefit would be small unless action were taken early since with time the radionuclides would tend to be transferred to soil.

The removal of contaminated topsoil would be the only practical measure that would be effective in reducing contamination levels[17,18] by more than 90%. The depth of topsoil that must be removed depends upon surface roughness: on smooth land, 1 in.; on bedded land, more than 6 in. (which would be impractical). Disposal of contaminated soil is a difficult problem. Thus there are strong physical and economic limitations. In any event it appears that topsoil removal would be used only for isolated small areas or for restricted areas of land that are most valuable for production of leafy vegetable crops. It should be recognized that this procedure offers no protection against subsequent contamination.

With shallow-rooted crops, deep plowing (30 cm) might be moderately effective; however, the experience has been that rooting tends to follow deep plowing, and here it has been necessary to use chemicals to inhibit rooting. In areas where the calcium content of the soil is low, the addition of lime might be moderately effective.

Modification of Farming System: A long-term overall reduction in ^{90}Sr contamination of food could theoretically be achieved by altering the farming system so that foods produced in the most highly contaminated areas were the less important sources of ^{90}Sr in the diet. An example would be the replacement of dairy cows by beef cattle on contaminated areas.

Principles of Dietary Modifications: It should first be remembered that, in regard to ^{90}Sr, we are primarily interested in remedial measures of a chronic nature, assuming that the input is to remain contaminated over long periods of time. We have pointed out that for manipulation of diets to produce a minimum body burden of radioactive strontium one should aim for a minimum value[19] of (OR$_{body/diet}$)/(% Ca in diet), where OR$_{body/diet}$ = (Sr/Ca of body)/(Sr/Ca of diet).

In experimental studies with rats, we have been able to reduce the strontium burden by a factor of almost 10 by adjustment of diets containing high levels of calcium, phosphorus, and magnesium.[20] Similar results have not been tested rigorously with human beings. It is possible to reduce the Sr/Ca ratio of milk by a factor of 2 to 4 by a similarly increased calcium feeding of dairy cows.[21] Such dietary interventions are far from feasible for two main reasons: (1) unknown possible side effects over long times and (2) difficulty of implementation. Also, supplemental calcium should originate from an uncontaminated source, i.e., inorganic as opposed to animal bones. A study of commercial calcium tablets showed many of them to have been derived from bone meal carrying a higher ^{90}Sr/Ca ratio than the contemporary diet.[22]

Decontamination of Milk: Extensive studies have been done cooperatively by the U. S. Department of Agriculture, the U. S. Atomic Energy Commission, and the U. S. Public Health Service which have culminated in demonstrating the feasibility of removing radiostrontium from milk by an ion-exchange process. It was possible to remove more than 90% of strontium from fluid whole milk in a plant processing 100,00 gal per 8-hr day without deterioration of quality.[23-25] It is also possible to remove ^{131}I by a modification, but this has little practical benefit when contrasted with alternatives that are available. Costs of decontaminating milk have been estimated at about 2 cents per quart. There are still some questions about the toxic effects of this milk when fed to newborn pigs which remain to be solved.[26]

Dietary Modifications: Of interest is the extent of reductions possible by modifications of dietary habits. Two situations are compared: (1) early after the contamination event when surface deposition is prominent and (2) at later times when the soil–plant–animal products pathway is more important. From our knowledge of discrimination processes, we have been able to predict the relative degrees of contamination among various types of foods. But we now have some data to support these ideas, and the following discussion is based primarily on survey data with calculated modifications based on experimentation.

Table 1 shows a typical pattern of contribution of calcium and ^{90}Sr to the diet during a period shortly after a contaminating event.[27] Dairy products and fruits and vegetables are the major contributors in terms of absolute amounts; the individual ratios of ^{90}Sr/Ca are compared later. Table 2 shows the effect of removing 90% of the ^{90}Sr from milk; there is less than 50% reduction in the ^{90}Sr/Ca of the total diet. However, for infants or others on a diet normally consisting almost entirely of milk,

Table 1

TYPICAL CALCIUM AND ^{90}Sr CONTRIBUTION TO TOTAL DIET, NEW YORK CITY, 1961 TO 1963

Product	Ca, g/year	^{90}Sr, pCi/year	^{90}Sr/Ca
Dairy	238	3784	
Grain	59	1050	
Meat, fish, and eggs	45	153	
Fruits and vegetables	64	2560	
Total	406	7547	18.6

Table 2

EFFECT OF MILK DECONTAMINATION ON CALCIUM AND ^{90}Sr DIETARY INTAKE, NEW YORK CITY, 1961 TO 1963

Product	Ca, g/year	^{90}Sr, pCi/year	^{90}Sr/Ca
Dairy	238	378	
Grain	59	1050	
Meat, fish, and eggs	45	153	
Fruits and vegetables	64	2560	
Total	406	4141	10.2

the net effect would be greater. The same general effect could be produced by elimination of milk from the diet and substitution of inorganic uncontaminated calcium. Table 3 shows what happens if milk is eliminated from the diet: two detrimental effects occur—a lowered calcium intake and a higher ^{90}Sr/Ca ratio. If fruits and vegetables[28] are rigorously processed and selected for a low ^{90}Sr/Ca ratio, only a small benefit (about 20%) can be attained (Table 4). Table 5 summarizes the possible effects of various treatments on the ^{90}Sr/Ca of the total diet. With the most heroic of efforts, only a factor of 3 appears to be attainable. The situation for 1967, which can be taken to represent a situation where the fallout rate was low, is also shown in terms of possible reductions.[29] The main points are that milk decontamination and manipu-

Table 3

EFFECT OF ELIMINATING MILK FROM DIET,
NEW YORK CITY, 1961 TO 1963

Product	Ca, g/year	^{90}Sr, pCi/year	^{90}Sr/Ca
Grain	59	1050	
Meat, fish, and eggs	45	153	
Fruits and vegetables	64	2560	
Total	168	3763	22.4

Table 4

PROCESSING AND SELECTING VEGETABLES FOR LOW ^{90}Sr CONTENT: EFFECT ON DIETARY INTAKE,
NEW YORK CITY, 1961 TO 1963

Product	Ca, g/year	^{90}Sr, pCi/year	^{90}Sr/Ca
Dairy	238	3784	
Grain	59	1050	
Meat, fish, and eggs	45	153	
Fruits and vegetables	39	966	
Total	381	5953	15.6

Table 5

COMPARISON OF RESULTS OF VARIOUS TECHNIQUES FOR REDUCING ^{90}Sr IN TOTAL DIET, NEW YORK CITY,
1961 TO 1963 AND 1967

	1961 to 1963	1967
(1) Normal	18.6	15.6
(2) Milk 90% decontaminated	10.2	10.4
(3) Milk eliminated	22.4	24.1
(4) Fruits and vegetables selected	15.6	15.6
(5) Combination of (2) and (4)	6.0	10.4

lation of fruits and vegetables would be comparatively less effective than when carried out under conditions of high fallout rate.

Food Allocation: An action that might be considered is the allocation of low ^{90}Sr foods to critical members of the population. These members include infants, young children, and pregnant and lactating women. There is usually about a 6-months supply of stored foods available, which would give time to organize other procedures.

Recent Work on Additives: Within recent years there have been two substances that have been shown to reduce the absorption from the gut of strontium much more than that of calcium—aluminum phosphate gel and alginates.

The effect of phosphate gels was first noted by Spencer, Lewin, and Samachson.[30] These gels are familiar to all of us—especially the older ones with worries—under trade names such as Gelusil, Digel, and Phosphaljel. However, not all commercial preparations are equally effective. Spencer,[30] using Phosphaljel produced by Wyeth Laboratories Division, American Home Products Corporation, reported average reductions in strontium uptake in man of about 87% as compared to reductions in calcium uptake of about 37%. Studies with dairy cows have shown little effectiveness in reduction in strontium levels in milk with amounts having to be fed that are impractical.[44]

There has been considerable interest in the use of alginates. The selective inhibition of strontium absorption following the administration of sodium alginate to rats was first reported by Skoryna, Paul, and Waldron-Edward, from Canada when they observed a 50 to 80% reduction of radiostrontium absorption with no significant reduction in calcium absorption.[31] Similar inhibition of radiostrontium absorption by sodium alginate has since been observed by others in rats and humans.[32-34]

Commercially available alginates are salts of naturally occurring compound polymers of mannuronic and guluronic acids (alginic acid) that are extracted from brown seaweed (Phaeophyceae). Sodium alginate is water soluble, and from a practical standpoint, it is already widely used in the food industries, including incorporation into such products as ice cream, jellies, jam, and puddings, as an emulsifying and stabilizing agent.

Alginates with a high guluronic acid content, such as those derived from certain *Laminaria* species, appear to be most effective. When these products are fed to rats at the rate of 10% of their diet, typical reductions in strontium absorption range from about 75 to 80%, whereas changes in radiocalcium absorption have varied between −29% and +33%.[32-34] Hesp and Ramsbottom in 1965 and Sutton in 1967 have reported a reduction in radiostrontium uptake of 64 to 89% when 10 g of sodium alginate derived from *Laminaria* species was fed to adult humans who had fasted overnight.[35,36] When sodium alginate,[32] derived from *Macroystis pyrifera*, which has a lower guluronic acid content, was administered as a jelly to human adults, strontium retention was reduced by about 56%, whereas radiocalcium retention was reduced by only 18%.

Humphreys and Tanaka[37,38] have described alginate derivatives, some of which appear to be more effective than sodium alginate. A derivative containing 95% L-guluronic acid when fed to rats at a rate of 10% of their ration reduced radiostrontium absorption by 84% with no inhibition of calcium absorption. When it was consumed by humans, a reduction in the absorption of ^{87m}Sr by 83 to 87% was indicated.[33,36] Tanaka,[38] after studying several degradation products of alginates, concluded that their strontium binding capacities in vivo are only partly dependent upon the presence of a high guluronic acid content.

In a very recent study,[39] the absorption of ^{47}Ca and ^{85}Sr was studied in four human volunteers with and without sodium alginate, and the alginate decreased the retention of ^{85}Sr by 70% and the retention of ^{47}Ca by 7%. The stable elements Na, K, Mg, and P were also studied, and no change was observed in their excretion pattern or plasma level. There has been some indication that alginate will interfere with iron metabolism because of its strong binding potential for ferric ion, but this issue is still equivocal.

Our own studies have shown that sodium alginates have a selective inhibition of strontium absorption in the bovine.[44] As with rats and humans, the source of the alginate is important in determining its effectiveness. With sodium alginate derived from *Laminaria* species, we have observed a reduction in milk radiostrontium levels of about 70 to 80% when 5 to 7% of the ration was sodium alginate. A serious problem of palatability of sodium alginate exists with cows. Most cows reject this material when included in their rations at levels above 5 to 7%. Some cows will not eat their feed when 1% sodium alginate is included.

We are presently attempting to see what the maximum reduction might be by using a combination of various factors that have been shown to be effective individually (calcium, PO$_4$, magnesium, Phosphaljel, and alginates). The possible effects on other essential trace minerals is a problem that would have to be explored before any long-term, large-scale application could be implemented.

Remedial Measures Against ^{137}Cs

Important Factors: The main feature about ^{137}Cs is that it tends to become trapped in the soil; so surface contamination is essentially the only circumstance in which this radionuclide becomes at all significant. The general methods that tend to reduce ^{131}I and radiostrontium would also tend to reduce ^{137}Cs exposures via milk. However, at early times ^{137}Cs could be an appreciable contaminant of meat as contrasted to the other radionuclides.

Use of Prussian Blue: As a countermeasure against ^{137}Cs, the feeding of Prussian Blue (ferric ferrocyanide) has been of recent interest. Nigrović[40,41] observed that oral administration of Prussian Blue reduced absorption of ^{137}Cs by as much as 99% in rats. In addition, it was observed that the excretion of parenterally administered ^{137}Cs was accelerated when Prussian Blue was fed.

Madshus et al.[42] have reported that, when young dogs were fed 1.5 to 3 g of Prussian Blue daily for 10 days followed by 11 days of whole-body counting, the ^{137}Cs biological half-time was reduced to 59% of that measured in control dogs. Two of these investigators then ingested 1 μCi of ^{137}Cs, and 10 months later they started to consume 3 g of Prussian Blue per day.[43] The biological half-time dropped from 110 to 115 days to about 40 days.

Our own studies[44] have confirmed the observations of Nigrović in respect to the effects of Prussian Blue fed to rats. Furthermore, this material was shown to be effective in the ruminant. Radiocesium levels in milk of cows have been reduced to about 1% of control levels when Prussian Blue was fed simultaneously with the ingestion of the radiocesium. When Prussian Blue was administered some time after the ingestion of ^{137}Cs or ^{134}Cs, the decline in radiocesium levels in milk with time was accelerated by as much as a factor of about 5. This effect has been observed at times of even 100 days after the ingestion of cesium.

Except for slight constipation in the human study, no side effects have as yet been observed following the ingestion of Prussian Blue. The binding mechanism of Prussian Blue for cesium in the gastrointestinal tract appears to be selective enough so that potassium metabolism is not greatly affected.[42]

IMPLEMENTATION OF REMEDIAL MEASURES

It is clearly recognized that the radiation dose to the critical tissue is the basic criterion. Levels of activity are often specified as an operational convenience but must always be related to dose.

It is important, in order to avoid confusion, to consider separately the two types of situations: (1) planned or controllable operating conditions and (2) uncontrolled situations. In the first situation the operations should be planned and executed so that certain agreed dose limits are not exceeded. The uncontrolled situations can only be remedied by action against the environmental contamination rather than against the source. Since the dose limits recommended for "planned conditions" are quite conservative, remedial action in an "uncontrolled situation" would usually not be justified if these limits are moderately exceeded.

Naturally, Public Health officials would like to have absolute numerical values specified for action levels since it would make their life much easier: at lower levels they could rest entirely easy in mind; at higher levels they could go into vigorous action. But this may not be feasible. The aim must be, if needed, to take early action, and this may well have to be done on the basis of the expected dose rather than on observed levels. This means that the trend in levels must be taken into consideration. Another point is that the same type of action may have different consequences depending upon the time and location. For example, a shift of dairy animals to stored feed may have very little disadvantageous impact if the farmers in a given area and in a given season happen to have adequate supplies available; on the other hand, such a remedial measure might mean a complete cessation of milk production if stored feed was not available. Thus it is hardly possible to specify universally applicable action levels, and it is difficult to propose any action levels before the envisaged situation has occurred. Nevertheless, it is most helpful if the consequences of various types of remedial action are explored beforehand so that decisions can be made without delay when an abnormal situation arises.

The philosophy and recommendations[45,46] for "Protective Action Guides" have been detailed by the Federal Radiation Council for ^{131}I, ^{89}Sr, ^{90}Sr, and ^{137}Cs. In general, action levels for accidental releases have been based on dosages of 2 to 10 rads for such exposure as may occur within the first 100 days or within a year. No specific levels are given for longer term effects except to indicate the need for evaluation if annual doses to the bone marrow may exceed 0.2 rad. These values are in general agreement with those stipulated by other countries. Numerical values for illustrative purposes are given in terms of radioactivity deposited and peak concentrations in milk that cause a dose of 1 rad. The Federal Radiation Council has also stressed the lack of value of remedial measures against worldwide fallout contamination.

GENERAL DISCUSSION

What then is the general impression about remedial measures? First, it appears that we are most fortunate since the situation most likely to require remedial measures, namely, ^{131}I contamination, can be coped with on a public-health basis without much difficulty. The circumstance that we cannot handle technologically on a large scale, namely, significant long-term ^{90}Sr contamination, seems unlikely to occur from any peacetime activity that can be envisioned. Only after a nuclear holocaust would ^{90}Sr contamination be critical, and this would occur during the recovery phase or after the catastrophic consequences of the external radiation had been experienced. At this time there might indeed be an essentially uncontrollable burden on the population.

Even though the development of feasible public-health methods for radionuclides other than ^{131}I appears unattainable, it is important that fundamental research continue. There may well be circumstances in which it is important that effective local action be taken: a good example of this was the decontamination following the H bomb affair in

Spain.[47] There are other examples of so-called "spin-off." Our studies over the years of strontium–calcium metabolism have led to the discovery and isolation by Wasserman of the calcium-binding protein that may be the carrier involved in the transport of calcium across membranes.[48,49] The study of milk storage, already mentioned in connection with remedial measures for ^{131}I, may contribute to our general distribution procedures.

Because a need for remedial measures is highly unlikely, it may be of interest to consider the public-relations implications of actual contamination that may occur. With the increased use of reactors for power, the possibilities of earth-moving operations, and other applications, there is bound to be some increase in environmental contamination. Is there a possibility that implementation of remedial measures would overcome public resistance to such endeavors? For example, consider that milk can be freed of ^{90}Sr at a cost of 2 cents per quart or less. Some have argued that at present levels of ^{90}Sr the widespread decontamination of milk would cost several millions of dollars for each case of leukemia prevented—money that could otherwise be used much more effectively for health improvement. Others have argued that people would be glad to pay 2 cents per quart for peace of mind and that very likely as a result the consumption of milk might indeed increase. However, it would be a good idea to be prepared. In a country that spends several times more on advertising of drugs than in operating its medical schools—who knows whether we can have logically ordered priorities.

In any event the American public is extremely sensitive in regard to any level and kind of environmental contamination. There is an urgent need to respond to the public demand by careful consideration and responsiveness to questions raised; there is a need to educate ourselves first, then our colleagues in other areas, and finally the administrators and the public.

REFERENCES

1. Frank A. Todd, Protecting Foods and Water Against Radioactive Contamination, in *Protection of the Public in the Event of Radiation Accidents*, Seminar Proceedings, Geneva, Switzerland, November 18–22, 1963, WHO Monograph Series, World Health Organization, Geneva, 1965.
2. The National Advisory Committee on Radiation, Radioactive Contamination of the Environment: Public Health Action, Report to the Surgeon General, U. S. Public Health Service, May 1962.
3. Merrill S. Read, Countermeasures Against Radionuclides in Foods, *Fed. Proc.*, 22(6): 1418-1422 (Nov.–Dec. 1963).
4. R. Scott Russell, Dietary Contamination: Its Significance in an Emergency, in Radiological Protection of the Public in a Mass Nuclear Disaster, Symposium Proceedings, Interlaken, Switzerland, May 26–June 1, 1968, pp. 279-306, H. Brunner and S. Pretre, Eds., Fachverband für Strahlenschutz, Würenlingen, Switzerland, 1968.

5. A. Preston and D. F. Jefferies, The ICRP Critical Group Concept in Relation to the Windscale Sea Discharge, *Health Phys.*, 16: 33-46 (1969).
6. F. W. Lengemann, Predicting the Total Projected Intake of Radioiodine from Milk by Man. I. The Situation Where No Countermeasures Are Taken, *Health Phys.*, 12: 825-830 (1966).
7. F. W. Lengemann, Predicting the Total Projected Intake of Radioiodine from Milk by Man. II. The Situation Where Countermeasures Are Employed, *Health Phys.*, 12: 831-835 (1966).
8. F. W. Lengemann and R. A. Wentworth, Predicting the Total Intake of Radioiodine of Humans Consuming Goats Milk, *Health Phys.*, 12: 1655-1659 (1966).
9. F. W. Lengemann, Predicting the Total Projected Intake of Radioiodine from Milk by Man: Modification of the Original Equation, *Health Phys.*, 13: 521-522 (1967).
10. F. W. Lengemann, R. A. Wentworth, and F. L. Hiltz, Predicting the Cesium-137 Intake from Milk of a Human Population After a Single Short-Term Deposition of the Radionuclide, *Health Phys.*, 14: 101-109 (1968).
11. C. L. Comar and F. W. Lengemann, General Principles of the Distribution and Movement of Artificial Fallout Through the Biosphere to Man, in *Radioecological Concentration Processes*, B. Averg and F. P. Hungate, Eds., Pergamon Press, Inc., New York, 1967.
12. C. L. Comar, R. A. Wentworth, and F. W. Lengemann, A Study of Metabolism of Selected Radionuclides Fed in Various Physical Forms to Dairy Cows, Report TRC-67-33, U. S. Naval Radiological Defense Laboratory, March 1967.
13. S. Hoover, U. S. Department of Agriculture, personal communication.
14. F. W. Lengemann and J. C. Thompson, Jr., Prophylactic and Therapeutic Measures for Radioiodine Contamination—A Review, *Health Phys.*, 9: 1391-1397 (1963).
15. C. A. Adams and J. A. Bonnell, Administration of Stable Iodine as a Means of Reducing Thyroid Irradiation Resulting from Inhalation of Radioactive Iodine, *Health Phys.*, 7: 127-149 (1962).
16. D. Ramsden, F. H. Passant, C. O. Peabody, and R. G. Speight, Radioiodine Uptakes in the Thyroid Studies of the Blocking and Subsequent Recovery of the Gland Following the Administration of Stable Iodine, *Health Phys.*, 13: 633-646 (1967).
17. R. F. Reitemeier, P. E. James, and R. G. Menzel, Reclamation of Agricultural Land Following Accidental Radioactive Contamination, in *Protection of the Public in the Event of Radiation Accidents*, Seminar Proceedings, Geneva, Switzerland, Nov. 18—22, 1963, WHO Monograph Series, World Health Organization, Geneva, 1965.
18. Agricultural Research Service, Protection of Food and Agriculture Against Nuclear Attack, U. S. Department of Agriculture, Handbook No. 234, p. 10, 1962.
19. K. Kostial, S. Vojvodic, and C. L. Comar, Effects of Dietary Levels of Phosphorus and Calcium on the Comparative Behavior of Strontium and Calcium, *Nature*, 208(5015): 1110-1111 (Dec. 11, 1965).
20. J. G. Ebel and C. L. Comar, Effect of Dietary Magnesium on Strontium—Calcium Discrimination and Incorporation into Bone of Rats, *J. Nutr.*, 96(3): 403-408 (November 1968).
21. F. W. Lengemann and C. L. Comar, Metabolism of Some Fission Products by Farm Animals, in *Agricultural and Public Health Aspects of Radioactive Contamination in Normal and Emergency Situations* (Papers Presented at the Seminar, Schevenigen, The Netherlands, 11—15 December 1961), pp. 92-115, Atomic Energy Series No. 5, Food and Agriculture Organization of the United Nations, Rome, 1964.
22. Calcium Tablets and Strontium-90, *Consumer Reports*, 26: 452-453 (1961).

23. Public Health Service, Full-Scale System for Removal of Radiostrontium from Fluid Milk, Environmental Health Series, Public Health Service Publication No. 99-RH-28, October 1967.
24. R. O. Marshall, E. M. Sparling, B. Heinemann, and R. E. Bales, Large-Scale Fixed-Bed Ion-Exchange System for Removing Iodine-131 and Strontium-90 from Milk, *J. Dairy Sci.*, 51(5): 673-678 (1968).
25. R. W. Dickerson, Jr., A. L. Reyes, G. K. Murthy, and R. B. Read, Jr., Development of a Pulsed-Bed Ion-Exchange Contactor for Removing Cationic Radionuclides from Milk, *J. Dairy Sci.*, 51(8): 1317-1324 (1968).
26. J. F. Loutit, personal communication.
27. J. Rivera and J. H. Harley, HASL Contributions to the Study of Fallout in Food Chains, USAEC Report HASL-147, Health and Safety Laboratory, July 1, 1964.
28. J. C. Thompson, Jr., R. R. Alexander, and C. L. Comar, Dietary ^{90}Sr Reductions Through Food Substitutions in the Fruit and Vegetable Category, *J. Nutr.*, 91(3): 375-382 (March 1967).
29. J. Rivera, Strontium-90 in Tri-City Diets: Results for 1966 and 1967 and Comparison with Predictions, USAEC Report HASL 193, Health and Safety Laboratory, Apr. 1, 1968.
30. Herta Spencer, Isaac Lewin, and Joseph Samachson, Preliminary Report — Inhibition of Radiostrontium Absorption in Man, *Int. J. Appl. Radiat. Isotop.*, 18: 779-782 (1967).
31. Stanley C. Skoryna, T. M. Paul, and Deirdre Waldron-Edward, Studies of Inhibition of Intestinal Absorption of Radioactive Strontium. IV. Estimation of the Suppressant Effect of Sodium Alginate, *Can. Med. Ass. J.*, 93: 404-407 (Aug. 28, 1965).
32. Joan Harrison, K. G. McNeill, and A. Janiga, The Effect of Sodium Alginate on the Absorption of Strontium and Calcium in Human Subjects, *Can. Med. Ass. J.*, 95: 532-534 (Sept. 3, 1966).
33. G. Patrick, T. E. F. Carr, and E. R. Humphreys, Inhibition by Alginates of Strontium Absorption Studied In Vivo and In Vitro, *Int. J. Radiat. Biol.*, 12: 427 (1967).
34. Krista Kostial, Tea Maljković, M. Kadić, R. Manitasević, and G. E. Harrison, Reduction of the Absorption and Retention of Strontium in Rats, *Nature*, 215(5097): 182 (July 8, 1967).
35. R. Hesp and B. Ramsbottom, Effect of Sodium Alginate in Inhibiting Uptake of Radiostrontium by the Human Body, *Nature*, 208(5017): 1341-1342 (Dec. 25, 1965).
36. Alice Sutton, Reduction of Strontium Absorption in Man by the Addition of Alginate to the Diet, *Nature*, 216(5119): 1005-1007 (Dec. 9, 1967).
37. E. R. Humphreys, Preparation of an Oligoguluronide from Sodium Alginate, *Carbohydrate Res.*, 4: 507-509 (January/February 1967).
38. Y. Tanaka, Deirdre Waldron-Edward, and Stanley C. Skoryna, Studies on Inhibition of Intestinal Absorption of Radioactive Strontium. VII. Relationship of Biological Activity to Chemical Composition of Alginates Obtained from North American Seaweeds, *Can. Med. Ass. J.*, 99: 169-175 (July 27, 1968).
39. T. E. F. Carr, G. E. Harrison, E. R. Humphreys, and Alice Sutton, Reduction in the Absorbtion and Retention of Dietary Strontium in Man by Alginate, *Int. J. Radiat. Biol.*, 14(3): 225-233 (1968).
40. V. Nigrović, Enhancement of the Excretion of Radiocesium in Rats by Ferric Cyanoferrate (II), *Int. J. Radiat. Biol.*, 7: 307 (1963).
41. V. Nigrović, Retention of Radiocesium by the Rat as Influenced by Prussian Blue and Other Compounds, *Phys. Med. Biol.*, 10: 81 (1965).
42. K. Madshus, A. Strömme, F. Bohne, and V. Nigrović, Correspondence Diminution of Radiocesium Body Burden in Dogs and Human Beings by Prussian Blue, *Int. J. Radiat. Biol.*, 10(5): 519-520 (1966).

43. Kjell Madshus and Aksel Strömme, Increased Excretion of ^{137}Cs in Humans by Prussian Blue, *Z. Naturforsch., B*, 23(3): 391-392 (1968).
44. R. A. Wentworth, unpublished.
45. Federal Radiation Council, Background Material for the Development of Radiation Protection Standards, Report No. 5, July 1964.
46. Federal Radiation Council, Background Material for the Development of Radiation Protection Standards — Protective Action Guides for Strontium-89, Strontium-90, and Cesium-137, Report No. 7, May 1965.
47. Lawrence T. Odland, Robert L. Farr, Kenneth E. Blackburn, and Amon J. Clay, Industrial Medical Experiences Associated with the Palomares Nuclear Incident, *J. Occup. Med.*, 10(7): 356-362 (July 1968).
48. R. H. Wasserman, R. A. Corradino, and A. N. Taylor, Vitamin D-Dependent Calcium-Binding Protein. Purification and Some Properties, *J. Biol. Chem.*, 243: 3978-3986 (1968).
49. R. H. Wasserman and A. N. Taylor, Vitamin D-Dependent Calcium-Binding Protein. Response to Some Physiological and Nutritional Variables, *J. Biol. Chem.*, 243: 3987-3993 (1968).

EFFECTS OF RADIATION IN MAN AND ANIMALS; RELATIONS AMONG RADIATION, VIRUSES, AND OTHER ENVIRONMENTAL HAZARDS; REPAIR OF RADIATION DAMAGE

After discussions of the origin, transport, and persistence of radionuclides in the biosphere, this session defines the potential hazards to man's health and well-being. Relevant biomedical research involves studies of cells, animals, and, when possible, man to learn the effects of external or internal irradiation and other environmental agents on longevity, carcinogenesis, and genetic mutations. Test results must be extrapolated to the population of radiation workers and to the general public in the form of radiation protection guidelines and limits that will permit the safe exploitation of nuclear energy and nuclear tools.

Recently an encouraging discovery has been made that repair of some radiation damage occurs. This increases the conservatism of existing protection criteria, which assumed the absence of repair. Since repair processes vary with the type of radiation, the dose, and the dose rate, careful study is required. Certain conditions of radiation exposure may prove to be much less hazardous than others. It may be possible to design such circumstances into our technology with beneficial results.

SOME BIOLOGICAL EFFECTS OF RADIATION IN RELATION TO OTHER ENVIRONMENTAL AGENTS

NORTON NELSON
Institute of Environmental Medicine, New York University Medical Center, New York City

ABSTRACT

The interactions between ionizing radiations and other environmental agents in causing hazards to man are not yet subject to orderly and quantitative presentation. We should eliminate the compartmentalization of research and set standards on different environmental hazards, lest we fail to recognize important and possibly synergistic interactions.

Responses to radiation are interdependent with age, hormonal status, and other factors. Enzymatic processes, which may be involved in defense against drugs or toxic compounds, can be affected by radiation exposure.

Possible additive or synergistic effects of radiation and chemical mutagens in producing genetic or somatic mutations are little understood. Activation of latent viruses, which then produce tumors, can be evoked by either radiation or chemical agents. Carcinogenesis by radiation or chemical agents presumably comes about via similar pathways. The statistical outcome in tumor incidence may show either additivity of radiation and chemical effects or, perhaps, a synergistic action. The first reasonably clear demonstration in man of interaction between radiation and a chemical carcinogen (tobacco) is seen in an enhancement of lung cancer incidence in uranium miners who smoke cigarettes.

My paper may stand in contrast to some of the very orderly and quantitative presentations that have been given at this symposium. The interaction of radiation with other environmental agents is not yet a systematic subject. I am not an expert in the field, but I am concerned about it. We should all become more concerned about it because I am sure we shall find instances in which these interactions will be very important.

At the present time the pattern is as follows. We are dealing with a variety of outputs from our technology which may or may not be hazardous. Those specialists who deal with the protection of the public health often work in compartments that are isolated one from the other. The air-pollution expert works with air pollution, and that almost invariably means chemical air pollutants; the health physicist or radiological protection specialist works with radiation. Other specialists are concerned about foodstuffs, and for them this generally, although not exclusively, means chemical constituents. Although there is a modest amount of overlap among the various professionals concerned with these different areas, this has been extremely modest. In general, standards for safety guidance for one contaminant are set without regard for the possible presence of other contaminants.

I am not sure that the situation is going to improve very rapidly because of the extraordinary difficulty of the problems. These are not confined to the interaction of radiation with other agents, whether biological or chemical, but are also very much involved in the interaction of one chemical agent with another and of one biological agent with another as well as the interactions of several agents, each with the others. So, the permutations go on and on. One can deal effectively only in very explicit situations where the issue can be cleanly and neatly defined. At the moment, general approaches are likely to be frustrating and a waste of time.

We have been particularly comfortable in dealing with the set of rules for the protection of the public health against radiation effects for a variety of reasons. In comparison with chemical contaminants, radiation is fairly new on the scene; so there are not accumulations of misinformation to confuse the picture. Biologically speaking, the modes of action of ionizing radiation are generally simpler than those of chemical contaminants. Different kinds of ionizing radiation have largely similar end actions on target tissues and biochemical molecules. Problems of transport to the target tissues or target molecules are relatively simpler than for the chemical contaminants that, after absorption, must pass through the body fluids to the tissue and on the way are subject to many possible biochemical alterations. Thus radiological protection standards, by and large, have been susceptible to more systematic and more quantitative development than have those in other fields.

Aside from the technical problem of standard setting, their philosophical basis from the social point of view is still ill defined.

In community air pollution we base one rationale on the attempt to define the most susceptible group in the population and then we set standards on the basis of an acceptable but reversible adverse effect on that most susceptible group. In terms of practical implementation, this procedure suffers from the difficulty, which may be even greater than in the radiation field, of defining the actual human response at very low levels of an atmospheric contaminant. This pattern has a plausible basis in that it recognizes that some acceptable cost is appropriate in view of the overall burden on the economy and society of ensuring a lower level of contamination.

In a field that is even older, that having to do with food contaminants, the philosophy is not well formulated. In many instances, standards for pesticides and food additives are based primarily on tests on laboratory animals for extrapolation to man; species differences in responses to chemical contaminants are generally much greater than they are to radiation. These tests are carried out on limited numbers of animals compared to the mega-mouse experiments that have been done on genetic effects of radiation. In the face of these uncertainties (the small numbers, the uncertainty of extrapolation to humans), an arbitrary safety factor, generally of 100-fold, is inserted in establishing, for example, a permissible pesticide residue. This is one way of guarding against possible mistakes.

Meanwhile our society is becoming more discriminating and insistent on increasingly stringent standards of environmental contamination. Accordingly, the joint influence of a variety of environmental contaminants will become more and more important. Part of this picture of increasing "fussiness" on the part of the public is related to the fact that our public-health practices have been sufficiently good so that the life-span has been increased, general health has improved, and the standards of medical care demanded by the public are higher. More of the population is advancing to older ages as the killing diseases of the infants and young people have been controlled. Concern for the older and perhaps more susceptible individuals is growing.

Let us consider some interactions of other agents with ionizing radiation. It is rather a disordered picture, primarily because relatively few attempts have been made to examine it systematically. The interaction between a chemical contaminant and radiation can be one of inhibition, one of no alteration in response, or one of increased response. The latter can be additive or synergistic.

We are all familiar with the fact that at very high doses of total-body irradiation the immunological responses and phagocytic activity that protect us from infection are damaged and that one of the main causes of death is an increased susceptibility to infection. Radiation and this infection can be regarded as coacting factors, although the radiation dosage level required is so high as to be outside our realm of interest.

There is good evidence that hormonal alterations can influence the response to radiation. Ovariectomy, for example, alters the response of irradiated rats to the induction of mammary tumors.[1] Similarly, one of the factors put forward for the heightened sensitivity of the thyroid to radiation in young people is the different hormonal status in children.[1]

There is some evidence that drug responses are altered by radiation. Barnes[2] found that the dose-response curve to amphetamine was significantly altered by 100 r of radiation, whether given at the end of the first hour or at the sixth hour after the drug. In a more subtle way, DuBois[3] has shown that a microsomal enzyme response is altered by radiation. A detoxifying enzyme, presumably a hydroxylase, which acts on a variety of agents, including some drugs and insecticides, appears to be affected. This enzyme system is clearly implicated in the metabolism of foreign chemicals, and the evidence suggests that ionizing radiation can also alter its detoxifying capability. These phenomena have been described at much higher levels of dosage than are of practical concern for normal peacetime circumstances.

Increase in the rate of aging resulting from radiation has been extensively studied. There are no corresponding detailed studies that I am aware of on chemicals in relation to nonspecific acceleration of aging, although shortened life-span is a routine observation in the toxicological evaluation of chemicals. Certainly, if mutations of the somatic cells are one of the responsible factors in this accelerated aging, then chemical agents and radiation might well have additive effects.

Curtis[4] has demonstrated the kinetics of changes in the number of mutations with time after irradiation. When carbon tetrachloride damage to the liver was superimposed on a single dose of radiation, the return toward a normal level of mutations in the liver was actually accelerated. The effect could be regarded as a beneficial response. A possible reason for this is that the liver damage associated with the carbon tetrachloride produced a very rapid tissue regeneration; possibly, during the rapid cell turnover, the nonmutated cells had a higher likelihood of survival and emerged supreme. Thus, in this particular instance, a chemical injury actually aided the elimination of mutations in the livers of these animals.

The point has been made that there has been a great deal of attention to radiation-induced mutations yet very little concern about chemical mutagens. This situation, I think, is changing. There is a rising concern about the possibility of chemical mutagens reaching the public through materials going into the foodstuffs or from other environmental sources. The Food and Drug Administration (FDA) is giving increased attention to chemical mutagens. It can be anticipated that concern for chemical mutagens will become a routine part of the evaluation of food additives, pesticides, and similar materials.

Evaluation of the mutagenicity of chemicals has a dimension not shared by radiation, namely, the intervening metabolic processing of these materials, which may be decisive for their mutagenic capabilities. Also, the number of compounds that one must be concerned about is very large. The FDA receives about one petition per day for licensing purposes. There are now some 5000 registered pesticide formulations on record. In the face of this volume, one can hardly imagine that there would be a mega-mouse experiment on each new chemical entering the dietary. There is an intense search for simpler procedures, ranging from chemical tests for biochemical damage to DNA, through systems employing microorganisms, to simplified mammalian tests. One simplified mammalian study is based on the production of dominant lethals in mice. This procedure permits tests using groups as small as 100 animals. On the other hand, its sensitivity is limited to fairly gross mutational effects, the dominant lethal; this type of study would not detect more subtle point mutations. One of the most extensive surveys on a variety of chemicals so far conducted uses this procedure; it includes some air pollutants, some food additives, some organic extracts of finished drinking water, some pesticides, and some pharmaceuticals and miscellaneous compounds.[5]

To the extent that mutagenic agents are capable of acting together, and there is a good reason to suppose that they will be, an additive joint action of chemical mutagens with radiation must be considered probable. There has been so far very little work that bears quantitatively on the interaction of chemical mutagens with radiation. Such joint action must be taken into account when the point is reached of setting safety levels on the total number of mutations considered permissible from all sources.

There is good evidence now that one of the causal mechanisms of cancer may be related to somatic mutations. Here also, one can easily envision an interaction between radiation, chemicals, and viruses as etiological agents.

Before discussing the problem of carcinogenesis as a result of somatic cell mutations, I will refer to what is probably a differing mode of action of some carcinogenic agents, that is, the activation of pre-existing or latent viruses in rodents. Relevant here is the work of Upton[6] and the work of Kaplan (see Upton reference[6]) demonstrating the stimulation of rodent leukemia by irradiation. Apparently the leukemia is of viral origin, and irradiation serves in some way to release and activate the responsible virus. Huebner,[7] of the National Cancer Institute, in as yet unpublished work has observed similar phenomena with methylcholanthrene and a nitrosamine. He attributes the tumors, which are lymphomas and fibrosarcomas, to the activation of a type C virus and suggests that the mechanism may be comparable to the activation of leukemia viruses by radiation.

If these chemicals can produce a response analogous to that produced by radiation, one wonders whether they would produce joint action with radiation. To the best of my knowledge, this experiment has not been done, but it is clearly a plausible one to pursue. It appears that the biological patterns are extremely similar.

For mammary cancer in rats, a similar mechanism may operate. The mammary cancer as an experimental laboratory model has some similarity to rodent leukemia in that the lesion has normally a fairly high rate of occurrence and is stimulated by doses of radiation that are also modest in terms of some other kinds of tumor induction.

Shellabarger[8] has examined the interaction of chemicals and radiation in mammary tumor induction. Animals were treated with methylcholanthrene, with X rays, or with both together. With comparable group sizes, there were 17 tumors with methylcholanthrene alone, 12 with X rays alone, and 30 (as compared to the expected 29) with both. Shellabarger concluded that the methylcholanthrene and the radiation were essentially additive, i.e., that each produced its own effect more or less independently although perhaps by the same mechanism. There was no stimulatory or synergistic effect. Although it has not to my knowledge been demonstrated that the mammary tumor is a virus-induced tumor, it has characteristics which suggest a viral origin. Thus the situation here may be analogous to that of the rodent leukemia.

There are many other tumors in which there is no reason to believe that a virus is involved. The critical event is presumed to be an alteration in the DNA molecule, leading to a mutated cell, which then, in its progressive divisions and proliferation, leads to malignancy. There is now an abundance of studies in the field of chemical carcinogenesis with quite specific information about the nature of the lesion on the DNA molecule produced by the chemical agent.

There is reason to suppose that the more classical kind of tumor produced by radiation, not involving viral etiology, e.g., carcinoma of epithelial tissues, may involve this mechanism of a mutated somatic cell through damage to DNA. In these cases, radiation doses of several thousand roentgens are required for tumor incidences of 10 to 20%. The biological mechanisms are sufficiently parallel that it would be logical to explore whether or not X rays in such systems would coact with chemical agents. I suspect that the answer would be affirmative.

The one instance in which there is now rather concrete evidence in man of the interaction of radiation with an environmental agent is in uranium mining. Smoking of cigarettes plays an important role in determining the outcome in individuals exposed by mining to the inhalation of radon daughter products. At moderate to high levels of occupational exposure, there is an unequivocal relation between inhalation of radon daughter products and increased lung cancer incidence. Saccomanno[9] found very substantial enhancement of lung cancer when comparing a cigarette-smoking population of miners to a smoking population of nonminers. In comparing nonminers who never smoked with nonsmoking uranium miners (obviously, the figures involve small populations and small numbers of tumors), the incidences of lung cancer are far below those in either of the preceding groups. This appears to be a most relevant illustration of the interaction of two agents, each of which appears to be carcinogenic in its own right.

Although this discussion could not be as thoroughly quantitative as one would like, it does suggest the desirability of studies of possible interactions between radiation and other agents. It would seem that areas most likely to pay off are those having to do with inheritable mutations and malignancies. I think in each instance there is now evidence to suggest that there may be similar mechanisms involved in the actions of radiation and of chemical mutagens. If we are to consider safe levels of population exposure to these agents, it is shortsighted not to consider all the significant sources of contribution to the ultimate cellular damage.

REFERENCES

1. J. Furth, in *Radiation Biology and Cancer: Twelfth Annual Symposium on Fundamental Cancer Research Conducted by the M. D. Anderson Hospital and Tumor Institute of the University of Texas*, pp. 7-25, University of Texas Press, Austin, 1959.
2. G. D. Barnes, Central Nervous System Drugs and X Irradiation: Their Interactive Effects, *Radiat. Res.*, 30: 351-358 (1967).
3. K. P. DuBois, Inhibition by Radiation of the Development of Drug-Detoxification Enzymes, *Radiat. Res.*, 30: 342-350 (1967).
4. H. J. Curtis, *Current Topics in Radiation Research*, M. Ebert and A. Howard, Eds., Vol. 3, pp. 139-174, North Holland Publishing Co., Amsterdam, 1965.
5. S. S. Epstein and H. Shafner, Chemical Mutagens in the Human Environment, *Nature*, 219: 385-387 (1968).
6. A. C. Upton, *Cellular Basis and Aetiology of Late Somatic Effects of Ionizing Radiation*, R. J. C. Harris, Ed., pp. 67-82, Academic Press, Inc., New York, 1963.
7. R. J. Huebner, personal communication.
8. C. J. Shellabarger, Effect of Methylcholanthrene and X Irradiation, Given Singly or Combined, on Rat Mammary Carcinogenesis, *J. Nat. Cancer Inst.*, 38: 73-77 (1967).
9. G. Saccomanno, Radiation Exposure of Uranium Miners, in *Radiation Standards for Uranium Mining, Hearings Before the Subcommittee on Research, Development, and Radiation of the Joint Committee on Atomic Energy, Congress of the United States, Ninety-First Congress, March 17 and 18, 1969*, Appendix 5, pp. 302-315, Superintendent of Documents, U. S. Government Printing Office, Washington, D. C., 1969.

DISCUSSION

DOBSON (LRL): In regard to uranium miners, cigarette smoking, and lung cancer, which is an extremely interesting interrelation, could you say a word about the possibility that there are different types of cancer involved. Is there a particular kind of tumor that seems to be related more to smoking?

NELSON: You are referring to the fact that oat-cell tumors appear to have a rather high occurrence in uranium miners. I feel that the type of tumor may have relatively little to do with the initiating events per se, but more with the pattern of differentiation and the rate of progression. This is purely speculative on my part. The histological distinction is associated with other factors, such as very rapid progression of the disease. In Saccomanno's series, those miners showing the oat-cell pattern had a distinctly shorter period from first definitive X-ray diagnosis to death or operative intervention.

DOBSON: Is there any information to suggest that the oat-cell type may be correlated with radiation exposure in the absence of smoking?

NELSON: I know of no evidence to suggest that is the case.

HATCH (LRL): We discussed yesterday the problem of pie cutting of radiation contributions from reactors, from testing, and from Plowshare applications. How soon do we need to extend our view of pie cutting to include the environmental contaminants on a par with radiation?

NELSON: I think the time is very near. It seems to me that the public is now alert enough and concerned about these problems to require action if we fail to do so ourselves.

HATCH: This seems especially important if the primary mechanisms of action are very similar.

NELSON: When the mechanisms are similar, the problem is eased immensely. It makes the quantitative determination of pie cutting and how to add up the dosage factors very much simpler than it would otherwise be. I suspect this might be the case where we are dealing with simple initiating mechanisms, for example, in the origin of primary malignancy, maybe in the viral-mediated tumors, and very probably in the interplay of chemical mutagens with radiation-induced mutation. These will be difficult, but there are other interactions that are going to be much more complicated.

EFFECTS OF SINGLE OR FRACTIONATED X IRRADIATION AND OF BONE-SEEKING RADIONUCLIDES ON MAMMALS: A REVIEW

LEO K. BUSTAD
Radiobiology Laboratory, University of California, Davis

ABSTRACT

In 1951 an experiment was begun to determine the late effects of single or fractionated whole-body X-ray exposure to young adult beagle dogs at the University of California, Davis. Reproductive capacity, based on the number of pups weaned in two successive litters, was utilized as a quantifiable means of measuring radiation effect. No decrement in reproduction was observed as a result of 100 r or 300 r X irradiation, even though the latter dose was acutely lethal to some dogs. All irradiated beagles exhibited life-span shortening, relative to controls, of about 9% for 100 r and 20% for 300 r, an equivalent of about 6%/100 r. Median survival time increased, however, in proportion to the length of the interval between fractionated X-ray exposures totaling 300 r.

In 1958 studies were begun on the toxicity of ^{90}Sr fed to beagles daily from midgestation to young adulthood. At the same time, comparable groups of dogs were injected with ^{226}Ra. Following the labeling period, skeletal ^{90}Sr deposition was reduced more rapidly in trabecular bone (half-time <1 year) than in cortical bone (half-time ~15 years). Almost none of the ^{90}Sr in teeth was lost. The average skeletal dose rate was about 6 rads per day at the highest feeding level; the mean marrow dose was 0.5 to 0.8 of bone dose.

Although the radiation dose to bone marrow was less than that to bone, the earliest change noted was in the leukocytes. Neutrophils showed the greatest response, almost 50% reduction by 18 months of age in the highest level group. The lymphocytes showed about 30% reduction in the same group. Although the erythrocyte and neutrophil precursors were apparently exposed to comparable radiation doses, peripheral erythrocyte numbers and packed cell volumes appeared unaffected except in animals that developed myeloproliferative disease. This disease has involved at least 14 dogs in the two highest ^{90}Sr groups and none in the ^{226}Ra groups. It presents a morphologic spectrum extending from myelofibrosis with myeloid metaplasia to granulocytic leukemia.

Long bones from dogs that received ^{90}Sr from early gestation had flintlike shafts that resisted breaking, narrowed marrow cavities, and thickened cortices. Radiation during development apparently depressed the remodeling process, affecting osteoclastic activity more than osteoblastic activity. The increase in hardness and thickness was not detected radiographically. In fact, even at the highest feeding levels, ^{90}Sr changes to date have been limited to endosteal and periosteal thickening. In contrast, extensive bone changes, including spontaneous fractures and osteogenic sarcoma, have been observed at the highest levels of ^{226}Ra.

The application of positron camera scanning has proven valuable in studies of bone-blood flow and erythropoietic activity; work in this area is continuing. Other continuing studies include evaluation of natural and radiation-induced aging effects and utilization of the marsupial *Marmosa mitis* in cytogenetic and immunologic investigations of radiation damage.

Our experience at the Radiobiology Laboratory at the University of California at Davis with beagle dogs will be emphasized in this discussion of some of the effects of X irradiation and bone-seeking radionuclides on mammals.

EFFECTS OF X IRRADIATION ON BEAGLES

Our study of the effects of fractionated whole-body X-ray exposure on female beagles was initiated in 1951 by Andersen and associates[1] at the University of California at Davis. This is, to my knowledge, one of only two long-term studies that has been essentially completed on the effects of gamma or X irradiation on the dog. (The other study is by George Casarett, University of Rochester.) Beagles were selected as the experimental subject because extensive physiological and medical knowledge about them was available; they had a broad genetic base, being a well-established breed; they were available in large numbers; and they possessed a short-hair coat, were of a medium size and calm disposition, and adapted well to colony housing. Also, the beagle is a long-lived breed with a low incidence of spontaneous tumors of bone and the hematopoietic system.

The study was initiated partially to answer the question of the long-term effects of fractionated irradiation to the crews of nuclear propelled aircraft. In this regard the experimental design utilized exposures of either 100 r or 300 r administered as single or fractionated doses shortly after puberty, at 10 to 12 months of age, according to the schedule shown in Table 1. During the early phases of the experiment, half the control and half the irradiated dogs were given the opportunity to whelp two litters. I will not discuss reproduction except to say that, on the basis of the first two litters from each of the bitches in the study, reproduction was not affected by the irradiation, even though more than half the animals at the highest level died within a few months after the radiation was administered as a single dose.[1-4]

Figure 1 shows that the survival of control and 100-r beagles was similar up to about 9 years postirradiation, whereas that of the 300-r beagles was lower at all times.[5] The median survival times for these control, 100-r, and 300-r groups were about 11.8, 10.5, and 9.2 years postirradiation, respectively. In terms of chronological age, the ob-

Table 1

EXPERIMENTAL DESIGN FOR X-IRRADIATION STUDIES OF
BEAGLES AT THE RADIOBIOLOGY LABORATORY

Subgroup	Exposure*	Total dose, r	Number of dogs
1	Control (sham irradiated)	0	57
2	25 r at 28-day interval		22
3	25 r at 14-day interval		25
4	25 r at 7-day interval		20
5	50 r at 28-day interval	100	21
6	50 r at 14-day interval		21
7	50 r at 7-day interval		20
8	100 r single		23
		Subtotal	152
9	75 r at 28-day interval		22
10	75 r at 14-day interval		23
11	75 r at 7-day interval		26
12	150 r at 28-day interval	300	25
13	150 r at 14-day interval		21
14	150 r at 7-day interval		23
15	300 r single		11
		Subtotal	151
		Total	360

*Radiation factors: 250 kvp, 30 ma, Thoraeus II filter (HVL, 2.65 mm Cu). Dose rate, 8.5 r/min, bilateral midline air dose at 140-cm distance. Female beagles, 8 to 12 months old when exposed.

served life-shortening relative to controls was about 9% for dogs exposed to 100 r and 20% for those given 300 r. On a lineal scale this represents a life-shortening effect of about 6% per 100 r.

Relative to the effects of fractionation, the interval between exposures was either 7, 14, or 28 days, and either two or four exposures were given. The total protraction of the dose — that is, the total elapsed time — varied from 7 to 84 days. Among the 100-r subgroups there was no correlation of life-span shortening with total elapsed time. However, among the 300-r subgroups there was a correlation, as shown in Fig. 2. For each additional day between first and last exposure (totaling 300 r), median survival time was increased by about 0.02 year. Thus, in the 7- to 84-day range of exposures, the life-span was extended by 0.17% per day for each extra day between the first and last exposure. In both the 300-r and the 100-r subgroups, the greatest life-span shortening was realized in those groups on the 14-day exposure schedule. This gives much fuel to the fire of the biomathematicians and cell synchronists. A detailed analysis of this study is given in Ref. 6.

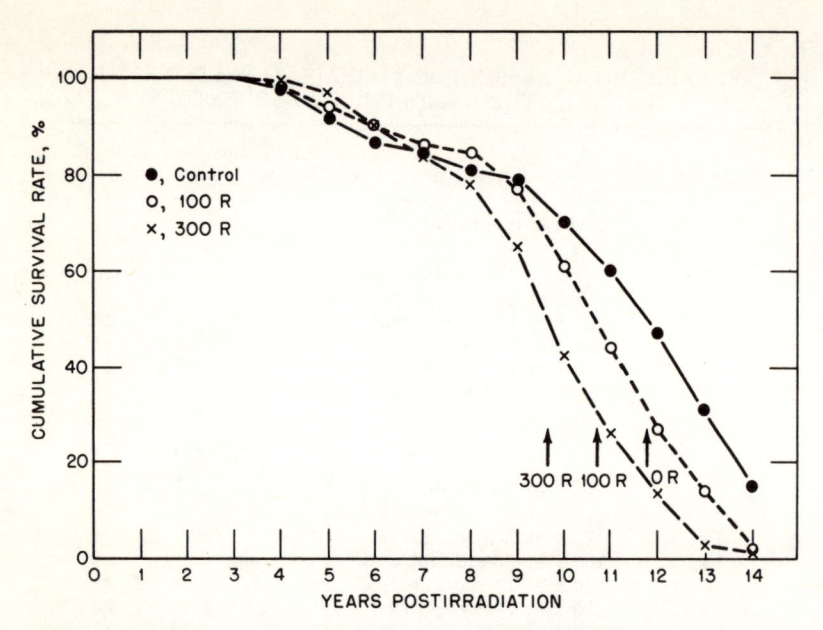

Fig. 1—*Cumulative survival rates for control and X-irradiated beagles. All dogs surviving 90 days post-first-irradiation are included. Arrows indicate median survival time for each group.*[5]

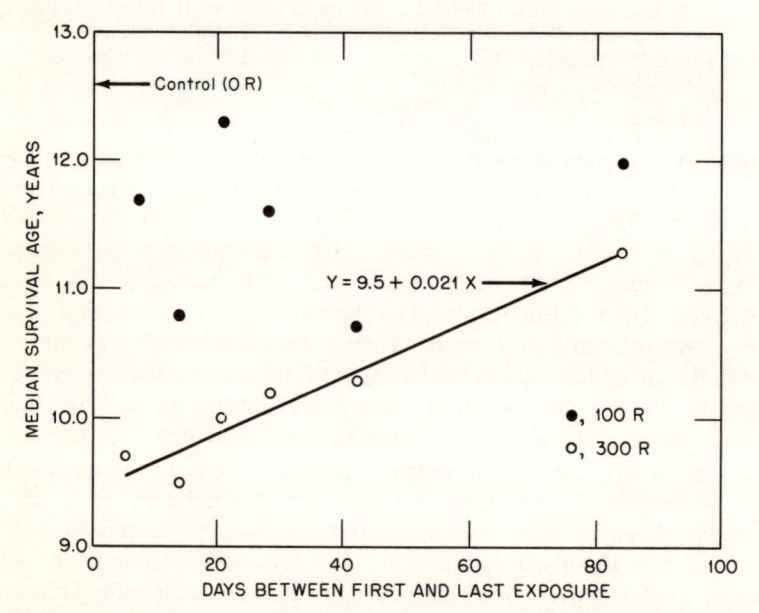

Fig. 2—*Median survival age following fractionated X-ray exposures totaling either 100 r or 300 r.*

Concomitant with the main life-span study, over 200 beagle pups were released to private owners in the Davis area on the conditions that they would take good care of the animals and submit an annual report of each dog's progress and, most important, its survival time. The survival rate to 1 year of age was 70%, with 16% of the deaths occurring before 1 month of age. Median survival time was 4.5 years of age. Most of the deaths were due to accidents involving motor vehicles. The cumulative survival rate of these "field dogs" compared to that of the control dogs at the Radiobiology Laboratory is shown in Fig. 3. If one begins with dogs alive at 1 year of age and corrects for accidental deaths, the median survival times of both the control and field dogs are the same (~12.5 years).

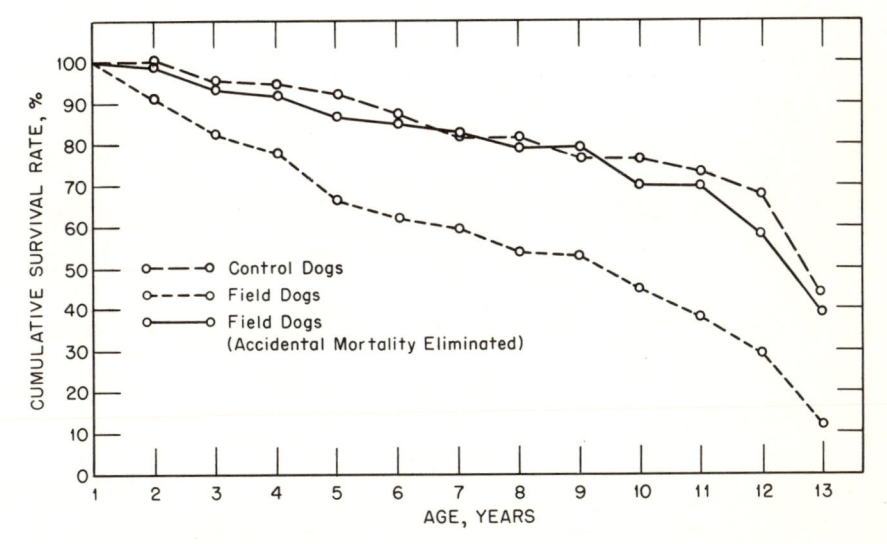

Fig. 3—*Survival of control animals in Radiobiology Laboratory compared with the field dogs.*

EFFECTS OF RADIONUCLIDES

A study of the effects of bone-seeking radionuclides was initiated at the University of California in 1958. As you may recall, this was a time when our country and the rest of the world were becoming very concerned about the long-term effects of low levels of fallout materials, especially ^{90}Sr. Realizing the potential of such contamination, the U. S. Atomic Energy Commission initiated several new studies including those on beagles at the University of Utah Radiobiology Laboratory[7] and the University of California at Davis[8] as well as studies on swine at Hanford

Laboratories.[9] The experimental design for the Davis project is shown in Table 2.

Considerations that influenced the ultimate experimental design were: (1) the lack of ^{90}Sr toxicity data in a long-lived species, (2) the desire to compare effects of continual ^{90}Sr ingestion with those seen

Table 2

EXPERIMENTAL DESIGN OF RADIONUCLIDE TOXICITY STUDIES

Radium-226 Injection Series
(Eight Semimonthly I.V. Injections Starting at 435 Days of Age)

Treatment code	Multiple of 1 level	Average μg/injection	μg ^{226}Ra/kg	Number of dogs
R00	0	0.00	0.000	81
R05	0.3	0.03	0.003	46
R10	1.0*	0.08	0.008	38
R20	6	0.5	0.047	41
R30	18	1.4	0.14	39
R40	54	4	0.42	41
R50	162	12	1.25	38

Strontium-90 Ingestion Series
(In utero to 540 Days of Age)

Treatment code	Multiple of 1 level	Average μCi/day	Diet μCi ^{90}Sr/g Ca	Number of dogs
D00	0	0.00	0.000	79
D05	0.3	0.03	0.007	75
D10	1	0.08	0.021	42
D20	6	0.5	0.123	64
D30	18	1.5	0.37	70
D40	54	4	1.11	56
D50	162	12	3.33	47

Strontium-90 Injection Series
(Single I.V. Injection at 540 Days of Age)

Treatment code	Multiple of 1 level	μCi ^{90}Sr/kg	Number of dogs
S20	6	3.7	19
S40	54	33	25

*This level was computed to represent the canine equivalent of 10 times the radiation protection guide value for man (0.1 μg ^{226}Ra).

following acute or subacute administration, as emphasized at the University of Utah and in the very early work at Argonne National Laboratory (Miriam Finkel, personal communication), and (3) the limited amount of quantitative data available on radium toxicity to human patients.

Concomitant with the main life-span study, over 200 beagle pups were released to private owners in the Davis area on the conditions that they would take good care of the animals and submit an annual report of each dog's progress and, most important, its survival time. The survival rate to 1 year of age was 70%, with 16% of the deaths occurring before 1 month of age. Median survival time was 4.5 years of age. Most of the deaths were due to accidents involving motor vehicles. The cumulative survival rate of these "field dogs" compared to that of the control dogs at the Radiobiology Laboratory is shown in Fig. 3. If one begins with dogs alive at 1 year of age and corrects for accidental deaths, the median survival times of both the control and field dogs are the same (~12.5 years).

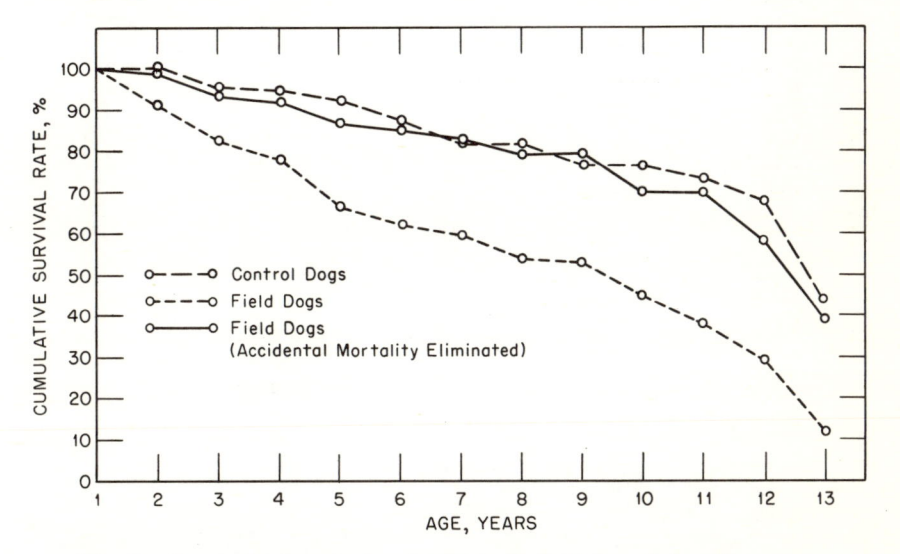

Fig. 3—*Survival of control animals in Radiobiology Laboratory compared with the field dogs.*

EFFECTS OF RADIONUCLIDES

A study of the effects of bone-seeking radionuclides was initiated at the University of California in 1958. As you may recall, this was a time when our country and the rest of the world were becoming very concerned about the long-term effects of low levels of fallout materials, especially ^{90}Sr. Realizing the potential of such contamination, the U. S. Atomic Energy Commission initiated several new studies including those on beagles at the University of Utah Radiobiology Laboratory[7] and the University of California at Davis[8] as well as studies on swine at Hanford

Laboratories.[9] The experimental design for the Davis project is shown in Table 2.

Considerations that influenced the ultimate experimental design were: (1) the lack of ^{90}Sr toxicity data in a long-lived species, (2) the desire to compare effects of continual ^{90}Sr ingestion with those seen

Table 2

EXPERIMENTAL DESIGN OF RADIONUCLIDE TOXICITY STUDIES

Radium-226 Injection Series (Eight Semimonthly I.V. Injections Starting at 435 Days of Age)				
Treatment code	Multiple of 1 level	Average µg/injection	µg ^{226}Ra/kg	Number of dogs
R00	0	0.00	0.000	81
R05	0.3	0.03	0.003	46
R10	1.0*	0.08	0.008	38
R20	6	0.5	0.047	41
R30	18	1.4	0.14	39
R40	54	4	0.42	41
R50	162	12	1.25	38

Strontium-90 Ingestion Series (In utero to 540 Days of Age)				
Treatment code	Multiple of 1 level	Average µCi/day	Diet µCi ^{90}Sr/g Ca	Number of dogs
D00	0	0.00	0.000	79
D05	0.3	0.03	0.007	75
D10	1	0.08	0.021	42
D20	6	0.5	0.123	64
D30	18	1.5	0.37	70
D40	54	4	1.11	56
D50	162	12	3.33	47

Strontium-90 Injection Series (Single I.V. Injection at 540 Days of Age)			
Treatment code	Multiple of 1 level	µCi ^{90}Sr/kg	Number of dogs
S20	6	3.7	19
S40	54	33	25

*This level was computed to represent the canine equivalent of 10 times the radiation protection guide value for man (0.1 µg ^{226}Ra).

following acute or subacute administration, as emphasized at the University of Utah and in the very early work at Argonne National Laboratory (Miriam Finkel, personal communication), and (3) the limited amount of quantitative data available on radium toxicity to human patients.

In our main experiment, radiostrontium feeding to the mother was begun 21 days after conception, and the pups became the main object of the experiment. After weaning, the pups were continued on the radiostrontium feeding until 18 months of age, which corresponds to young human adulthood. Six different levels of ^{90}Sr, covering over a 500-fold dose range, were utilized. A similar range of exposures was utilized for ^{226}Ra administration and was related to the dosage regimen at the University of Utah. At Davis, however, the ^{226}Ra was given in fractionated doses from 14 to 18 months of age, rather than in a single dose. Also, to provide comparison with the ^{90}Sr studies at the University of Utah, a small group of dogs 18 months old was injected with ^{90}Sr at two different levels. As a means of interspecies comparison, the spectrum of effects in beagles consequent to ^{226}Ra administration can then be compared with that observed in men and women who received radium several decades ago. The results of the ^{226}Ra studies will be compared with the ^{90}Sr effects observed in the dogs, hopefully providing a firm basis for extrapolation of the possible ^{90}Sr hazards to man. Considerations, of course, must be given to differences in the type of radiation, the dose rate, and the species.

Hematological Changes

The first changes following chronic ingestion of ^{90}Sr by beagles are seen in the blood, chiefly in the leukocytes and to a lesser extent in the thrombocytes. Although the erythrocyte precursors are apparently exposed to comparable radiation doses, the peripheral erythrocyte numbers and packed cell volumes appear unaffected except in animals that develop a myeloproliferative disease. In an obvious dose—effect relation that is nonlinear at the three highest levels, circulating neutrophils show the greatest response: almost 50% reduction by 18 months of age in dogs at the highest level of ^{90}Sr (Fig. 4). The maximum depression is noted near the end of the strontium feeding period, when values are about 40% for leukocytes and about 30% for lymphocytes. Recovery is evident in some of the groups.

The effects of radium vs. strontium are more pronounced but of somewhat shorter duration (Fig. 4). Interestingly, the curves for the time course of the cellular concentration in the peripheral blood are reasonable portrayals of the inverted image of the dose rate (Fig. 5).

Utilization of a probit analysis permitted estimation of the various doses of ^{90}Sr and ^{226}Ra effective in causing a 25% reduction in the peripheral neutrophils.[10,11] Although the physical characteristics of ^{90}Sr and ^{226}Ra differ, as do their modes and times of administration, the probit analysis technique allows comparison of the two bone seekers in terms of equal hematologic effects at equal times (ages). Such a com-

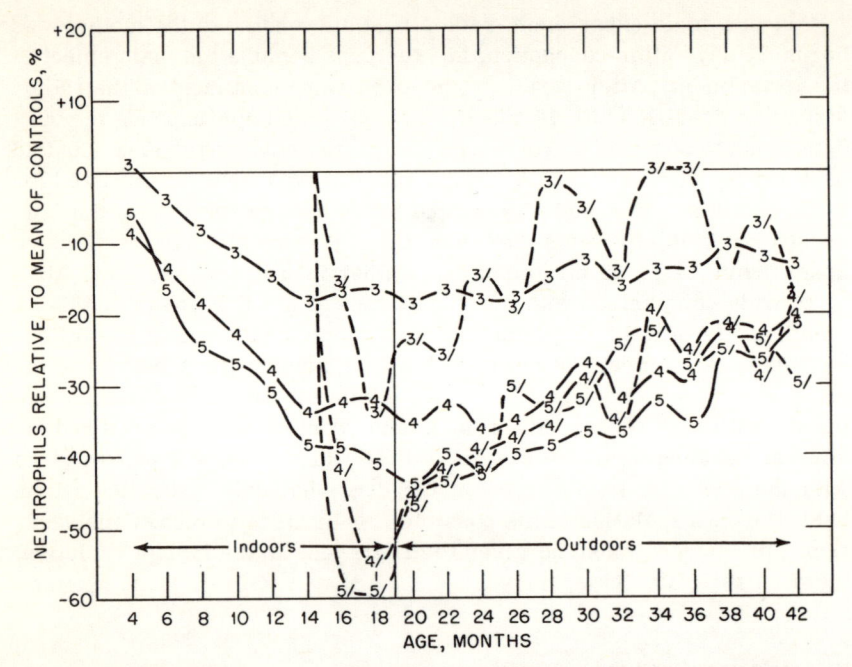

Fig. 4—Change in neutrophil numbers as a function of time in highest level ^{90}Sr (3, 4, 5) and ^{226}Ra (3/, 4/, 5/) groups.

parison has predictive value and permits evaluation of similarities in response (Fig. 6).

In the animals exposed to ^{90}Sr for an extended time, the most interesting observation is the apparent dose-related incidence of myeloproliferative disorders.[11-13] Ten cases of myeloproliferative disease have been confirmed in dogs fed the highest level of ^{90}Sr (~12 μCi/day) and in four at the next highest level (~4 μCi/day). Thus, although the cases are limited in number, they are distributed approximately in proportion to the dose rates, that is, differing by a factor of about 3. The age at onset has ranged from 14 to 72 months, with cumulative radiation doses of from 1000 to 10,000 rads to the bone marrow and to the bone up to the time of death.

These cases present a morphologic spectrum linking myelofibrosis with myeloid metaplasia to granulocytic leukemia. Anemia, poikilocytosis, and anisocytosis, hypochromasia, and terminal thrombocytopenia are consistent features in the afflicted animals. Terminal leukocyte counts range from 3000 to over 40,000 cells/mm³, with various degrees of shift to the left. Splenomegaly is the salient gross finding in most dogs and is highly correlated with the degree of tissue involvement. Major histologic lesions are pronounced granulocytic

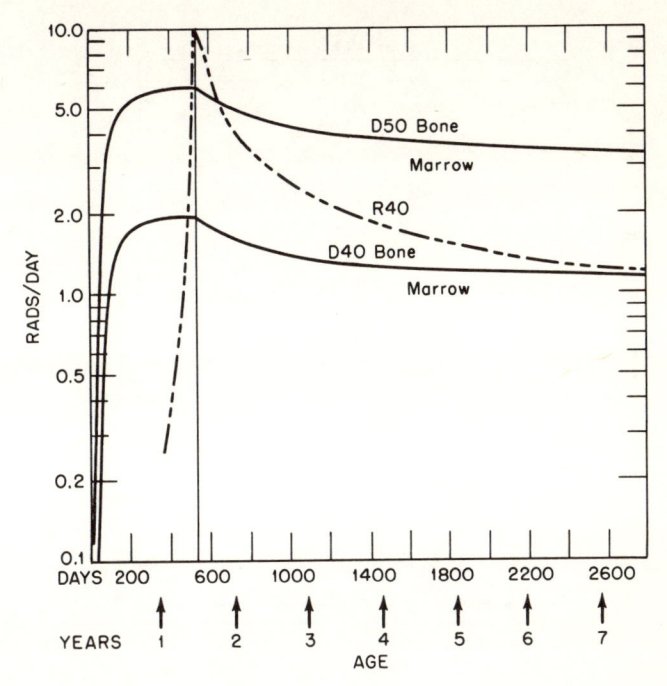

Fig. 5—Radiation dose as a function of age in bone and bone marrow of the two highest levels of ^{90}Sr feeding (D40 and D50) compared with the dose to bone in the next-to-highest level of ^{226}Ra (R40).

proliferations in bone marrow and spleen with concomitant erythroid and megakaryocytic depletion. Many organs show varying degrees of involvement, with the liver and lymph nodes commonly involved. In the most acute cases, the spleen and bone marrow contain cell populations composed mostly of blast cells. The radiation-induced myeloproliferative disorder should serve to shed light upon the fundamental pathogenic relations between myelofibrosis with myeloid metaplasia and granulocytic leukemia in man.

The incidence of this disease has not yet abated, and some of our current effort is devoted to an understanding of the mechanism. In this regard, ^{59}Fe kinetic studies have been completed in five dogs, four at the highest levels of strontium and one at the lowest level of strontium. The last mentioned dog died of an aplastic anemia, and one of the others died of myeloid leukemia; the rest are still alive. Preliminary analysis of iron kinetics by Marvin Goldman and Marie Bulgin suggests some explanations for the apparent erythroid depression. A defect in primitive cell production which causes a reduction in marrow cellularity is often seen. The myeloproliferative cases usually present myeloid to erythroid ratios greater than 1 and a marrow defect between the baso-

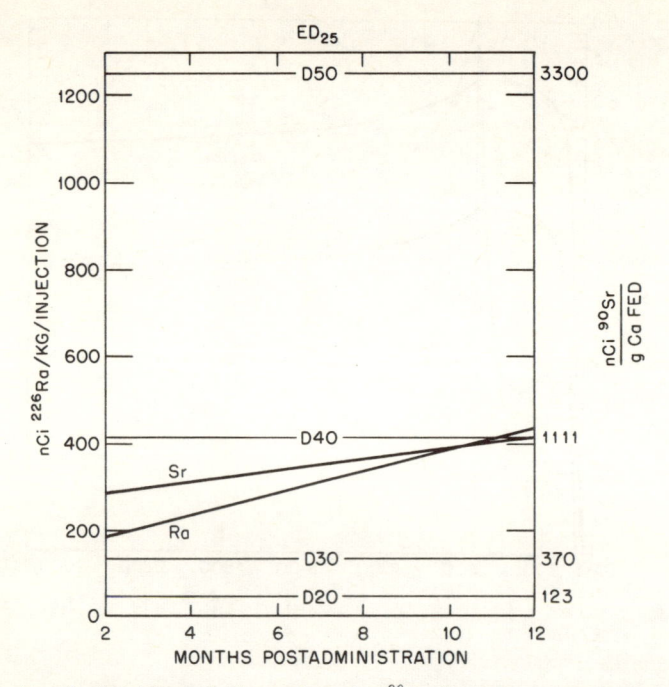

Fig. 6 — Probit interpolation values for ^{90}Sr diets necessary to produce 25% neutrophil depression at ages indicated. Horizontal lines indicate feed level used, e.g., D50 = 3330 nCi ^{90}Sr/g Ca, or ~12 μCi/day. (From L. K. Bustad et al., in Delayed Effects of Bone Seeking Radionuclides, p. 258, University of Utah Press, Salt Lake City, Utah, 1969.)

philic rubicytes and metarubricytes. In the latter case, ferrokinetics indicate a slight decrease in plasma ^{59}Fe clearance into marrow and a decrease in labeled red-cell synthesis.[14]

Utilizing total-body scintillation camera scanning of positron emitting ^{52}Fe, in cooperation with D. C. VanDyke at the Donner Laboratory, we have evaluated the change in erythropoietic activity in the bone-marrow compartment.[11,15] With this technique it is obvious that the erythropoietic activity in an older dog exposed to ^{90}Sr at the highest level is severely compromised (Fig. 7) (M. Goldman and M. Bulgin, unpublished observations).

Bone

The whole-body retention of ^{90}Sr and its distribution varies among individuals and with age and time after the cessation of radionuclide administration.[16] On the basis of whole-body monitoring data, at least two exponential terms describing retention are evident; one with a long-term component whose mean half-period is about 15 years and one with a short-term component having a half-period of <0.3 year. The former

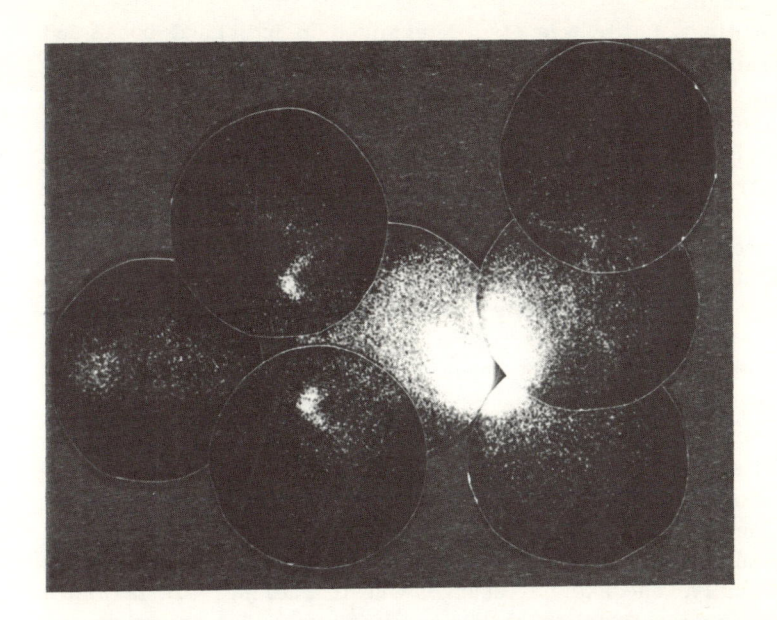

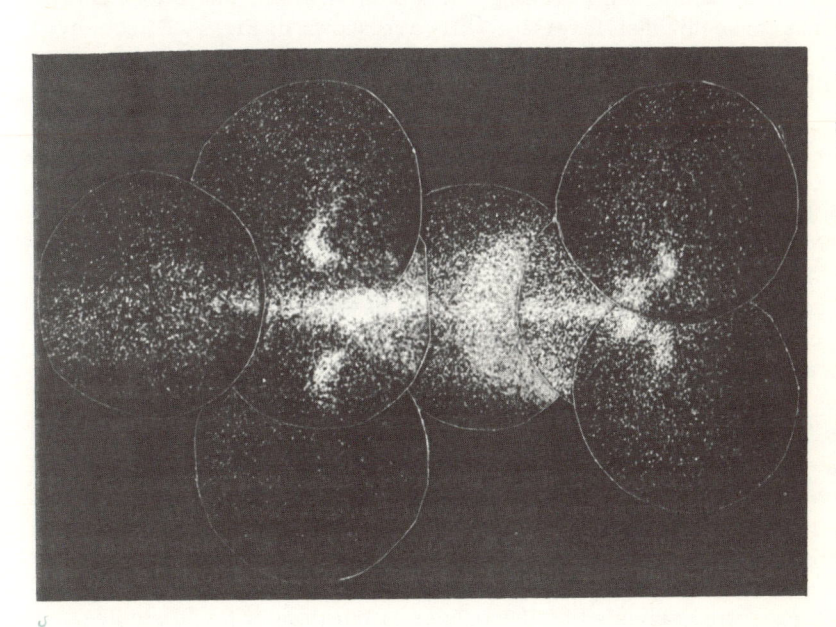

Fig. 7.—Positron scintillation camera survey of ^{52}Fe distribution in a low- (left) and high-level ^{90}Sr-fed animal (right), indicating loss of active bone marrow in the appendicular skeleton.

accounts for about 80% of the maximum body burden acquired after 1.5 year on a ^{90}Sr diet.[17]

Distribution of ^{90}Sr was also determined in individual bones and teeth.[17] Trabecular bone corings were obtained from femora, humeri, and lumbar vertebrae; cortical bone was obtained from the mid-shafts of the femora and tibiae. The estimated half-period for ^{90}Sr retention postadministration was 15 years for cortical bone and slightly over 1 year for trabecular bone. There was little loss of label from teeth.

The long bones of dogs fed high levels of ^{90}Sr daily from early gestation show an increased hardness, narrowing of the marrow cavity, and thickening of the cortex. Microradiographs indicate fewer than normal hypomineralized osteons and a smooth rather than a scalloped endosteal surface (Fig. 8). Apparently, continuous irradiation from beta-emitting ^{90}Sr in developing bone alters the remodeling process. It is suggested by McKelvie[18,19] that osteoclastic activity is depressed more than osteoblastic activity.

The effects of ^{90}Sr on bone are not, however, easily demonstrated by conventional radiography.[20] With the application of a coding system of 1 to 7, denoting a range of injury from normal to malignant, 20 bone areas, corollary to those studied in the dial painters,[21] were evaluated radiographically. The skeletal changes due to radium were far more severe than those seen following ^{90}Sr administration. The injury scores for the three highest levels of ^{226}Ra are shown in Fig. 9. Effects even from the highest (D50) level of ^{90}Sr are below the plot of the lowest radium level shown (R30); that is, ^{90}Sr injury to bone would rate an injury score of less than 5. Thus far the changes seen following ^{90}Sr administration are restricted to random distributions of endosteal and periosteal thickening in long bones. The periosteal changes occur predominantly in the mid-tibia; the endosteal changes, distal to the "knee" and "elbow."[22,23]

The bone changes at the highest level of radium are extensive and include "lead lines" and poorly calcified new bone at rib ends, trabecular coarsening, endosteal cortical thickening and sclerosis in the long bones, periosteal thickening, osteolytic lesions, fractures, and some bone tumors. Severity of injury increases, of course, with dose and with age. We have found the use of positron-emitting ^{18}F in combination with total-body scanning with a scintillation camera (Anger camera) to be exceedingly valuable in early detection of bone abnormalities.[11,15] Using ^{18}F to determine bone-blood flow, we have detected abnormal bone-blood flow in regions where there was no radiographic evidence of a lesion until several weeks later[15,24] (Fig. 10). (We are most appreciative of the cooperation extended by the Donner Laboratory in these studies.)

We have also observed a radium effect in cartilage. In a biochemical study of collagen, neutral sugars and mucopolysaccharides from

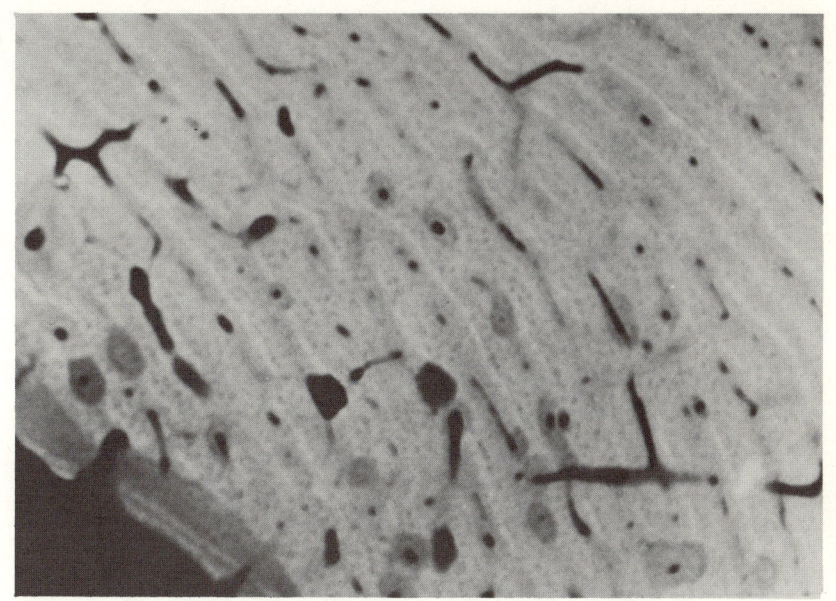

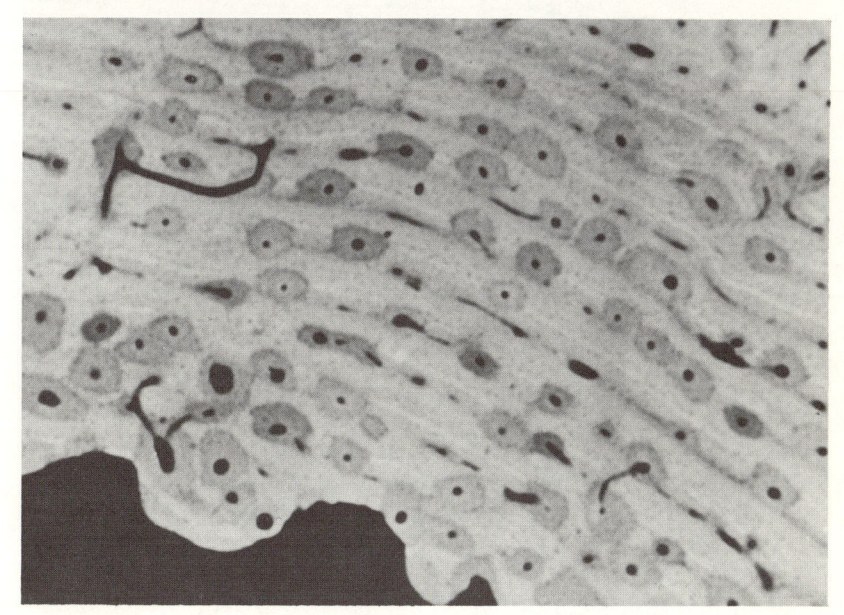

Fig. 8—Microradiographs of irradiated (left) and control (right) femurs. (40×).

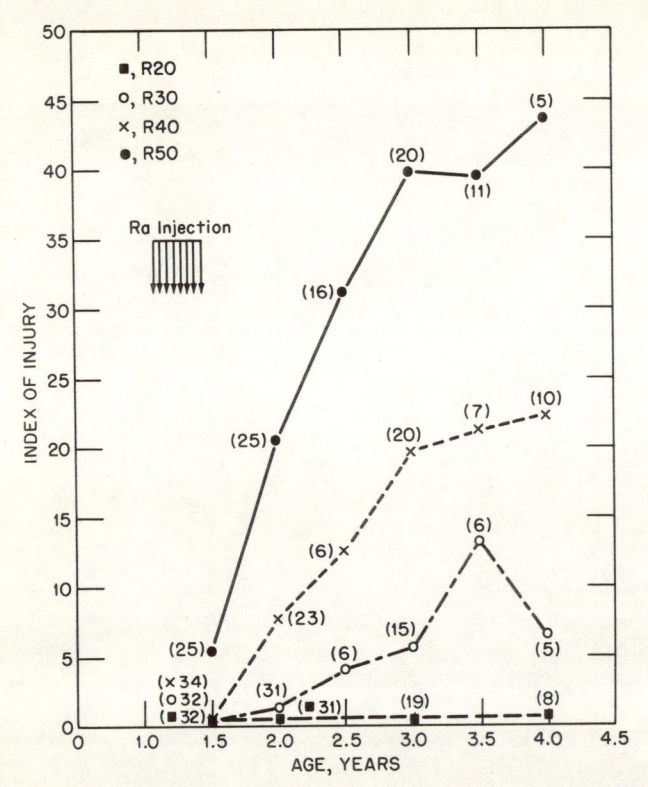

Fig. 9—Index of injury for dogs at the three highest levels of ^{226}Ra injection. The injury score for the highest level of ^{90}Sr feeding falls below that for the lowest ^{226}Ra level shown.[23] The number of dogs in each age group is shown in parentheses.

ribs, costal and articular cartilage, Tsai and coworkers[25] observed marked reduction in hexosamines and hexuronic acid levels.[25] When hexosamine was fractionated into galactosamine and glucosamine, the former showed a change parallel to that of total hexosamine; no effect was seen in the glucosamine (Fig. 11). A fall in the galactosamine level in costal cartilage with advancing age is also observed in the dog.[26]

Since bone tumors have been observed in beagles in the University of Utah studies,[28] a very important question arises relative to the paucity of bone tumors in our ^{90}Sr groups. As Goldman[15] has pointed out, the pattern of ^{90}Sr labeling following an acute intravenous administration to a young adult dog in the Utah studies may be more effective than that resulting from daily feeding during the growth period. If long periods are necessary for bone tumors to develop, it may be that areas containing the most ^{90}Sr for the longest time are the least cellular and

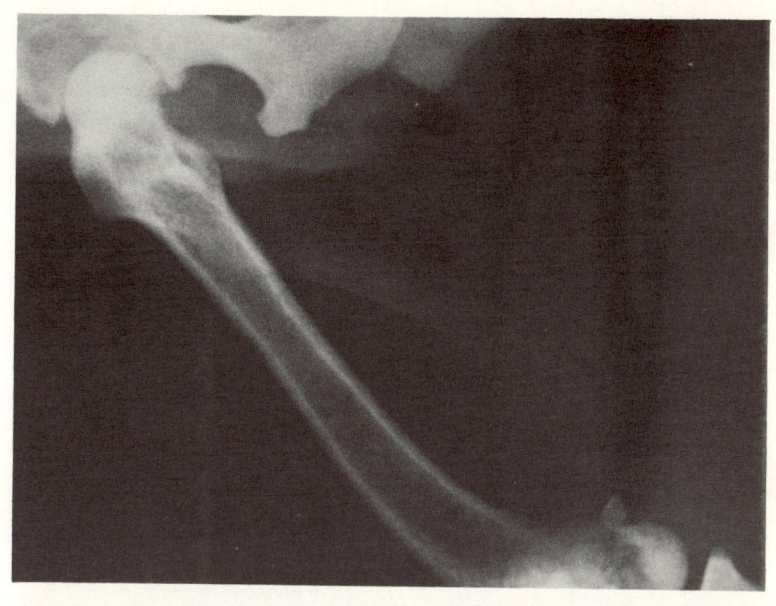

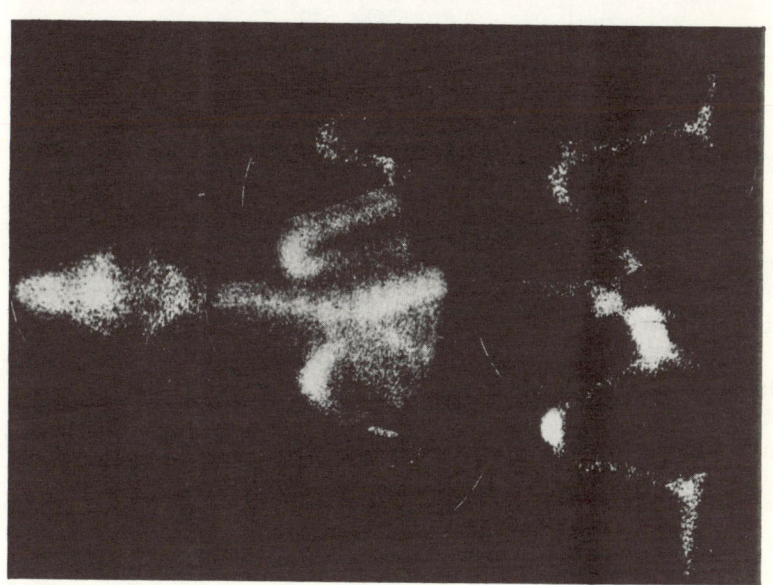

Fig. 10—Fluorine-18 scan of ^{226}Ra-induced lesions demonstrates three rib fractures (left), periosteal lesion in left humerus, and osteosarcomas in pelvis and left femur (left). Two months later an osteosarcoma was detected in the left femur (right).[24]

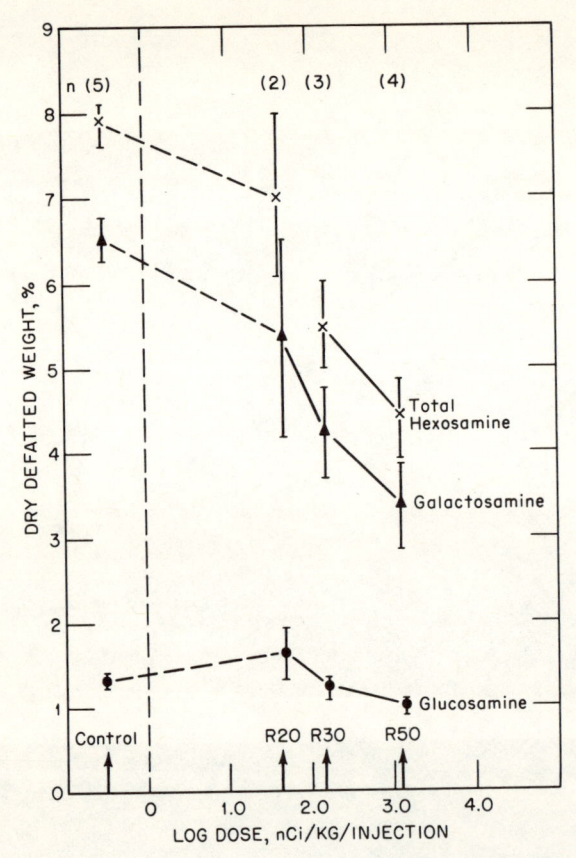

Fig. 11—Change[27] in total hexosamine and in galactosamine and glucosamine in costal cartilage as a function of the dose of ^{226}Ra. (From Huan-Chang C. Tsai et al., Health Phys. (in press).

that fewer cells are at risk. The more active (trabecular) regions of bone lose their ^{90}Sr more rapidly, thus sparing the more cellular regions by the decreasing dose rate resulting from rapid loss of ^{90}Sr. No doubt, as the colony ages, we will observe more bone tumors in our ^{90}Sr-fed animals at the highest levels. It appears, however, that our method of radionuclide administration (daily administration from conception to adulthood) results in a greater hazard to bone marrow than to bone.

It is, of course, very important to determine the most critical period during development when a bone-seeking radionuclide would be most potentially hazardous. We are examining this problem in two ways. In the first study Wright[29] is feeding three strains of inbred mice (RFM, C57BL, and BALB/c) ^{89}Sr for 180 days beginning either at conception, weaning, or adulthood. Leukemias and no bone tumors have been seen to date in the RFM strain, whereas bone tumors are the predominant neoplasm in the other two strains. Differences in sensitivity to radionuclide exposure starting at conception or weaning are not yet obvious, but adult exposure groups appear to be less sensitive.

In the second study, we are using protracted ^{60}Co gamma-ray exposure to simulate the radiation dose from ^{90}Sr to bone and marrow. Initial exposures will be given to animals in utero, at early life, or at adulthood. The time of rapid growth of bone and bone marrow is expected to be the critical period relative to the development of the myeloproliferative disease.

Aging Studies

In addition to those changes with age in bone and in the hematopoietic system which are receiving attention in our main studies, we have a unique opportunity to study natural and radiation-induced aging in the dog. In our large colony of beagles on life-span studies, we are evaluating a number of parameters including changes in ^{40}K content of the body with time and, in cooperation with B. Strehler of the University of Southern California, cellular pigment changes in the brain. Additional physiologic function studies are being developed.

Marsupial Studies

As a sort of postscript, I will tell you of some preliminary studies with a very interesting animal, *Marmosa mitis*.[30] Marmosa is a very widely distributed genus in Central and South America. Our animals are from Colombia, S. A. They are small (80 to 120 g) pouchless marsupials with a very simple chromosome pattern (Figs. 12 and 13).

A method for culturing peripheral lymphocytes[32] from this species has been developed and is being used to monitor a small number of animals[33] receiving dietary ^{90}Sr.

Attempts are also being made to transmit radiation-induced neoplasms from the dog to marmosa by inoculation of tissue or cell-free preparations into 3- to 5-day-old embryos.

We believe that marmosa will prove to be a very good model in toxicity studies since they have an immunologically incompetent, external fetus that is accessible 14 days after conception; 14 large, karyometrically distinguishable chromosomes; and, according to preliminary studies by M. Shifrine (unpublished observations), only two immune globulins in their serum.

In long-term radiation studies on mammals, we are attempting to create a firm basis for meaningful extrapolation to man. A companion goal in these studies is to exploit some of the unique biologic characteristics of several species in order to formulate models applicable to both basic and applied biology and medicine.

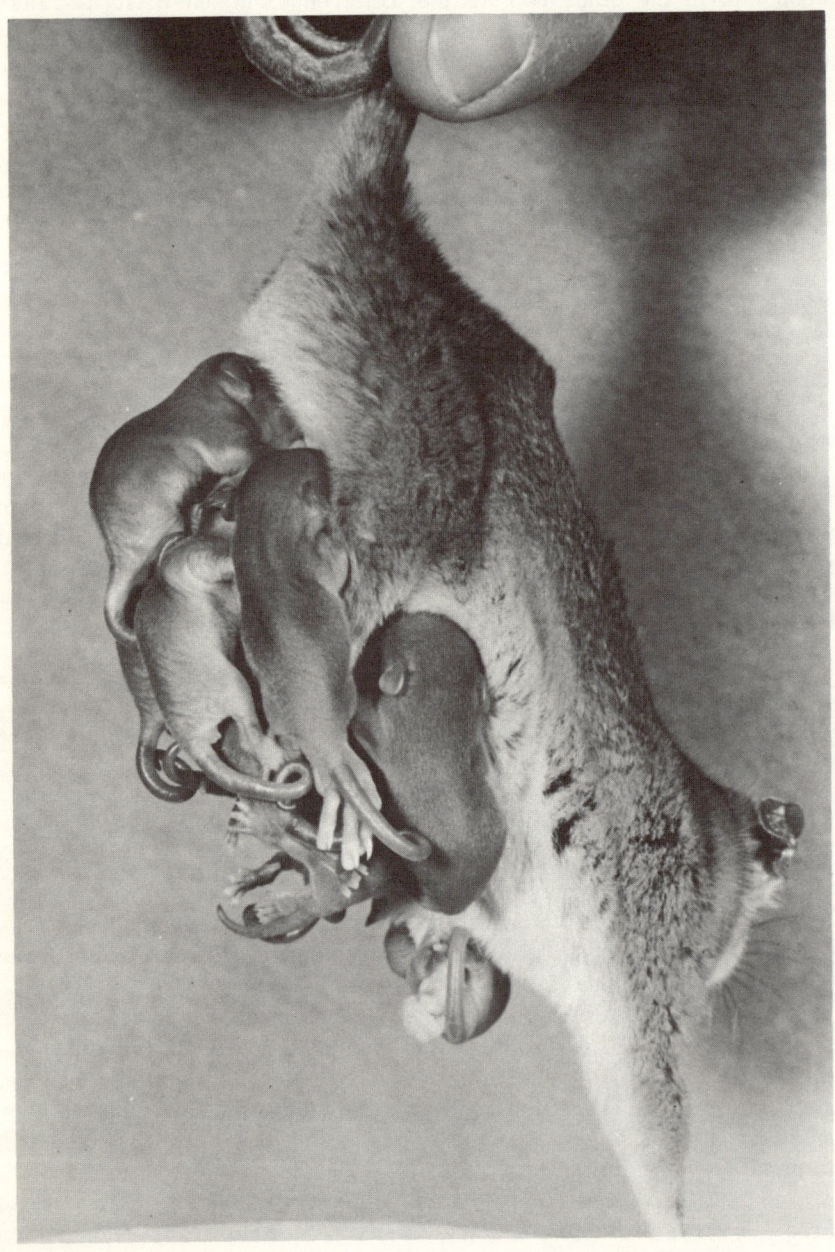

Fig. 12—*Female* Marmosa mitis *with 32-day-old young.*[30]

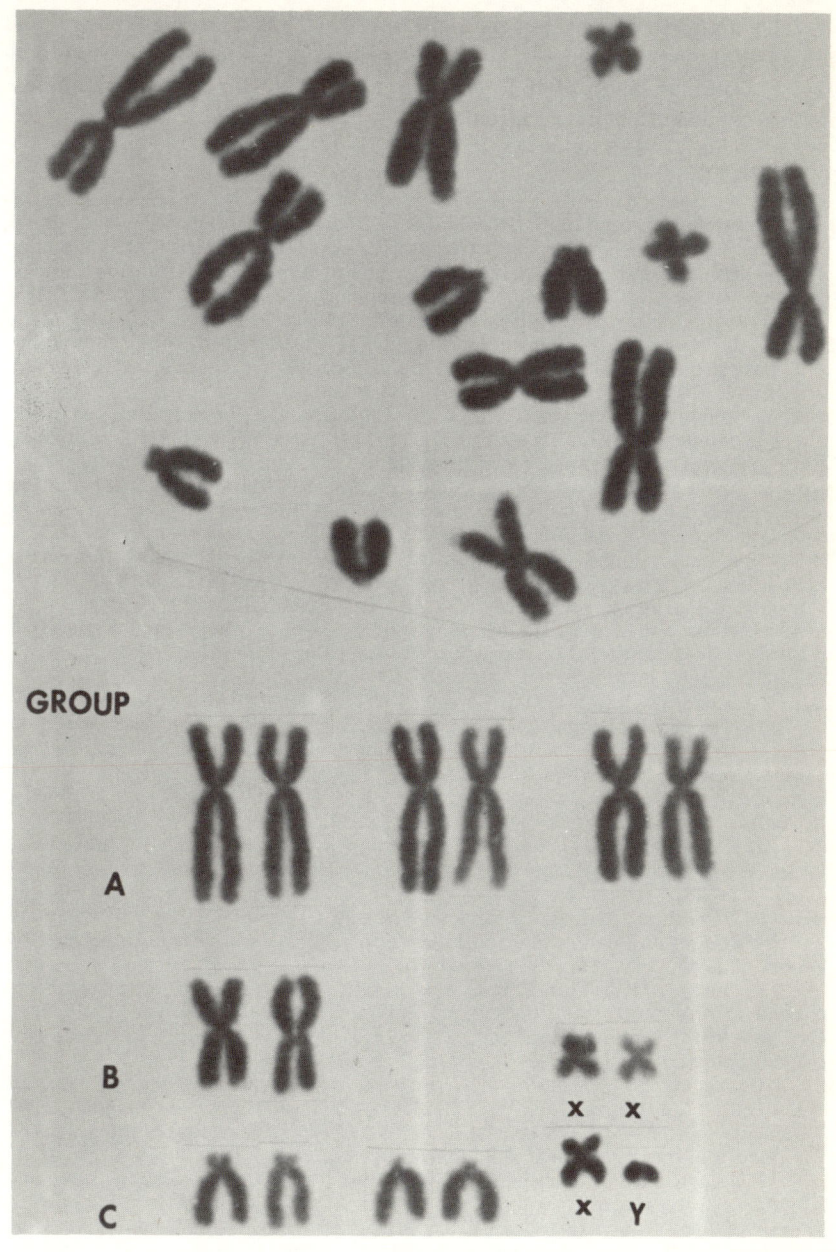

Fig. 13—Karyotype of Marmosa mitis.[31]

ACKNOWLEDGMENTS

The author appreciates the help of all his associates at the Radiobiology Laboratory whose work is reviewed. Special thanks are due Marvin Goldman and Leon Rosenblatt and Ellen Haro for their assistance in manuscript preparation.

REFERENCES

1. A. C. Andersen and L. S. Rosenblatt, Effects of Fractionated Whole-Body X-Ray Exposures on Reproductive Ability and Median Survival of Female Dogs (Beagles), pp. 11.1-11.13, in Dose Rate in Mammalian Radiation Biology (D. G. Brown, R. G. Cragle, and T. R. Noonan, Eds.), USAEC Report CONF-680410, Agricultural Research Laboratory, 1968.
2. A. C. Andersen, F. T. Shultz, and T. J. Hage, The Effect of Total-Body X Irradiation on Reproduction of the Female Beagle to 4 Years of Age, *Radiat. Res.*, 15: 745-753 (1961).
3. A. C. Andersen, Reproductive Ability of X-Irradiated Female Beagles, 1966 Annual Report, USAEC Report UCD-472-113, pp. 5-7, Radiobiology Laboratory, University of California, Davis, 1966.
4. A. C. Andersen, Effects of Single and Fractionated Whole-Body X Irradiation on Female Beagles, 1967 Annual Report, USAEC Report UCD-472-114, pp. 3-6, Radiobiology Laboratory, University of California, Davis, 1967.
5. L. S. Rosenblatt and A. C. Andersen, Survival of Control and X-Irradiated Beagles, 1968 Annual Report, USAEC Report UCD-472-115, pp. 2-6, Radiobiology Laboratory, University of California, Davis, 1968.
6. A. C. Andersen and L. S. Rosenblatt, The Effect of Whole-Body X Irradiation on the Median Life-Span of Female Dogs (Beagles), *Radiat. Res.*, 39: 177-200 (1969).
7. T. F. Dougherty, Study of the Long Term Biological Effects of Internal Irradiation in Adult Beagles, in *Some Aspects of Internal Irradiation*, pp. 3-6, T. F. Dougherty, W. S. S. Jee, C. W. Mays, and B. J. Stover, Eds., Pergamon Press, Inc., New York, 1962.
8. A. C. Andersen and M. Goldman, Pathologic Sequelae in Beagles Following Continuous Feeding of Sr-90 at a Toxic Level, ibid., pp. 319-328.
9. R. O. McClellan, L. K. Bustad, W. J. Clarke, N. L. Dockum, J. R. McKenney, and H. A. Kornberg, Bone-Seeking Radionuclides in Miniature Swine, ibid., pp. 341-348.
10. L. S. Rosenblatt and M. Goldman, The Use of Probit Analysis to Estimate Dose Effects on Postirradiation Leukocyte Depressions: A Preliminary Report, *Health Phys.* 13: 795-798 (1967).
11. L. K. Bustad, M. Goldman, L. S. Rosenblatt, D. H. McKelvie, and I. I. Hertzendorf, Hematopoietic Changes in Beagles Fed Sr-90, in *Delayed Effects of Bone Seeking Radionuclides*, pp. 279-291, C. W. Mays, Ed., University of Utah Press, 1969.
12. M. Goldman, D. L. Dungworth, J. F. Wright, J. E. West, J. W. Switzer, and H. Tesluk, Myeloproliferative Disorders in Sr-90-Burdened Beagles, 1968 Annual Report, USAEC Report UCD-472-115, pp. 72-74, Radiobiology Laboratory, University of California, Davis, 1968.
13. D. L. Dungworth, M. Goldman, J. W. Switzer, and D. H. McKelvie, Development of a Myeloproliferative Disorder in Beagles Continuously Exposed to Sr-90, *Blood* (in press).
14. Marvin Goldman and Marie S. Bulgin, Erythropoietic Alterations in Beagles with Sr-90-Induced Myeloproliferative Disorders, 1969 Annual Report, USAEC Report UCD-472-116, pp. 73-77, Radiobiology Laboratory, University of California, Davis, 1969.

15. Marvin Goldman and D. C. VanDyke, Bone-Seeking Radionuclide Effects as Demonstrated by Scintillation Camera Scanning, 1968 Annual Report, USAEC Report UCD-472-115, pp. 66-67, Radiobiology Laboratory, University of California, Davis, 1968.
16. Marvin Goldman and R. J. Della Rosa, Studies on the Dynamics of Strontium Metabolism Under Conditions of Continual Ingestion to Maturity, *Strontium Metabolism*, pp. 181-194, J. M. A. Lenihan, J. T. Loutit and J. H. Martin, Eds., Academic Press, Inc., New York, 1967.
17. R. J. Della Rosa and Marvin Goldman, Whole-Body Sr-90 Retention and Distribution in Trabecular and Cortical Bone of Beagles, 1969 Annual Report, USAEC Report UCD-472-116, pp. 33-38, Radiobiology Laboratory, University of California, Davis, 1969.
18. D. H. McKelvie, Shirley Coffelt, and Adamina Scholes, Bone Changes in Beagles Uniformly Labeled with Strontium-90: A Preliminary Report, 1967 Annual Report, USAEC Report UCD-472-114, Radiobiology Laboratory, University of California, Davis, 1967.
19. M. Goldman, R. J. Della Rosa, and D. H. McKelvie, Metabolic, Dosimetric, and Pathologic Consequences in the Skeletons of Beagles Fed Sr-90, *Delayed Effects of Bone Seeking Radionuclides*, pp. 61-77, C. W. Mays, Ed., University of Utah Press, Salt Lake City, Utah, 1969.
20. R. Jean Romer Williams, R. J. Hanson, and D. H. McKelvie, Radiographic Changes in Skeletons of Beagles Administered Strontium-90 and Radium-226, 1967 Annual Report, USAEC Report UCD-472-114, pp. 60-62, Radiobiology Laboratory, University of California, Davis, 1967.
21. R. D. Evans, The Effect of Skeletally Deposited Alpha-Ray Emitters in Man, pp. 142-180, in Radium and Mesothorium Poisoning and Dosimetry and Instrumentation Techniques in Applied Radioactivity, Annual Progress Report for 1966, USAEC Report MIT-952-3, Physics Department, Radioactivity Center, Massachusetts Institute of Technology, 1966.
22. R. Jean Romer Williams and R. J. Hanson, Radiographic Changes in Skeletons of Beagles Administered Sr-90 and Ra-226, 1968 Annual Report, USAEC Report UCD-472-115, pp. 63-65, Radiobiology Laboratory, University of California, Davis, 1968.
23. R. Jean Romer Williams, R. J. Hanson, Marvin Goldman, and L. S. Rosenblatt, Radiographic Changes in Skeletons of Beagles Administered Sr-90 and Ra-226, pp. 41-44, 1969 Annual Report, USAEC UCD-472-116, Radiobiology Laboratory, University of California, Davis, 1969.
24. M. Goldman, R. Jean Romer Williams, and Marie S. Bulgin, F-18 Scanning for Visualization of Ra-226-Induced Bone Lesions, 1969 Annual Report, USAEC Report UCD-472-116, pp. 39-40, Radiobiology Laboratory, University of California, Davis, 1969.
25. Huan-Chang C. Tsai, R. J. Della Rosa, and Nancy Nix, Biochemical Studies on Bone and Other Connective Tissues. 1. Biochemical Survey of the Organic Matrix of Bone and Cartilage, 1968 Annual Report, USAEC Report UCD-472-115, pp. 45-47, Radiobiology Laboratory, University of California, Davis, 1968.
26. Huan-Chang C. Tsai and Nancy Nix, Sr-90 and Ra-226 Effects on the Mucopolysaccharides of Costal Cartilage, 1969 Annual Report, USAEC Report UCD-472-116, pp. 45-49, Radiobiology Laboratory, University of California, Davis, 1969.
27. Huan-Chang, C. Tsai, R. J. Della Rosa, L. S. Rosenblatt, and Nancy Nix, Radium-226 Effects on the Mucopolysaccharides of Cartilage, *Health Phys.*, (in press).
28. T. F. Dougherty, Research in Radiobiology, Semiannual Report of Progress in the Internal Irradiation Program, USAEC Report COO-119-235, pp. 38-43, University of Utah, 1966.

29. J. E. Wright, Pathologic Effects of Continuous Sr-89 Ingestion in Mice: A Preliminary Report, 1969 Annual Report, USAEC Report UCD-472-116, pp. 96-99, Radiobiology Laboratory, University of California, Davis, 1969.
30. L. K. Bustad, H. G. Wolf, and R. D. Barnes, *Marmosa mitis,* a Small Marsupial for Studies in Radiation Biology, 1968 Annual Report, USAEC Report UCD-472-115, pp. 104-105, Radiobiology Laboratory, University of California, Davis, 1968.
31. C. D. Scott and R. D. Barnes, Cytogenetic Studies of *Marmosa mitis,* 1968 Annual Report, USAEC Report UCD-472-115, pp. 106-107, Radiobiology Laboratory, University of California, Davis, 1968.
32. H. G. Wolf, Leslie Siemon, A. L. Philbrick, and Angela Foin, A Method for Culturing Peripheral Lymphocytes from *Marmosa mitis,*1968 Annual Report, USAEC Report UCD-472-115, pp. 108-109, Radiobiology Laboratory, University of California, Davis, 1968.
33. H. G. Wolf, A. Kimiko Klein, and Angela T. Foin, Hematologic and Cytogenetic Changes in Marmosa Ingesting Sr-90, 1969 Annual Report, USAEC Report UCD-472-116, pp. 119-120, Radiobiology Laboratory, University of California, Davis, 1969.

DISCUSSION

CASSEN: Is there any perceptible difference in the causes of death between your irradiated and control dogs?

BUSTAD: There is very little difference. According to Andersen in our laboratory, the female beagle manifests over a 50% incidence of mammary tumors by 10 to 12 years of age. These tumors do appear somewhat earlier and in somewhat higher incidence in the irradiated series. Andersen will soon be publishing some information on this. Probably among the chronic diseases there was a slightly greater percentage in the controls; but the controls lived longer. There were not really any major differences in the cause of death.

CASSEN: Have other cancers or leukemia occurred?

BUSTAD: Yes, this is a controversial issue. I mentioned a myeloproliferative syndrome that is accompanied by anemia. There is a reduction in the neutrophil component; however, there are blast cells that may appear in the blood stream. There is a myeloid metaplasia with a filling in of the bone marrow with these cells. A condition sometimes appears that resembles granulocytic leukemia. Some people are quite excited about this condition as to where in the spectrum of leukemia it belongs. It varies a lot. Some people say that it is not really like granulocytic leukemia because it does not always kill the dog with a great increase in the granulocyte component. The highest white blood cell count we have seen is around 45,000. Of course, you must remember that the bone marrow is being irradiated. There are some people who do not agree: William Dameshek, Arthur Upton, Gene Cronkite, Birute Biskis, Tom Fritz, Bob Jones, Bill Clarke, and Ed Howard. They see a similar condition in the swine at Hanford, and they feel that the nature of it is still open to discussion. We are transferring some of this material to *Marmosa mitis* and also to fetal dogs to see whether there might be some virus involved in the induction process, as was previously discussed by Nelson.

LOUGH: I am puzzled about ^{18}F. I have been informed that this radioisotope localizes in bone tumors and in old or new fractures. I would like to know about its appearance in the vascular bed as well as in the tumor tissue.

BUSTAD: It is essentially a function of the vasculature. In an area where you have a fracture, of course, there is a great increase in the blood supply; the same applies for a tumor. Fluorine-18 is a good indicator of the bone-blood flow.

LRL PARTICIPANT: You mentioned the use of thermoluminescent dosimetry studies of the bone. Can you elaborate a little bit about how and when the dosimeters are emplaced and how the doses compare with calculations?

BUSTAD: This was the work of Marvin Goldman from our laboratory and Bill Spiers, an eminent radiation physicist at Leeds in England. What they did was to take the bones from our dogs after death and remove the bone marrow; then they impacted the thermoluminescent material in the marrow cavity, left it for a while, and then dumped it out and measured the dose.

DOBSON (LRL): May I ask whether your beagles were drinking fresh milk or whether they were on pasture that they showed such high levels of ^{131}I?

BUSTAD: They were essentially on "pasture." They were out in the environment, and they do not spend much time in their beer barrels (individual houses). Fallout could get on their feed dishes, it could fall into their food; some of it fell on them and they may have licked it off. I do not know the principal route there. Some of the contamination we showed was probably on the skin, even though we had washed the dogs and given them a good shampoo before counting them.

FACTORS AFFECTING THE RADIATION INDUCTION OF MUTATIONS IN THE MOUSE*

WILLIAM L. RUSSELL
Biology Division, Oak Ridge Laboratory, Oak Ridge, Tennessee

ABSTRACT

Research on the genetics of mice at the Oak Ridge National Laboratory is reviewed. Emphasis is placed on the specific gene locus method for testing the effects of physical and biological factors on the nature and frequency of radiation-induced mutations in mice. The review is limited to those findings considered relevant to the estimation of genetic hazards of radiation for man. Rates of radiation-induced mutations at seven gene loci tested varied more than 30-fold. There was a difference in distribution of induced rates of mutation in oocytes and in spermatogonia. Both sexes showed a marked effect of radiation dose rate on mutational frequency. Although spermatogonia did not exhibit a threshold dose rate for mutation induction, oocytes appeared to approach such a threshold at low doses. The comparative effects of fission neutrons and gamma X radiation on oocytes and spermatogonia are discussed. The departure from a linear relation between mutation frequency and dose suggests that low doses of radiation do not pose the genetic hazard previously anticipated. Other topics reviewed are dose fractionation, radiation quality, and effects of the interval between irradiation and conception on mutation frequency. The results indicate that, under some circumstances, mammalian germ cells can repair much of the mutational or premutational damage induced by radiation. Thus the genetic hazard will be less per unit dose of radiation when the exposure is spread out in time, is delivered in small dosage, or when an interval occurs between a radiation of the female germ cells and conception.

Whenever man invents new tools and new sources of energy, he always has to cope with a new set of problems that he has introduced. Man's harnessing of nuclear energy has forced us to focus our attention on the health problems arising from the biological effects of ionizing radiation. Fortunately the earlier uses of ionizing radiation, particularly

---

*This paper is a modified reprint of the paper given by Dr. Russell at the Brazilian Academy of Science, Rio de Janeiro, 1967.

in medicine, had already stimulated extensive research. Thus the mutagenic effect of X rays was first reported by Muller 15 years before man's first initiation of a self-maintaining nuclear chain reaction. Furthermore, public concern over the genetic effects of radioactive fallout from test explosions of nuclear weapons led to the expansion of genetic studies several years before the achievements of reactor development made atomic energy economically competitive with other sources of power.

Thus, we now have a considerable body of knowledge on the induction of mutations by ionizing radiation. This seems to be an appropriate time and occasion for a review of studies on mammalian radiation genetics begun at Oak Ridge over 20 years ago.

In the planning phase of the mammalian radiation genetic studies at Oak Ridge, we considered three possible main approaches to the study of the radiation induction of point mutations. (Major chromosome aberrations are not discussed here; they are reviewed elsewhere.[1])

1. The scoring and analysis of mutations at specific gene loci.
2. Determination of mutation frequencies in a whole segment of the genome, e.g., the X chromosome, or a marked portion of an autosome.
3. Empirical measurements of overall effects in descendant generations. For example, tabulating effects on life-span, productivity, and other vital statistics, no attempt being made to detect the underlying mutations or even to measure mutation frequencies as such.

For various reasons, some of which are detailed below, the specific-locus method was chosen as the one to concentrate on at first. It has proved to be so successful that it is still used in the major part of our current research. The second method has not been used by us but has been tried in various forms by other investigators. We have employed the third method to some extent,[2,3] realizing that complete measures of genetic hazards can be obtained only with its help. Information on individual mutations, or on blocks of mutations, will never be complete enough for a synthesis of the total phenotypic damage to be expected. However, the method usually does not provide an easy road to clear-cut findings. Many investigators trying to measure a mutational effect on a quantitative character have ended up with inconclusive results.[4] The main reason for the difficulty probably lies in the extensive variability usually found in quantitative traits. On this background a small shift in the mean as a result of newly occurring mutations is not likely to be statistically significant even with fairly large sample sizes.

The specific-locus method[5] has the disadvantage of requiring large numbers of animals, but it has many compensating advantages. Results are clear-cut and repeatable. Recessive mutations are detected in the first generation offspring. A whole range of recessive mutations from those with slight effects to those causing embryonic lethality are recovered and can be carried as stocks for further investigation. Other advantages will become apparent in later sections of this paper.

In our hands the specific-locus method has been used for comparative purposes. Because of the limited number of loci studied (seven in our work) and the wide variability in mutation frequency among these loci, the method is not, in our view, a suitable means for obtaining estimates of the average mutation rate for all loci, or the total rate for the species. It is true that our data have been used for such estimates by national and international committees, but our own publications have been concerned primarily with comparisons, such as mutation frequencies at different doses, dose rates, and cell stages. When one is comparing the mutation frequencies at two different dose rates, for example, a sample of seven loci seems adequate when the same loci are used on each side of the comparison. Furthermore, in such comparisons the wide variability among the loci proves to be an added advantage: one can see whether or not the distribution of mutation rates among the loci is different on the two sides of the comparison. For example, in cell-stage comparisons, where it does differ, this provides evidence of a qualitatively different response of the cell stages compared. Thus the specific locus method is useful in detecting qualitative differences in response as well as quantitative ones.

In our program, then, the specific-locus method has been used for comparative purposes, namely, to test the importance of various physical and biological factors that might affect the frequency of occurrence of, or the nature of, the mutations induced by ionizing radiation. Several new and unexpected effects, some of them quite dramatic, have turned up.

This paper reviews the information obtained in our laboratory with the specific-locus method. The review omits technical details, as well as many of the tables and graphs presented elsewhere. It is limited to those findings which are considered important in the estimation of genetic hazards of radiation in man. The subheadings refer to the various major factors that have been found to influence radiation-induced mutation.

SEX AND CELL STAGE

The spermatogonia in the male and dictyate oocytes in the female are the cell stages of prime consideration in the estimation of genetic hazards of radiation.[6] Our work on other cell stages is, consequently, not discussed here. It has been reviewed elsewhere.[7-10] The differences in response of spermatogonia and oocytes to the other factors affecting radiation-induced mutation are often quite striking. Since this biological factor cuts across all the other factors studied, its effects are discussed in the appropriate sections dealing with each of these factors.

GENE LOCUS

Radiation-induced mutation frequency varies markedly with gene locus. In spermatogonia, where the data are most extensive, the difference between loci with the highest and lowest mutation rates for the seven loci tested is more than 30-fold.[10]

Information on the distribution of spontaneous mutation rates among the loci is not yet extensive. As far as it goes, it shows some differences from that for induced rates in spermatogonia, but the general pattern appears to be similar.

The distribution of induced rates in oocytes also differs in some respects from that in spermatogonia. The most striking difference is a qualitative one. One of the special features of our particular specific-locus method is the inclusion of two loci that are closely linked: the dilute (d) and short-ear (se) loci. (Crossover frequency, 0.16%.) The advantage of this is that deficiencies involving both loci, provided they are viable in the heterozygote, can be distinguished from mutations involving only one of the two loci. It turns out that in spermatogonia induced deficiencies of this kind are extremely rare compared with the sum of mutations at the two individual loci.[10] On the other hand, in oocytes the deficiencies are comparable in frequency with the total of single mutations at the two loci.[10]

The overall frequency of recessive lethals is higher than the frequency of viables in the induced mutations in both spermatogonia and oocytes. This is also true for the limited sample of spontaneous mutations observed in the male. In all cases, however, there are marked differences among the loci. Some loci have given almost exclusively lethal mutations. Other loci yield a predominance of viables.[8]

Another aspect of the distribution of mutation rates among loci will be discussed in the section on dose rate.

DOSE RATE

Our first experiment to test the effect of dose rate for X- and gamma-ray induced mutation frequency in spermatogonia gave a clear-cut positive result.[9] Mutation frequency for a given dose of radiation at low dose rate was much below that for the same dose at high dose rate. This has been repeatedly confirmed by us[11] and has been checked independently.[12] The effect also occurs in oocytes.[9,11]

The range of dose rates now explored in spermatogonia extends from approximately 1000 r/min to 0.001 r/min. From 1000 r/min to

90 r/min, there is no significant change.[13] Mutation frequency then drops as the dose rate is lowered to 9 r/min and drops still further at 0.8 r/min to a frequency between one-third and one-quarter of that at 90 r/min. From then on, through tests at 0.009 r/min and 0.001 r/min, there is no further reduction in mutation frequency.[11]

The response of oocytes is quite different. Over the range of dose rates tested from 1000 r/min to 0.009 r/min, there is a continuous drop in mutation frequency. The difference is not significant over the 1000 r/min to 90 r/min range,[14] but from there downward the mutation frequency drops rapidly from a value that is higher than that in spermatogonia to one that is very much lower.[11]

Other publications[9,10,15,16] have discussed the evidence for the view that the dose-rate effect is due to a capacity of the spermatogonia and oocytes to repair mutational or premutational damage and that this capacity is saturated or damaged at high dose rates. If this is true, it uncovers a pathway through which many factors, including biological ones, could influence the mutational outcome of a radiation exposure. The difference in response of spermatogonia and oocytes could be an example of this: the oocytes may have a greater capacity for repair than the spermatogonia.

Whatever the explanation of the dose-rate effect is, the experimental data so far give no indication of a threshold dose rate in spermatogonia. The mutation frequency at 0.001 r/min, the lowest dose rate tested, is still appreciable. In oocytes, on the other hand, the mutation frequency at 0.009 r/min is extremely low. Even with a dose of 400 r, it is not significantly greater than the spontaneous mutation rate in males. (A reliable figure for the spontaneous rate in females is not yet available.) Thus the answer to the question of whether or not there is a threshold dose rate for mutation induction may turn out to be "No," for mouse spermatogonia, and "Yes, for all practical purposes" in mouse oocytes.

An interesting finding that may have a bearing on the preceding problem is that the distribution of mutation rates among the seven gene loci in spermatogonia is not affected by dose rate.[10] I have suggested elsewhere[15] that this indicates that the mutations which are repaired and those which are not may be qualitatively alike. Thus repair or failure to repair could be simply a matter of probability. Under favorable conditions (low dose rate in oocytes in resting dictyate stage), the probability of repair could be almost 100%. In dividing spermatogonia, on the other hand, there might always be some stages in the cell cycle in which the probability of repair is low. This at least provides one plausible hypothetical mechanism that could account for a threshold dose rate in oocytes and a lack of threshold in spermatogonia.

In dose-rate tests with fission neutrons, spermatogonia showed no dose-rate effect on mutation.[17] Oocytes showed a dose-rate effect which is much smaller than that obtained with X and gamma rays and which is on the border line of statistical significance.[18] More work is needed here.

DOSE

Of particular interest here are the departures from a linear relation between mutation frequency and dose. At a dose of 1000 r of 90 r/min X radiation, a curious phenomenon was observed: the mutation frequency not only departed from a linear relation with the frequencies at lower doses, it was actually lower than that obtained at 600 r.[19] The experiment was repeated and gave the same result.[11] A parallel phenomenon was observed with fission neutrons for doses above about 100 rads.[17] Since this phenomenon has been observed only at relatively high doses, its direct implications for human genetic hazards are presumably limited. However, it is possible that its cause involves a mechanism of more general interest. Thus we have suggested that the explanation of the effect might be the selective elimination at high doses of the more mutationally sensitive cells in the spermatogonial population. If this is the case, then the question arises as to whether some selective elimination is taking place at much lower doses. The fact that 50% of the spermatogonial cells are killed with a dose of 22 r of gamma rays[20] certainly provides a cogent basis for the question.

In specific terms the question raised above is whether the mutation frequency in spermatogonia at low doses might be higher than expected from a linear relation with the frequencies at, say, 300 r and 600 r. In our first paper on the effect of dose rate, we posed a question that raises the possibility of just the opposite kind of result.[9] We postulated that, if the repair mechanism responsible for the dose-rate effect can operate at low dose rates, it might also operate at high dose rates provided the total dose is low enough. If so, the mutation frequencies with low doses of acute irradiation would turn out to be lower than expected from a linear relation with the frequencies at high doses. We are now testing this expectation[21] with a dose of 50 r. However, we chose to do this first in oocytes, partly because the repair mechanism appears to be more effective than in spermatogonia, and partly because the possible complications of cell selection are minimized owing to the fact that there is not much killing of the oocytes in the late follicle stages that provide the offspring whose mutation rates are compared.

The outcome to date of the 50-r experiment in females is shown in Table 1, where the data are compared with results from experiments at 400 r. The mutation frequency at 50 r is only about one-third of that which would have been predicted from the 400-r frequency on the basis of a linear relation with dose. The difference is highly significant statistically.

Table 1

MUTATION FREQUENCY IN FEMALE MICE EXPOSED TO
SMALL AND LARGE DOSES OF 90 R/MIN × IRRADIATION

Dose, r	Number of offspring	Number of mutations at 7 loci	Mean number of mutations per locus per roentgen* × 10^8
50	169,038†	11	18.6‡
400	14,842	23	55.3

*The extremely low spontaneous rate is ignored in the calculation.

†Restricted to conceptions occurring in the first 7 weeks after irradiation to match the 400-r experiment in which all of the data fell within this period.

‡Significantly below the frequency per roentgen at 400 r (P = 0.0017).

Thus, in females at least, the genetic hazard from low doses of acute irradiation may be considerably less than had been anticipated. The finding of an appreciable effect in this direction with a dose as high as 50 r provides reasonable grounds for hope that the reduction effect may be even greater in the lower range of doses that human beings would normally encounter.

DOSE FRACTIONATION

One type of dose-fractionation experiment can be considered an extension of the work on low doses and low dose rates. In a recent experiment of this kind,[22] a reduction in mutation frequency was observed. This has great importance for the estimation of hazards. The results are shown in Table 2. Eight fractions of 50 r of 90 r/min X radiation spaced 75 min apart reduced the mutation frequency in oocytes to only a little more than one-third of that obtained with a single exposure of 400 r. This confirms the reduced effect of small doses described in the preceding section and indicates that, if a repair process is involved, this process can continue to operate, at least to a considerable degree, even when the 50 r doses are spaced fairly close together in time.

Other dose-fractionation experiments have provided evidence on basic mechanisms. For example, in oocytes, two doses of 200 r of acute X rays given 24 hr apart yielded a mutation frequency not significantly different from that obtained with a single 400-r exposure.[15,16] This result, taken in conjunction with one of the dose-rate experiments, furnished strong evidence against the view that the dose-rate effect could be explained on the basis of two-hit aberrations.

In other special cases, fractionation greatly augments mutation frequency. In spermatogonia two doses of 500 r of acute X rays spaced

Table 2

MUTATION FREQUENCY IN FEMALE MICE EXPOSED TO SINGLE AND FRACTIONATED DOSES OF 90 R/MIN × IRRADIATION

Dose, r	Number of offspring	Number of mutations at 7 loci	Mean number of mutations per locus per roentgen* × 10^8
400 r single exposure	14,842	23	55.3
400 r fractionated†	27,906	19	24.3‡

*The extremely low spontaneous rate is ignored in the calculation.
†Eight doses of 50 r spaced 75 min apart.
‡Significantly below the frequency from the single exposure (P = 0.0062).

24 hr apart[23] gave more than five times the mutation frequency obtained with a single dose of 1000 r. This last phenomenon has raised interesting questions about the mechanism responsible for it, but it seems unlikely that this mechanism will be operating at the dose levels important in human hazards.

RADIATION QUALITY

Results with X and gamma rays have been quite similar. The only other kind of radiation tested by us has been fission neutrons. Some of the comparisons of the effects of neutrons and of X and gamma rays are discussed in the other sections of this paper. The remaining important ones are presented briefly here.

In general, for a given absorbed dose, neutrons prove to be far more mutagenic than X and gamma rays, namely, of the order of 5 or 6 times both for oocytes and for the rising part of the dose curve for spermatogonia.[17,18] This is for acute irradiation. Since no neutron dose-rate effect has been observed for spermatogonia, and only a relatively small one, compared with X and gamma rays, for oocytes the relative biological effectiveness of neutrons at low dose rates is much higher than at high dose rates.[17,24]

The distributions of mutations among the seven loci is quite different for neutron and X irradiation of spermatogonia. The general order of ranking of rates is similar, but the differences between rates at different loci are smaller with neutrons, and the dilute-short-ear deficiencies are not so rare.[14] Thus, as might have been expected, the array of mutations induced by neutron irradiation is qualitatively different from that induced by X rays. This should be kept in mind in the estimation of hazards. The RBE's (relative biological effectiveness) alone are an inadequate measure of relative risks.

INTERVAL BETWEEN IRRADIATION AND CONCEPTION

In recent work with neutron irradiation of females, we found that the interval between irradiation and conception has a tremendous effect on mutation frequency.[18] Offspring born from conceptions occurring in the first 6 or 7 weeks after irradiation with the dose used by us have a high mutation frequency (59 mutations in 89,301 offspring). Mutation frequency then drops dramatically. In that same experiment, offspring from all later conceptions gave 0 mutations in 120,483 young. Even the upper 99% confidence limit of this zero frequency is below the spontaneous mutation rate in males.

What is the cause of this startling change in mutation frequency? Offspring conceived in both time intervals came from cells that were dictyate oocytes at the time of irradiation. (We postpone mating until the day after irradiation to avoid any conceptions from cells irradiated in postdictyate stages.) From conceptions occurring in the early time interval, a female would normally produce two litters. The only distinction between these and the later litters that have the low mutation frequency is that the later litters must have come from oocytes in earlier phases of the dictyate stage. The obvious possibilities are: (1) that these earlier phases of the dictyate are less sensitive to mutational damage, (2) that they have a much greater capacity for repair of mutational or premutational damage, or (3) that cell selection occurs.

We pointed out that, if the effect was a result of selection, the mechanism might conceivably be one that was peculiar to neutron irradiation, i.e., to the concentration of ionizations along the proton tracks. It was obviously important to find out whether the phenomenon also occurred with X rays. Unfortunately, with X rays the doses that are mutagenic enough to permit scoring of mutation frequency with moderate sample sizes also cause the onset of sterility in the females before they have had a third litter. We therefore had to go down to the low dose of 50 r and face the problem of raising inordinately large numbers of offspring to get enough mutations. The problem was compounded further by the discovery, during the experiment, that even for conceptions in the first 7 weeks after irradiation the mutation frequency with 50 r is lower than would have been anticipated from a linear relation with the results at higher doses. (See the earlier section on "Dose.") Of course this discovery was, in itself, of first importance, but it has made the testing of the effect of the time interval even more cumbersome.

Table 3

MUTATION FREQUENCY IN FEMALE MICE AT TWO INTERVALS AFTER EXPOSURE TO 50 R OF 90 R/MIN × IRRADIATION

Interval between irradiation and conception	Number of offspring	Number of mutations at 7 loci
First 6 weeks	155,882	11
More than 6 weeks	86,668	0*

*Significantly below the frequency in the earlier interval (P = 0.0077).

The data obtained to date in this experiment are shown in Table 3. The evidence is now fairly strong that reduction in mutation frequency in the later period after irradiation occurs with X rays as well as with neutrons. The phenomenon appears to be a general one.

Additional information is now available on its possible cause. Oakberg[25] has studied ^{3}H-uridine incorporation in mouse oocytes. He finds a changing pattern of incorporation during the growth of the oocyte. In the eight stages of dictyate oocyte growth distinguished by him in terms of degree of follicular development, he observed that stage 1 oocytes had a turnover rate similar to that of ovarian stromal cells. Stages 2 to 4 showed heavy labeling. Rate of incorporation slowed somewhat in stage 5, was very low in early stage 6, stopped altogether in late stage 6, and remained zero in stages 7 and 8. Oakberg suggests that the supply of late stage 6 and of stage 7 and 8 oocytes, where the metabolic activity measured by him is low, may be sufficient to provide the first two postirradiation litters, in which mutation frequency is high. Litters conceived more than 7 weeks after irradiation could have been derived from oocyte stages that were metabolically active at the time of radiation exposure. Oakberg concludes: "It seems likely that metabolic activity would be closely correlated with capacity for repair. Thus the data on ^{3}H-uridine incorporation suggest that changing capacity for repair of genetic damage may be an important factor in the change in mutation frequency with time after irradiation as observed by Russell."

Whatever the cause, the phenomenon is obviously of potentially great importance in the estimation of genetic hazards. Of course it is not yet known whether the oocyte stages in the human female respond in the same way, but this is certainly a strong possibility. Studies such as those made at Hiroshima and Nagasaki can be reevaluated, with attention being given to the fact that most of the data came from conceptions occurring at a considerable time interval after radiation exposure.

CONCLUSIONS

When we started our program 20 years ago, it was generally believed that point mutation rate is linearly related to radiation dose, that it is independent of dose rate and dose fractionation, and that there is no repair of radiation-induced mutational damage and no threshold dose or dose rate. Most of these and corollary views continued to hold sway for some time: see, for example, the 1958 Report of the *United Nations Scientific Committee on the Effects of Atomic Radiation*.[26] The results from our program summarized in this paper, as well as others not mentioned, demonstrate that the problem of radiation mutagenesis is far more complex than had been imagined. For example, 10 years ago the question: "Is there any dose-rate effect on point mutation induction?" would have been a straightforward "No!" Now the answer would be: "It depends, apparently on species and certainly on cell stage. The mouse shows no dose-rate effect in spermatozoa, but a marked one in spermatogonia and oocytes. However, the response in these last two stages is quite different ...."

The problem of arriving at permissible doses for the human population involves additional complexities. Since there appears to be no threshold dose rate for mutation induction in spermatogonia, any radiation exposure involves some genetic risk. Thus permissible doses have to be worked out in roughly the same way that an engineer would use in attempting to justify a hydroelectric project, namely, by estimating a cost/benefit ratio. Thus, even if we had exact, detailed and complete knowledge of the genetic risks of radiation, we would still have the problem of balancing these against highly nebulous appraisals of what the benefits of radiation will be.

Of course, our knowledge of the genetic risks is very far from complete. Our meagre information on measures of overall damage in descendant populations was mentioned at the beginning of this paper. Most of the data obtained in our own program reported here deal with comparative rather than with total risks. The findings are, however, of considerable practical value. Their main application to the genetic-hazard problem is threefold. First, they point the way for additional, potentially important comparative tests. Second, they indicate the most efficient biological and radiation conditions for maximizing the mutagenic effects. (This is particularly useful in planning experiments, such as those measuring effects on quantitative traits, where the mutational damage is difficult to detect.) Third, they can be applied directly to radiation protective procedures by indicating which of two or more possible procedures is likely to minimize the genetic risk. This last point was emphasized as follows in the 1966 Report of the *United Nations Scientific Committee on the Effects of Atomic Radiation*.[27] "Although absolute measures of risk are still very uncertain and will probably remain so for some time, major advances have been made in our knowledge of the relative risks under various conditions of radiation exposure and for different biological variables such as the reproductive-cell stage. These findings are of considerable practical value. Thus it is useful to know that the genetic hazard will be less per unit dose of radiation when the exposure is spread out in time, is delivered in small dosage, or when a long interval occurs between irradiation of the female germ cell and conception. These factors must be clearly borne in mind when making comparative risk estimates."

REFERENCES

1. Liane B. Russell, *Prog. Med. Genet.*, 2: 230-294 (1962).
2. W. L. Russell, *Proc. Natl. Acad. Sci., U. S.*, 43: 324-329 (1957).
3. U. H. Ehling, *Genetics*, 54: 1381-1389 (1966).
4. Proceedings of the Symposium, The Effects of Radiation on the Hereditary Fitness of Mammalian Populations, *Genetics*, 5: 1019-1217 (1964).
5. W. L. Russell, *Cold Spring Harbor Symp. Quant. Biol.*, 16: 327-336 (1951).
6. W. L. Russell, *Proc. Amer. Philosoph. Soc.*, 107: 11-17 (1963).
7. W. L. Russell, L. B. Russell, and E. F. Oakberg, Radiation Genetics of Mammals, in *Radiation Biology and Medicine*, W. D. Claus, Ed., Chap. 8, Addison-Wesley Publishing Company, Inc., Reading, Mass., 1958.
8. W. L. Russell and L. B. Russell, The Genetic and Phenotype Characteristics of Radiation-Induced Mutations in Mice, *Radiat. Res.*, Supplement 1, 296-305 (1959).
9. W. L. Russell, L. B. Russell, and Elizabeth M. Kelly, *Science*, 128: 1546-1550 (1958).
10. W. L. Russell, in *Genetics Today*, Proceedings of the 11th International Congress of Genetics, Vol. 2, The Hague, Netherlands, 1963, pp. 257-264, S. J. Geerts, Ed., Pergamon Press, New York, 1965.
11. W. L. Russell, The Effect of Radiation Dose Rate and Fractionation on Mutation in Mice, in *Repair from Genetic Radiation Damage*, pp. 205-217, 231-235, Sobels, Ed., Pergamon Press, New York, 1963.
12. Rita J. S. Phillips, *Brit. J. Radiol.*, 34: 261-264 (1961).
13. W. L. Russell and Elizabeth M. Kelly, Mutation Frequency in Mouse Spermatogonia at High Radiation Dose Rate, USAEC Report ORNL-3922, pp. 84-85, Oak Ridge National Laboratory, Oak Ridge, Tennessee, 1966.
14. Unpublished.
15. W. L. Russell, *Japan J. Genet.*, 40: (Suppl.) 128-140 (1965).
16. W. L. Russell, Repair Mechanisms in Radiation Mutation Induction in the Mouse, USAEC Report BNL-50058, pp. 179-189, Brookhaven National Laboratory, 1967.
17. W. L. Russell, *Nucleonics*, 23: 53-56, 62 (1965).
18. W. L. Russell, *Proc. Natl. Acad. Sci., U. S.*, 54: 1552-1557 (1965).
19. W. L. Russell and L. B. Russell, *Progress in Nuclear Energy, Biological Sciences*, Vol. 2, pp. 179-188, J. F. Loutit, Ed., Pergamon Press, New York, 1959.
20. E. F. Oakberg, *J. Exp. Zool.*, 134: 343-356 (1957).
21. W. L. Russell and Elizabeth M. Kelly, *Genetics*, 52: 471 (1965).
22. W. L. Russell and Elizabeth M. Kelly, Mutation Frequency in Female Mice Exposed to High-Intensity X Irradiation Delivered in Small Fractions, USAEC Report ORNL-3999, pp. 88-89, Oak Ridge National Laboratory, 1966.

23. W. L. Russell, *Proc. Natl. Acad. Sci., U. S.,* 48: 1724-1727 (1962).
24. A. L. Batchelor, Rita J. S. Phillips, and A. G. Searle, *Nature,* 201: 207-208 (1964).
25. E. F. Oakberg, Evelyn C. Lorenz, Roselynn A. Dynesius, and Diane W. Slover, ^{3}H-Uridine Labelling of Mouse Oocytes, USAEC Report ORNL-4100, pp. 115-116, Oak Ridge National Laboratory, 1967.
26. *United Nations Scientific Committee on the Effects of Atomic Radiation,* Report to the General Assembly, Official Records: Thirteenth Session, Supplement No. 17, A/3838, United Nations, New York, 1958.
27. *United Nations Scientific Committee on the Effects of Atomic Radiation,* Report to the General Assembly, Official Records: Twenty-First Session, Supplement No. 14, A/6314, United Nations, New York, 1966.

LATE EFFECTS OF EXTERNAL IRRADIATIONS IN ANIMALS AND THE PREDICTION OF LOW-DOSE EFFECTS

DOUGLAS GRAHN
Division of Biological and Medical Research, Argonne National Laboratory, Argonne, Illinois

ABSTRACT

The late effects of whole-body exposure to ionizing radiation are well defined in terms of life shortening in experimental animals. In mice, for example, single exposures will produce a life shortening of 28 days/100 r, whereas lifetime exposures at dose rates below 25 r/day will induce only a loss of 4 days/100 r accumulated. Life-table statistics offer a sensitive approach to such data and also provide a rational basis for interspecies extrapolation. Present data would suggest that man would incur a loss of 1 day/r for low dose-rate protracted exposures and 5 to 10 days/r for brief high-dose-rate exposures.

Tumor death rates are less well developed in mice, though they are precise for man. Induction probabilities appear to be about 10^{-6} per rad per man-year at risk for leukemia, thyroid, and bone cancers. Estimation of exact risk at extremely low doses remains obscure owing to the interaction of biological and environmental factors.

The late effects of whole-body exposure to ionizing radiation are best defined quantitatively in terms of life shortening and/or the specific pathologic changes that accompany or lead to death. The effects of single doses of low LET radiations are well documented, and the basic life-shortening parameter[1-3] for young adult mice is about 28 days/ 100 r. To this would be added components attributable to specific pathology, such as leukemia, sex differences, age factors, and LET factors.[3] Fractionated or terminated exposures[1] that do not exceed a 1000 r total dose or a 50- to 100-day protraction period also induce about the same life-shortening effect per roentgen, though some dose-rate effect begins to appear as daily exposure levels drop below 25 r/day.

Protracted, but terminated, exposures have a more complicated effect when daily dose levels[1] are above 25 r, protraction periods are greater than 100 days, and total doses are greater than 1500 r. Under steady pressure of injury, the rat and mouse appear to develop a state of near equilibrium for injury and recovery. This does not occur for several weeks to months, but when this equilibration sets in, the rate of injury accumulation drops sharply from 10 to 30 days of life lost per roentgen to a value close to 4 days per roentgen. This latter figure is the minimum effect seen in mice under duration-of-life daily irradiation at dose rates below 25 r/day. The state of our knowledge concerning the effects of exposures terminated before appreciable mortality has occurred or before the last 25% of the population has died out is poor compared to our understanding of what can be called the limiting exposure conditons — single doses or lifetime daily doses.

The duration-of-life exposure regime provides our most dependable prediction equation for the life-shortening effects.[1,4,9] The logarithm of the mean after survival (MAS) is linearly related to daily dose in roentgens per day. The form of the exponential relation is simply

$$MAS_D = MAS_0 e^{-\beta D} \qquad (1)$$

where D is the daily dose level and β is the regression of ln MAS on D. The value of β for the average mouse is -0.038 or 3.8 days lost per roentgen accumulated; 3.8% lost per roentgen per day.

The most informative approach to the analysis of radiation effects is through the basic statistics of the life table.[2,5-9] Although all degrees of sophistication can be employed, one needs only the basic death-rate estimates for all causes and for major specific causes to define the radiation risks in the population.

It has been generally shown that populations subjected to a single dose of radiation will have their death rates elevated above the control, but the death-rate regression will be parallel to the control.[2,6,8] There is an exponential increase in the intercept value with increasing single dose. Daily irradiation causes the death rates to progressively diverge from control, but now the intercept is unchanged.[2,6,8,9] The increase in the death-rate slope is an exponential function of daily dose.[9]

Actual populations do not ideally adhere to these expectations; there may be deviations from parallel displacement from single doses, and there are nonlinear components in the daily dose response. An example of the latter is given in Fig. 1. A major cause of the nonlinearity at the higher dose levels (above 6 r/day) is the occurrence of leukemia. If this cause of death is removed from the population, the data can be fitted with either first- or second-degree equations with about equal reduction of the residual variance. Data adjusted in this way and fitted by linear equations are shown in Fig. 2.

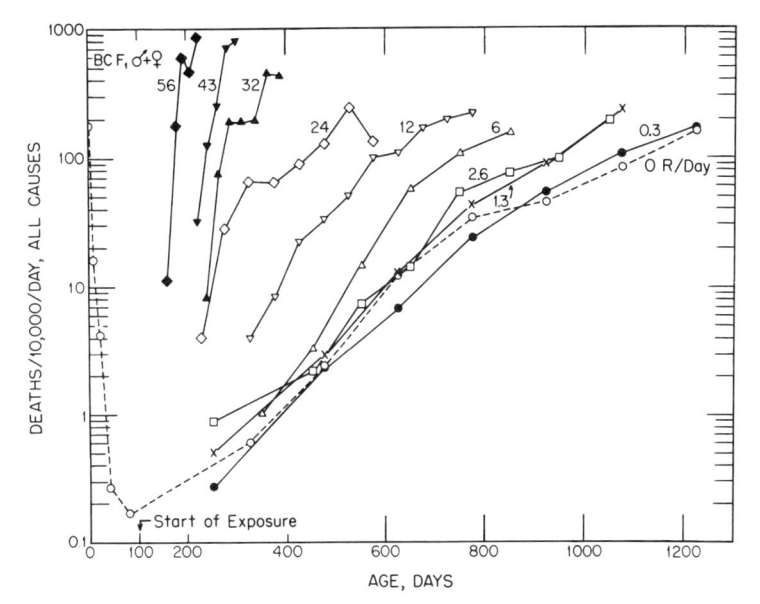

Fig. 1—*Age-specific mortality rates for all causes of death for daily ^{60}Co gamma-radiation dose levels as indicated. Data from BCF_1 (C57BL/6 × BALB/c) hybrid mice, both sexes in equal numbers, 100 days of age at start of exposure. See Ref. 9 for details.*

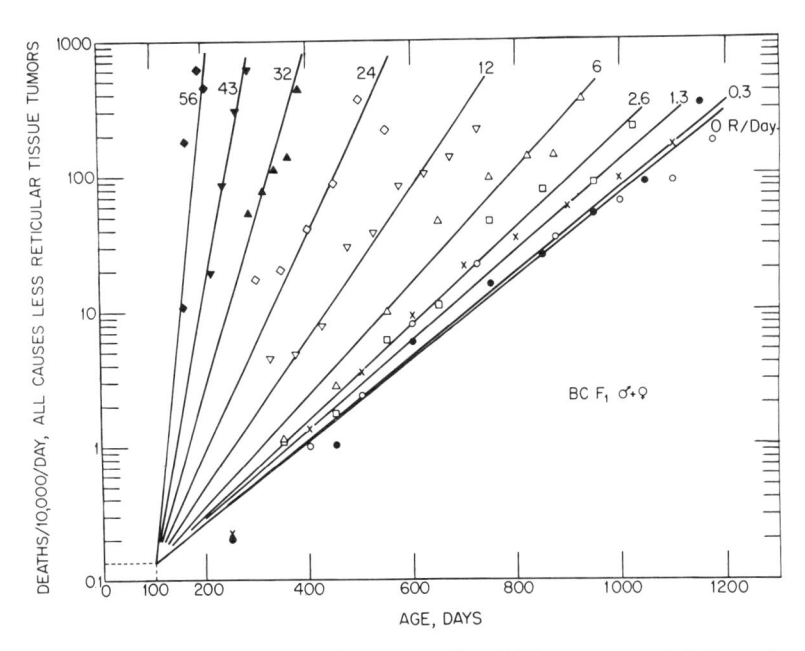

Fig. 2—*Age-specific mortality rates for BCF_1 mouse populations in which all deaths from reticular tissue tumors have been removed. Data fitted with linear equations forced through a common 100-day intercept of 13.5×10^{-6} deaths per mouse-day.*

The death-rate regressions themselves are exponentially related to dose in roentgens per day. Figure 3 shows two basic relations of the survival statistics and death-rate slopes of populations under daily gamma irradiation. The exponential decline in survival time, noted above, and the exponential increase in mortality-rate slope are both evident. Median survival time can be predicted from the mortality-rate slope by the relation

$$\text{MST} = \frac{1}{ke^{\chi D}} \ln \left[\frac{1 + 0.693\, ke^{\chi D}}{r} \right] \qquad (2)$$

where k = control slope
 r = common intercept in deaths per mouse day
 D = daily dose in roentgens per day
 χ = regression of slope on dose

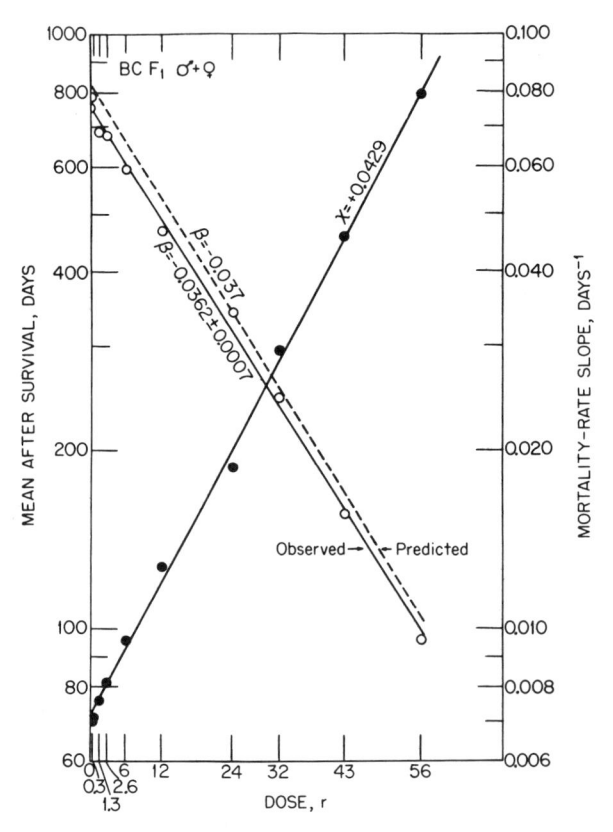

Fig. 3—*Log MAS vs. daily dose and log mortality-rate slope vs. daily dose; BCF₁ mice, sexes combined, leukemia decremented.*

One final prediction equation is available from these relations; this predicts the relation between MAS and the ratio of death-rate slopes to the control slope: k_D/k_0. This is a power function (linear on a log−log graph) and conforms to the equation

$$MAS_D = MAS_0 \ [k_D/k_0]^{-0.831} \tag{3}$$

A 50% reduction in MAS is induced by a dose of about 19 r/day in the mouse, and this is associated with 10-fold increase in the average death rate. Thus when k_D/k_0 equals 2.303, then $0.693/-\ln (\ln 10) = -0.831$. This equation, which is independent of dose rate, can be used to estimate dose, estimate change in survival, or estimate excess mortality, depending upon the information available. In the case of U. S. radiologists, for example, their 5-year reduction in life expectancy and changes in death rate over other medical specialists suggest they were exposed to a dose between 50 mr and 150 mr/day for a 30 to 35 year professional lifetime.[9]

The analysis of deaths from specific causes is also readily managed through actuarial techniques.[5,9,10] In this instance there are no preexisting expectations of the response of life-table parameters as there are for the case of all causes of death. Many of the specific dose responses are nonlinear and phasic in nature. In spite of that, the analytical quality of the method is far superior to the usual observation of incidence rates. A few examples will serve to demonstrate this.

The final incidence of several tumor types is given in Fig. 4. In no instance is the relation between incidence and daily dose a simple one that could readily lead to a prediction of response over a wide range of doses. Nevertheless, it is evident that there is a decided increase in tumor yield at all the lowest doses where life-shortening factors are minimal.

In contrast, the death rates from reticular-tissue tumors (leukemias), ovarian tumors and cysts, and pulmonary tumors all reveal the presence of excess mortality at all radiation levels and usually some progression of mortality rate with dose (Figs. 5 to 7). No single model of dose-response relations can be used to describe these data except that the excess mortality can be derived mathematically and related to dose. Although such analysis has only begun, we can show that pulmonary tumor death-rate ratios progressively (and exponentially) rise with dose level.[9] It is fully anticipated that some form of "integrated risk analysis" that estimates the excess in death rate, regardless of existing age differences in risk period or complex nonlinear components, will reduce the mortality experience to terms useful in prediction equations.

Prediction of response at extremely low doses continues to be a problem, not just for the mouse, on which we have extensive data, but

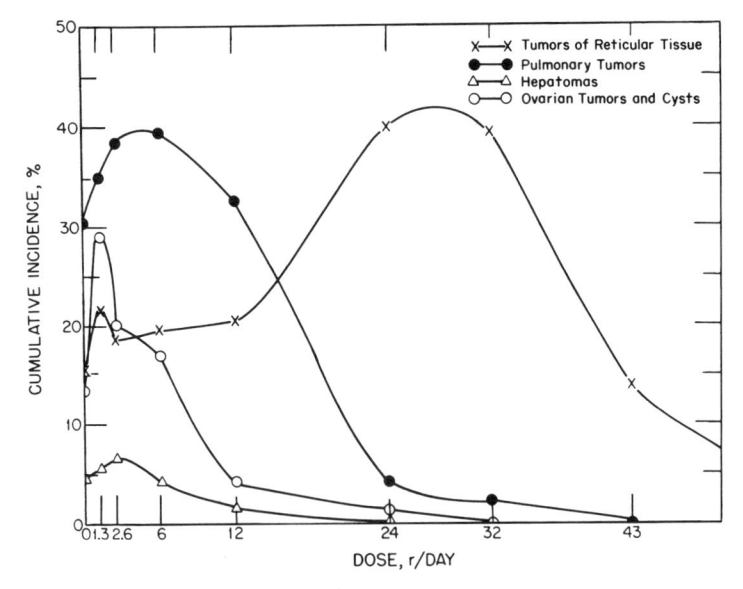

Fig. 4—Final incidence of reticular tissue tumors, hepatomas, and ovarian tumors and cysts for strains A/Jax, BALB/c, C57BL/6, and BCF₁ combined. Pulmonary tumors from combined data of strains A, BALB, and BCF₁ only.

seriously so for other species including man. There are several reasonable approaches to the problem. One approach is to use the exponential equation, Eq. 1, that describes life shortening as a function of daily dose. The life-shortening term, β, which is -0.038 days/r for the mouse, can be converted to terms appropriate for man by applying the ratio of life expectancies or, preferably, the ratio of control death-rate regressions.[9] The ratio of man to mouse is generally about 30 to 1. The life-shortening term would then be about 1.1 days/r accumulated. The dose that would reduce man's life expectancy (from 20 years of age) by 50% would be about 0.65 r/day. The life-shortening estimate for man of approximately 1 day/r is somewhat below commonly quoted estimates that range from 5 to 30 days/r. Some of this range is due to the inclusion of single-dose effects that are greater than those from protracted exposure, however, some is also due to inadequate experience among animal populations exposed to low daily doses. The single-dose response would, in fact, be about 5 to 10 times greater than the low daily dose value, or 5 to 10 days/r.

The greater problems in extrapolation and prediction in man may not only be those relating to the methodological details of converting life-table statistics. Prediction and observation are going to be harassed by a multitude of biological, environmental, and socioeconomic variables. For example, random noise in any large, un-

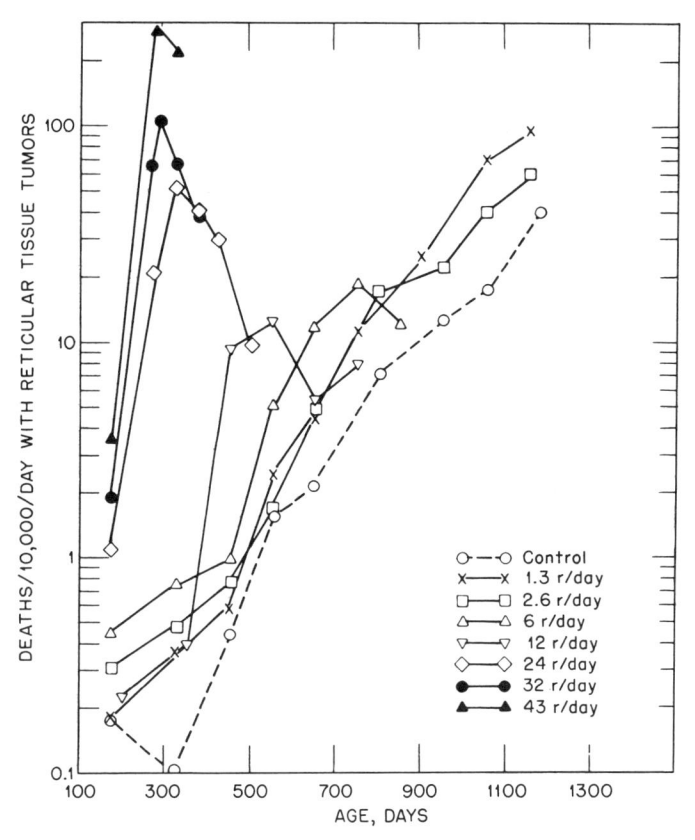

Fig. 5—Age-specific mortality rates for reticular tissue tumors; combined data by sex and strain (A/Jax, BALB/c, C57BL/6, BCF$_1$).

controlled population can simply swamp the effects of low levels of insult that do not increase end points by 3 to 5%. There is no simple solution to noise levels; careful attention to concomitant variables and accuracy of ascertainment are imperative. Socioeconomic variables, at least in the United States, can be quite well controlled statistically by taking full advantage of available census data.[11,12] Typical of these variables are medium income, years of attained education, and occupations. The effect of some of these on neonatal mortality rates in major divisions of the United States is shown in Fig. 8.

Another serious problem is that of confounded variables; the case where one effect can be reasonably related to two or more causes. An example of this is also seen in the neonatal death rates in the United States as a function of altitude or background radiation (Fig. 9). A careful analysis of causes ultimately revealed that altitude is the primary variable in the change of neonatal death rate and that this is

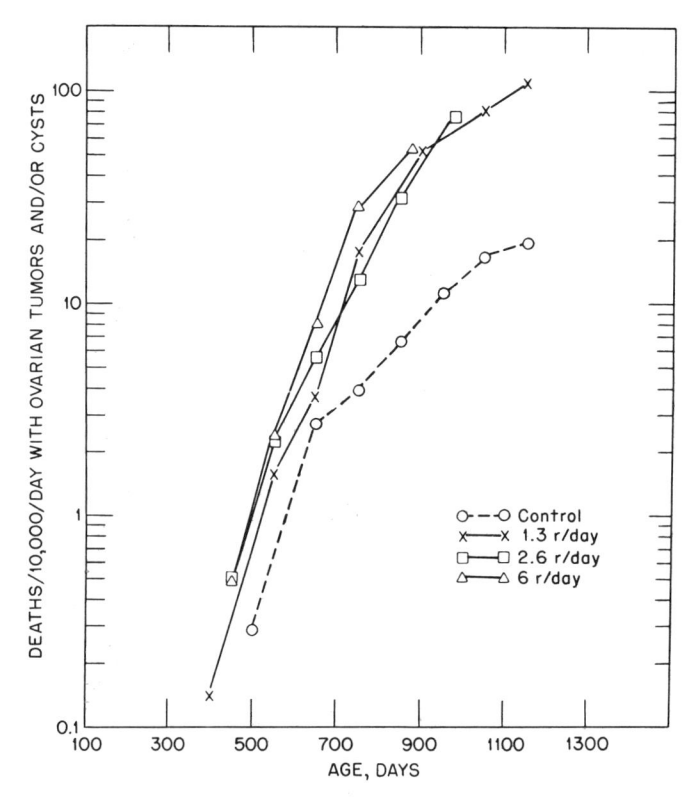

Fig. 6 — *Age-specific mortality rates for ovarian tumors and cysts; combined data by strain.*

closely related to weight at birth.[11] The latter reflects the slight oxygen deficit of mountain habitation; birth weight declines with increasing altitude, and this is followed by a higher probability of neonatal death.

Accuracy of ascertainment of the end point is also critical. If one chooses to use population statistics, the chosen end point should have a proved accuracy in initial ascertainment and in the record-keeping routines. An unhappy example of incomplete ascertainment that led to inappropriate conclusions was seen in one particular effort to associate worldwide variation in congenital malformation deaths among infants to background radiation.[13] In that case, much of the variation could be attributed to the inaccuracy and incompleteness of recording, not radiation. For example, most equatorial and subtropical countries have inadequate vital statistical procedures, whereas Northern European nations have developed highly efficient methods of record taking. The increase in background radiation with increasing geographic latitude was therefore a circumstantially correlated variable, not a

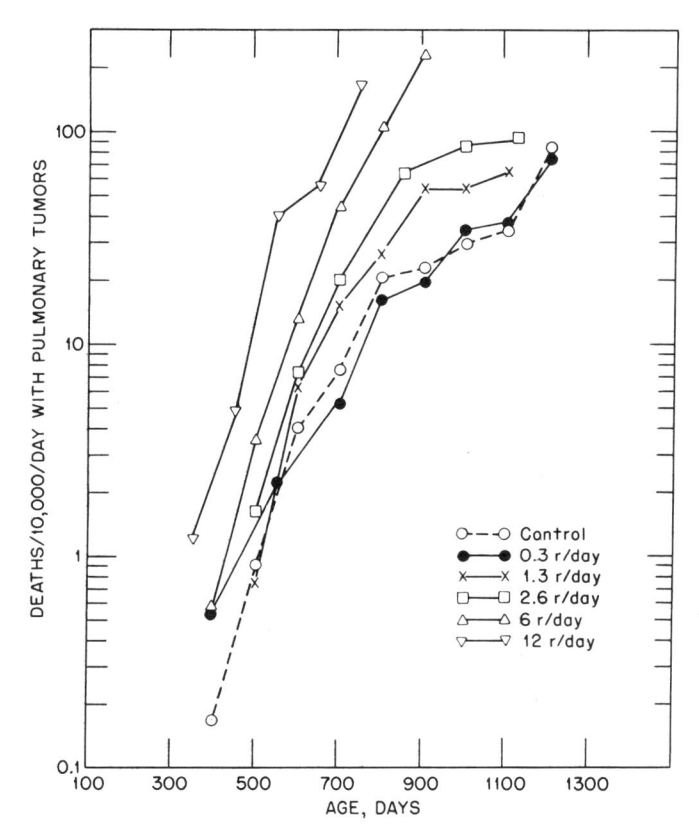

Fig. 7—Age-specific mortality rates for pulmonary tumors; combined data by sex and strain (A/Jax, BALB/c, BCF$_1$).

causative variable. There continue to be efforts to correlate background-radiation changes with variations in fetal, neonatal, and infant mortality that unfortunately still do not properly allow for confounded biological and socioeconomic factors.[14]

A summary of problems relating to the observation and prediction of biological response to low levels of environmental stress — radiation or otherwise — indicates the following factors to be pertinent.

1. Relevance of the biological end point to the stress in question.

2. Existence of other independent causative factors; the confounded variables.

3. Quality of measurement of alleged primary causative factor.

4. Influence of secondary biological variables, such as sex, age, genetic, or racial factors.

5. Influence of secondary environmental or socioeconomic variables, such as geologic environment, income, education, temperature, humidity, and diet.

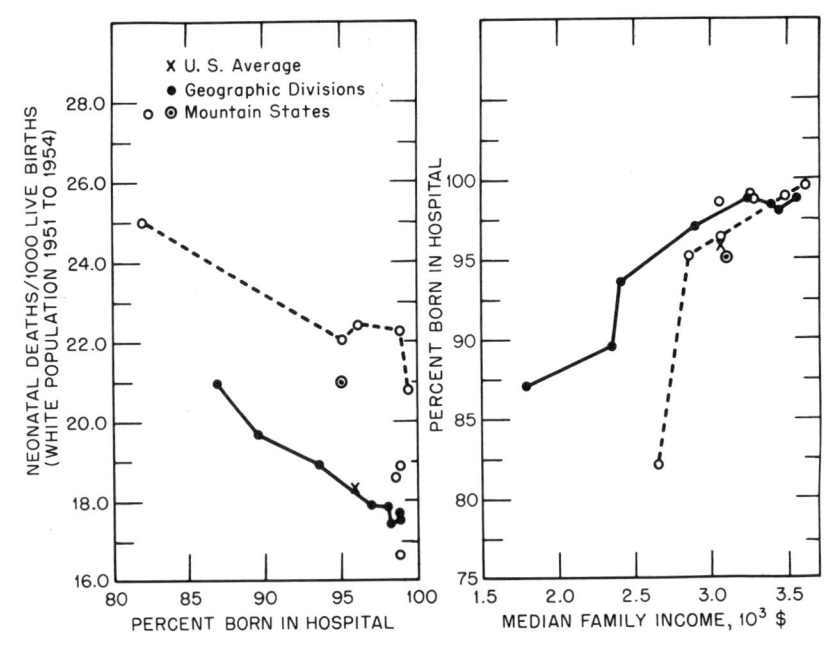

Fig. 8 — *U. S. neonatal death rate for major geographic subdivisions and mountain states vs. births occurring in hospital, correlation between income and hospital birth. As income is a direct function of attained level of education, neonatal mortality can be described as a function of the general level of education in the community. The same trends exist in the general U. S. white population as in the mountain states, but the latter are displaced upward owing to additional geographic factors.*

6. Quality of ascertainment of chosen end point; random noise and signal-to-noise ratio for the event in question.

The prediction of the late effects of low levels of ionizing radiation on animal and human populations has developed to a varying degree for different end points. It has been best developed for general life shortening; for man the prediction would be 1 day/r for low-dose-rate protracted exposures and 5 to 10 days/r for high-dose-rate brief exposures. The estimation of tumor induction rates is less well developed. Though leukemia mortality rates in man have been explored in detail, the probabilities for other tumor types are still quite vague. Generally, the induction probability seems to be about 10^{-6} per rad per man-year at risk for leukemia, thyroid and bone cancers.[15] Ultimately, the most accurate predictions of low-dose effects will have to be in terms of life-table parameters; risks can then be evaluated in relation to both age interval and end point. The continuously changing nature of biological responses to environmental stress will then be properly recognized.

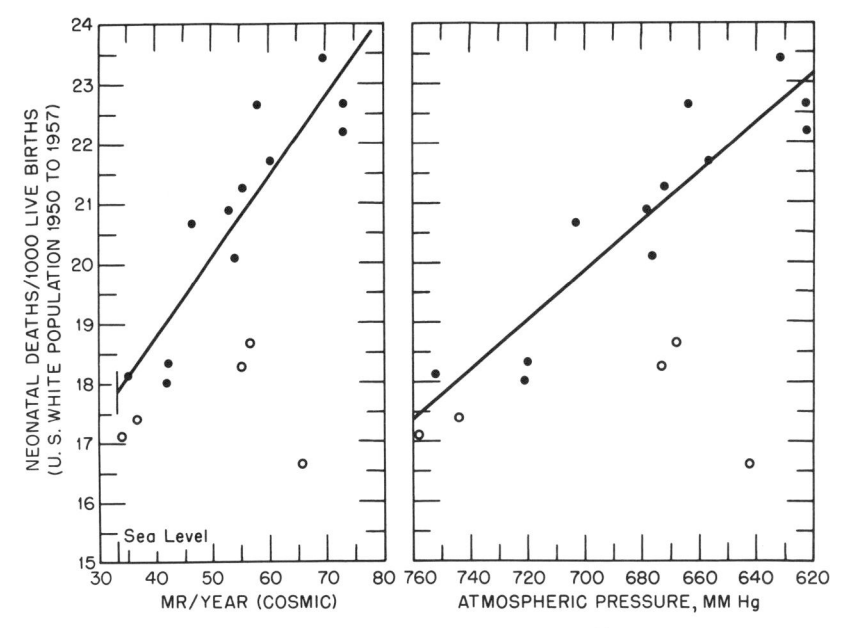

Fig. 9—U. S. neonatal death rate as a function of (1) cosmic radiation and (2) atmospheric pressure or altitude. Death-rate data adjusted for socioeconomic differences. ●, states with commercially useful uranium or helium deposits plus Nebraska and minus Utah. ○, in order of appearance from sea level: Delaware, Illinois—Indiana, Idaho, Montana, Utah. See Ref. 11 for details.

REFERENCES

1. D. Grahn and G. A. Sacher, Fractionation and Protraction and the Late Effects of Radiation in Small Mammals, in *Dose Rate in Mammalian Radiation Biology*, D. G. Brown, R. G. Cragle, and T. R. Noonan, Eds., USAEC Report CONF-780410, pp. 2.1-2.27, 1968.
2. G. A. Sacher, The Gompertz Transformation in the Study of the Injury—Mortality Relationship: Application to Late Radiation Effects and Aging, in *Radiation and Ageing*, P. J. Lindop and G. A. Sacher, Eds., pp. 411-441, Taylor & Francis Ltd., London, 1966.
3. D. Grahn, Genetic Control of Physiological Processes: The Genetics of Radiation Toxicity in Animals, in *Radioisotopes in the Biosphere*, R. C. Caldecott and L. A. Snyder, Eds., pp. 181-200, University of Minnesota, Minneapolis, 1959.
4. G. A. Sacher and D. Grahn, Survival of Mice Under Duration-of-Life Exposure to Gamma Rays. I. The Dosage—Survival Relation and the Lethality Function, *J. Nat. Cancer Inst.*, 32: 277-321 (1964).
5. A. M. Brues and G. A. Sacher, Analysis of Mammalian Radiation Injury and Lethality, in *Symposium on Radiobiology*, J. J. Nickson, Ed., pp. 441-465, John Wiley & Sons, Inc., New York, 1952.
6. G. A. Sacher, On the Statistical Nature of Mortality, with Especial Reference to Chronic Radiation Mortality, *Radiology*, 67: 250-257 (1956).

7. H. B. Jones, A Special Consideration of the Aging Process, Disease, and Life Expectancy, *Advan. Biol. Med. Phys.*, 4: 281-337 (1956).
8. N. I. Berlin, An Analysis of Some Radiation Effects on Mortality, in *The Biology of Aging*, B. L. Strehler, Ed., pp. 121-127, American Institute of Biological Sciences, Washington, D. C., 1960.
9. D. Grahn, Biological Effects of Protracted Low-Dose Radiation Exposure of Man and Animals, in *Colloquium on Late and Subtle Effects of Radiation*, R. J. M. Fry, D. Grahn, and M. L. Griem, Eds., Taylor & Francis Ltd., London, in preparation.
10. A. C. Upton, M. A. Kastenbaum, and J. W. Conklin, Age-Specific Death Rates of Mice Exposed to Ionizing Radiation and Radiomimetic Agents, in *Cellular Basis and Aetiology of Late Somatic Effects of Ionizing Radiation*, R. J. C. Harris, Ed., pp. 285-297, Academic Press, Inc., New York, 1963.
11. D. Grahn and J. Kratchman, Variation in Neonatal Death Rate and Birth Weight in the United States and Possible Relations to Environmental Radiation, Geology, and Altitude, *Amer. J. Hum. Genet.*, 15: 329-352 (1963).
12. D. Grahn, Methodological Problems in the Use of Standard Vital Statistical Data in the Study of Neonatal Mortality and Birth Weight, in *Genetics and the Epidemiology of Chronic Diseases*, J. V. Neel, M. W. Shaw, and W. J. Schull, Eds., pp. 321-335, U. S. Department of Health, Education, and Welfare, Public Health Service Publication No. 1163, 1965.
13. J. P. Wesley, Background Radiation as the Cause of Fatal Congenital Malformation, *Int. J. Radiat. Biol.*, 2: 97-118 (1960).
14. E. J. Sternglass, Evidence for Low-Level Radiation Effects on the Human Embryo and Fetus, in *Radiation Biology of the Fetal and Juvenile Mammal*, Richland, Wash., May 5-8, 1969, Melvin R. Sikov and D. Dennis Mahlum, Eds., AEC Symposium Series (CONF-690501), 1969.
15. A. C. Upton, Effects of Radiation on Man, *Annu. Rev. Nucl. Sci.*, 18: 495-528 (1968).

DISCUSSION

GOFMAN (LRL): What do you consider a "low radiation dose" in man—the total dose, say in a 30-year lifetime, the cumulative dose, exclusive of natural background?

GRAHN: The cumulative dose—less than a kilorad.

GOFMAN: Twenty rads per year is a low dose?

GRAHN: Yes. In other words, the occupational limits are truly low doses.

GOFMAN: In those circumstances you would be the best person to have holding the hand of the Plowshare people. In the somatic area you really do not worry at those levels? The whole area of the Plowshare problem is way below 20 rads per year. However, I am totally unconvinced that such a level is not a problem.

GRAHN: For some end points there may be effects that would trouble you. One thing came out of these data that we should be a little wary of. All the late-life leukemias which up to now have been considered to be fairly insensitive to change by radiation exposure actually showed a progressive elevation of the death rate at 800 to 1100 days of age. So now we do find some evidence that late-life leukemias, reticulum cell sarcomas, etc., are affected by doses below

1 rad/day for a mouse. My "kilorad" limit may have to be pulled down a little.

PARKER: If I understood you correctly, you said your female mice chicken out on litter bearing if they see an X ray. W. L. Russell gave us data on his mice, which were merrily going along having litters. Can you tell us why the southern mice are so much more sexy than the northern ones?

GRAHN: It is not a contradiction but a matter of time after the exposure. The irradiated female will litter for about $2\frac{1}{2}$ litters over the first 50 days postexposure, then she will quit. From there on out the somatic interactions become important.

COHEN (LRL): I believe on your charts (Fig. 9) you plotted data points at 520 mb. That is equivalent to an altitude of over 15,000 ft.

GRAHN: It could not have been quite that high. The highest point I had was Leadville—Climax. There are a few people in Climax and 8000 in Leadville. They actually have about 50 births a year in Leadville. The altitude is 10,800 ft.

FINKLEA: Do you associate the dependence of your infant mortality on altitude with a radiation effect?

GRAHN: No, I was not trying to develop the whole argument here; I was just trying to use it as a vehicle to demonstrate problems of prediction.

FINKLEA: Looking at the Mormon population and what is known of the physiology of smoking, it is possible that some of the variations in altitude dependence could better be explained on the basis of a respiratory effect or hypoxia.

GRAHN: Yes. If you look at the data on altitude physiology, the effect on the fetus is largely one of hypoxia. The mother becomes unable to maintain sufficient placental transfer of oxygen to support the normal weight accumulation of the fetus.

FINKLEA: Twenty cigarettes per day will convert about one-fifth of circulating hemoglobin into carboxy hemoglobin. Birth weights in Baltimore and other places where smoking mothers have been studied are less than those of babies from nonsmokers. Mothers with various cardiovascular deficiencies or valvular defects also have small babies.

GRAHN: The smoking effect is not very big. The altitude effect is large and consistent. This is still true after correction for the fact that average income and average education in Utah is a notch above the neighboring states. They are also a little bit younger population.

FINKLEA: Certainly the smoking effect should be greatly accentuated with increasing altitude, particularly with the increased oxygen demands of pregnancy.

GRAHN: Yes, I guess a nonlinear relation with altitude in smokers.

RADIATION REPAIR MECHANISMS IN MAMMALIAN CELLS

J. E. CLEAVER
Laboratory of Radiobiology, University of California Medical Center,
San Francisco, California

ABSTRACT

Mammalian cells use several biochemical mechanisms to repair or tolerate DNA damage. Breaks caused by X rays in the DNA chain are rejoined rapidly; damage to DNA bases caused by ultraviolet light is repaired by removal of the damage and synthesis of a replacement region. Only a small fraction of the damage caused by ultraviolet light (pyrimidine dimers) is excised, and this particular repair system may be inefficient in mammalian cells. A human hereditary disease, xeroderma pigmentosum, appears to be defective at the excision step of repair. Unexcised damage interferes with DNA replication such that newly synthesized strands contain numerous gaps; the number of gaps increases as a function of the amount of damage. The gaps are joined by a process that can be inhibited by caffeine. The correlation of a high incidence of cancer with defective repair in xeroderma pigmentosum indicates that unrepaired DNA damage may be implicated in some forms of carcinogenesis.

During the first half of this century the emphasis in radiobiology was placed on the means whereby radiation damages and kills cells and animals. A subtle shift in emphasis has taken place over the past 10 years, and now the current and very fashionable interest is in the question of why radiation damage does not always kill. Originally we considered that many cells in a population survive irradiation because they receive no damage to critical target molecules. This consideration was based on the random distribution of absorbed energy and led to the target and hit theories of radiobiology. In their simplest form, these theories said, "If radiation hits a critical region of a cell or animal, it kills; if it misses, then the organism survives." Another reason for survival could be that the amount of radiation damage received is insufficient for killing. Damage may be insufficient because a cell has many copies of important molecules and can simply discard damaged ones and synthesize replacements or because the cell can recognize damage and render it innocuous. This latter possibility, by which we imply the operation of repair mechanisms, is a very interesting and important one.

The subject of repair has become so fashionable, unfortunately, that it is now a standard way to interpret incomprehensible results. Everything that occurs in irradiated organisms is interpreted by some people as evidence for repair systems. To prove that we do indeed observe a repair process, we must at least show that the process (1) is a response to damage, (2) restores the original structure, and (3) contributes to the survival of irradiated cells. It may not be possible to satisfy all these criteria in a single experiment, but they should be applied to any claim concerning repair processes.

Unbeknown to man until recently, living creatures have long been aware of the hazards of radiation and have evolved biochemical mechanisms to modify and repair radiation and other damage. The importance of such mechanisms is seen in their widespread occurrence in most living creatures. I will concentrate my discussion on the repair in mammalian cells (human and rodent). These processes are typical of those found in the smallest organism, in Mycoplasma,[1] in bacteria,[2] and in other microorganisms[3] and higher organisms.[4,5] In addition to such long-established characteristics of living creatures as motility and reproduction, we may well add the characteristic of self repair. Creatures that have lost the ability to repair[5] are very sickly indeed, as will be shown later.

CELL KILLING BY ULTRAVIOLET LIGHT AND DRUGS

Repair obviously involves biochemical mechanisms that function after radiation damage has occurred. Therefore we must distinguish among the welter of things that occur in irradiated organisms, those which represent repair leading to survival and those which represent death and general cellular breakdown. Damage to whole tissues by radiation or other agents is usually repaired by synthesis of new cells to replace dead ones.[6] In this discussion, however, I am concerned with intracellular repair in individual cells from animals or man.

Some insight into repair in irradiated cells is obtained by the use of drugs given to cells after irradiation. Many bacteria and mammalian cell types show a synergism between ultraviolet (UV) light and acriflavin or caffeine (Fig. 1) when these drugs are supplied after irradiation.[7,8] We can see several ways in which such synergism could arise.

1. An increased permeability of irradiated cells which allows more of the drug to enter irradiated cells.

2. Interaction between the drugs and radiation products to produce a poison.
3. Alterations in cell growth rates by the drugs that indirectly modify the expression of radiation damage.
4. Inhibition of biochemical repair systems by the drugs.

In all likelihood, caffeine and acriflavin interfere with specific biochemical repair systems. The stages at which these drugs act will be discussed later.

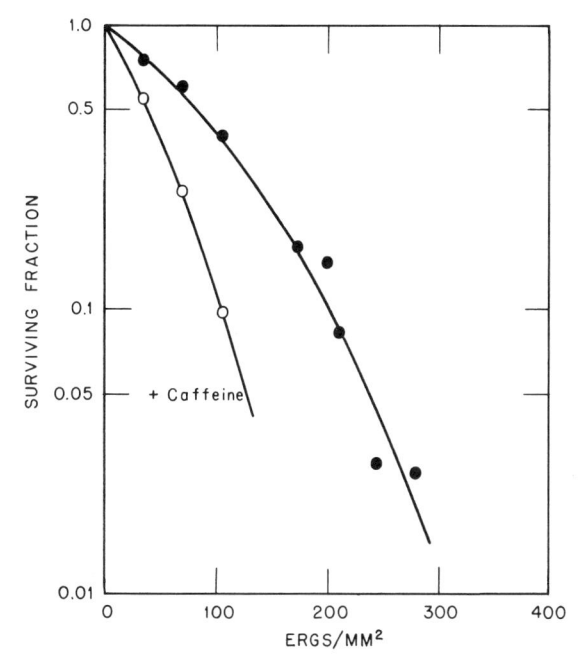

Fig. 1 — Survival curves for Chinese hamster (DFAF) cells irradiated with ultraviolet light and grown in Eagle's basal medium, 10% fetal calf serum, and supplemented with 10^{-3} M caffeine. (J. E. Cleaver, unpublished experiments.)

IMPORTANT BIOLOGICAL MOLECULES AND REPAIR

The response of a cell to radiation depends on the nature of the molecules damaged and the damage itself. Most molecules in a cell are present in numerous copies, e.g., sugars, amino acids, phospholipids, and enzymes. Damage to a large fraction of these molecules can be handled by simply throwing away the damaged ones and synthesizing new ones. Only molecules which are crucial for cell survival and which are present in few copies must be repaired rather than replaced. The genetic material, deoxyribonucleic acid (DNA) consists mainly of molecules that are unique in the information they carry. The discovery of repetitive nucleotide sequences in DNA of higher organisms does not invalidate this argument since in most mammalian species at least half the DNA is in the form of unique sequences.[9] It is not surprising, therefore, that radiation repair mechanisms are concerned exclusively (as far as we know) with damage to DNA.

NATURE OF RADIATION DAMAGE TO DNA

We can distinguish, in an approximate manner, three kinds of chemical change in DNA that could interfere with its function (Fig. 2). These changes can be caused by radiation, drugs, or carcinogenic agents.

1. Chain breaks: single- or double-chain breaks are the main results of ionizing radiation.[10,11] These breaks can be very complex and may involve some damage to the bases adjacent to the break itself (Fig. 3).

2. Base damage without chain breakage: this is the main result of irradiation with UV light[12,13] or treatment with certain drugs[14] or carcinogens.[15]

3. Cross-linking: this may occur between strands, between adjacent DNA molecules, or between DNA and protein.[16,17] This damage is much more difficult to characterize than that described in the preceding paragraph because of the large number of possible compounds that can be formed and can be a result of UV light, X rays, or chemical agents.

It is important to note that most of these forms of damage involve mainly one DNA strand and that the information in DNA is coded in duplicate in the base sequences on opposite strands. The reason for such redundancy in stored information could well be to protect genetic information from loss due to chemical or radiation damage.

The most famous damage to DNA is the dimer formed between adjacent pyrimidine molecules in DNA strands after irradiation[12,13] with UV light (Fig. 4). This is very important for bacterial radiation damage but less so for mammalian cells.[13] Next I shall use UV light as an example of an agent that causes predominantly base damage as opposed to X rays which cause predominantly chain breaks.

POSSIBLE MECHANISMS OF REPAIR

The repair of DNA damage can be considered as a straightforward engineering problem. We have a double-stranded molecule with infor-

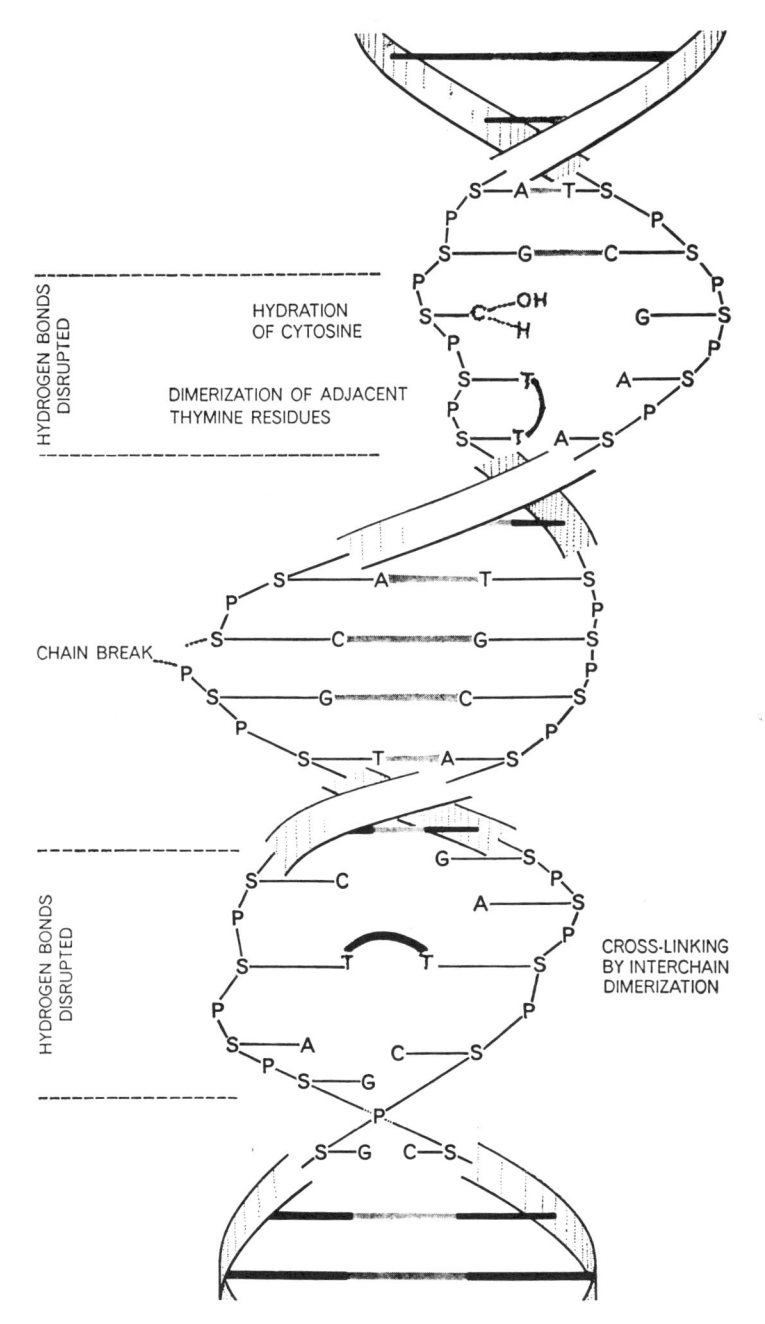

Fig. 2—*DNA molecule illustrating possible forms of radiation damage, chain breakage, base damage, and cross-linkage.* [From R. A. Deering, Sci. Amer., 207 (6): 144 (December 1962).]

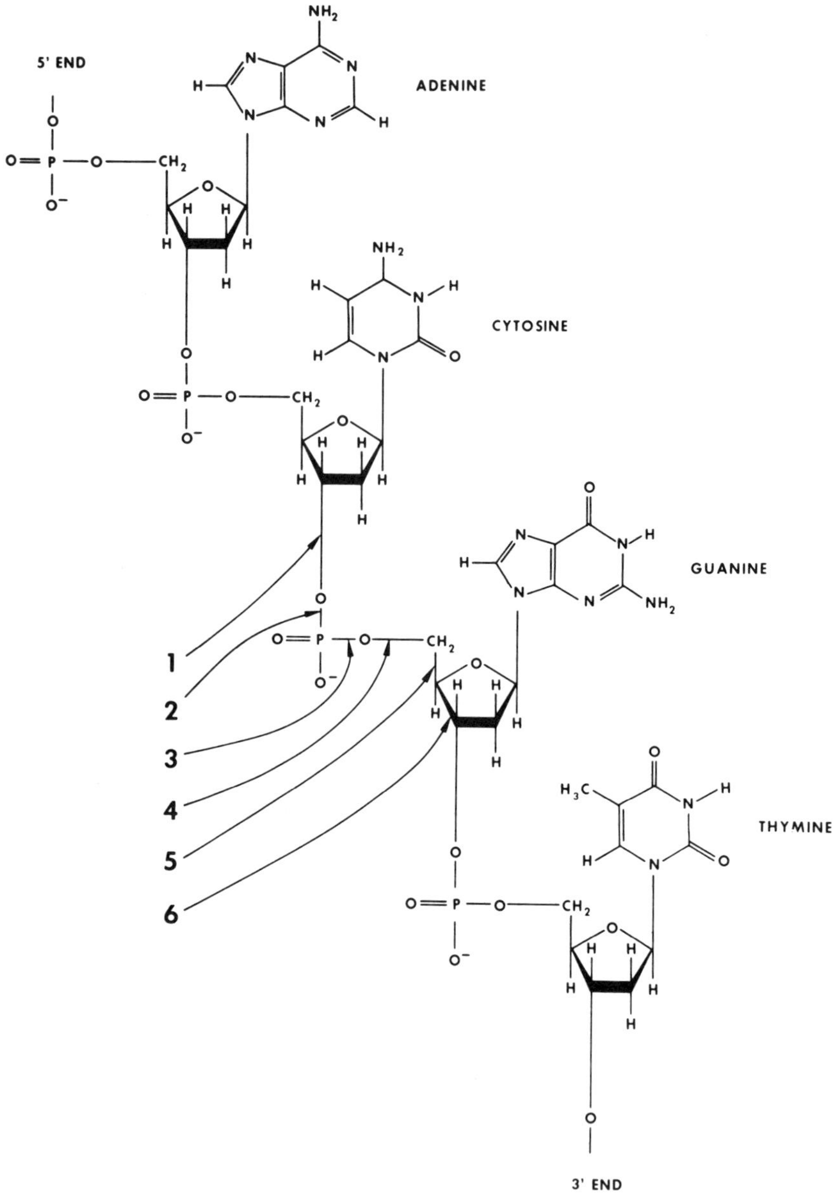

Fig. 3—*One DNA polynucleotide chain indicating the six different bonds (1 to 6) that compose the linear continuity of the chain. Breakage of any of these bonds will interrupt the chain to produce a single-strand break in DNA.*

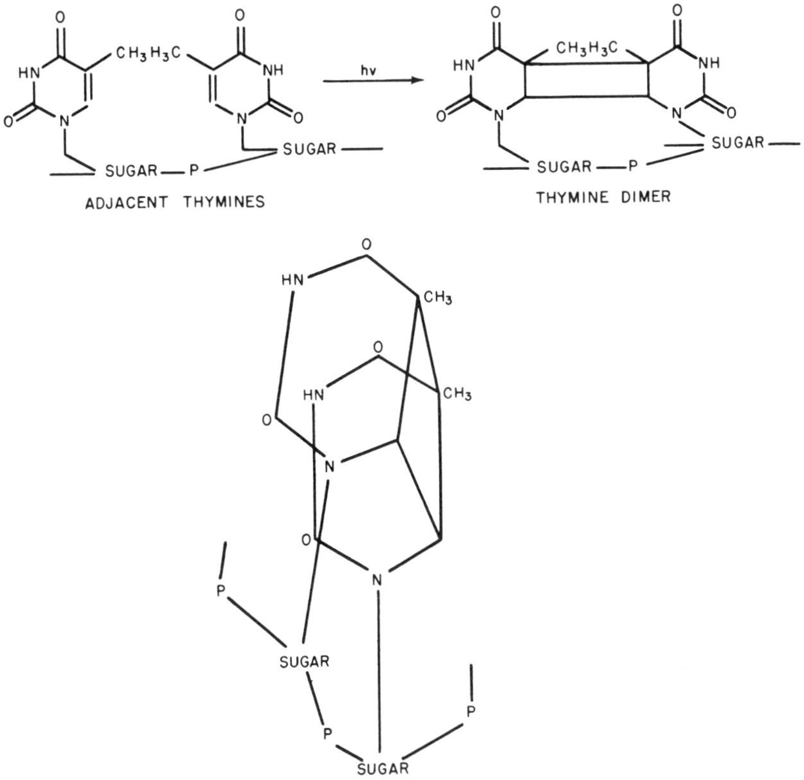

Fig. 4— The thymine dimer formed between four adjacent thymines on a polynucleotide chain. [Top: from R. B. Setlow, in Mammalian Cytogenetic and Related Problems in Radiobiology, *p. 292, C. Pavan et al., Eds., Pergamon Press, Inc., 1964. Bottom: from R. B. Setlow, Science, 153: 379-386, Fig. 1 (1966).]*

mation coded in duplicate on opposite strands, and we have to repair the damage it has suffered without excessive loss of information. There are several ways this can be done, and, with few exceptions, mammalian and bacterial cells use them all.

1. The damage can be corrected in situ if it is not very extensive. This can be done for the thymine dimer. It is split into two monomers by an enzyme that uses energy from visible light (photoreactivation[18]). This enzymatic process is present throughout biological species except for mammals.[19,20] Since we are concentrating on mammalian cells, I will say no more about this process.

2. Chain breaks[21,22] that do not involve damage to bases adjacent to the breaks can be rejoined enzymatically by polynucleotide ligase if the break leaves a 3'hydroxylgroup and a 5'phosphate group (Fig. 3). If

bases are also damaged, they will have to be replaced, and rejoining will then require a complex sequence of enzymatic steps.[23,24]

3. Base damage must be corrected by cutting out the damaged regions and replacing the bases. The correct base sequence is then determined by the intact opposite strand (Fig. 5). This process may be involved in correcting base damage from UV light, drugs, or X rays.

4. Damage may be ignored until the cell has to separate the DNA strands to replicate the DNA. Then, if damage is on one strand only, the opposite undamaged strand may be used to synthesize both new strands and so minimize, though not repair, the effects of base damage.

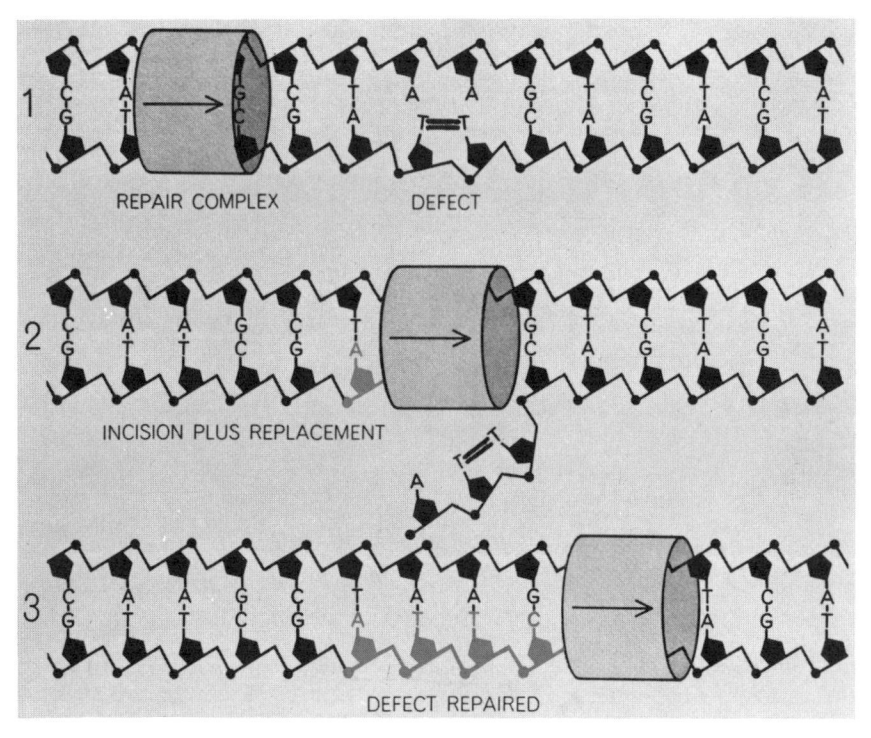

Fig. 5 — Possible scheme for the repair of damage to DNA bases by excision of damaged regions and insertion of new regions. [From P. C. Hanawalt and R. H. Haynes, Sci. Amer., 216 (2): 42-43 (February 1967).]

REPAIR OF SINGLE-STRAND BREAKS

Breaks in the polynucleotide strands of DNA can be conveniently studied by denaturing the molecule with strong alkali and measuring the molecular weights of the resulting single-strand pieces. In such measurements, low molecular weights imply that there were many breaks in the single strands of the original molecules; high molecular weights imply there were few breaks. The molecular weights[25] can be measured by placing whole cells onto an alkaline sucrose density gradient and determining the sedimentation rate of DNA molecules (Fig. 6). The pH of the alkaline (12.0 to 12.5) is sufficiently high for most cellular constituents (proteins and RNA) to be denatured and degraded

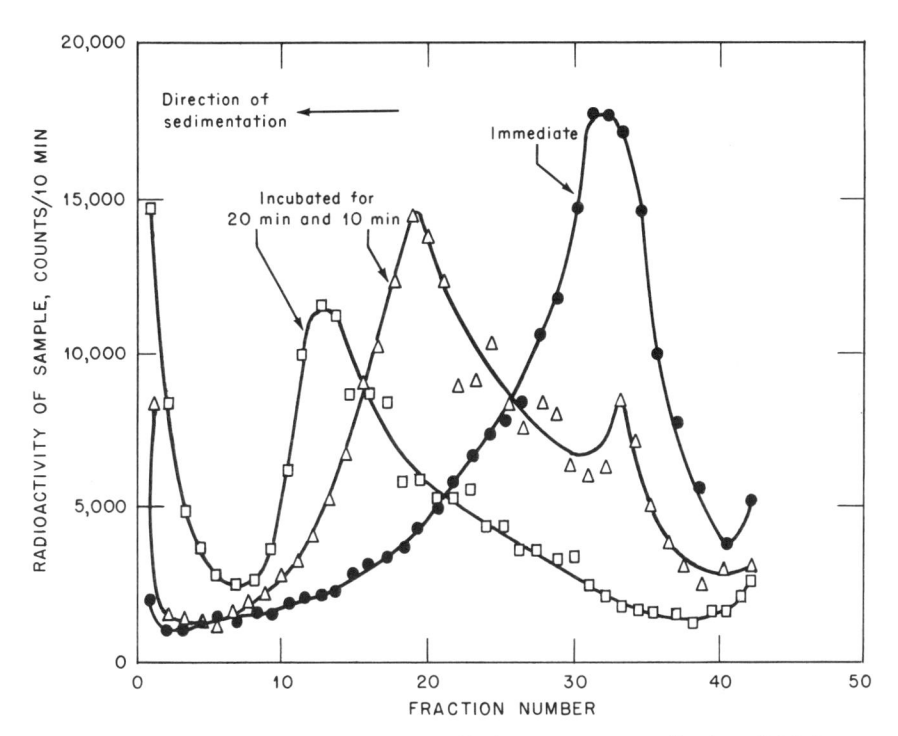

Fig. 6—Sedimentation profiles in alkaline sucrose gradients, pH 12.5, of DNA from mouse lymphoblasts (L5178Y) at various times after irradiation with 30 krads of X rays under nitrogen. [From J. T. Lett, I. Caldwell, C. J. Dean, and P. Alexander, Nature, 214: 790 (1967).]

into small molecules and for DNA to be denatured into single strands. In such a gradient the DNA sedimentation rate during centrifugation is a function of the molecular weight (Fig. 6).[25] After irradiation with X rays, the sedimentation rate is reduced; this indicates that the DNA now contains single-strand breaks, and the denatured single strands have a reduced molecular weight (Fig. 7). If cells are allowed to grow after irradiation for 10 or 20 min at 37°C, the sedimentation rate increases, which is an indication that the breaks have been rejoining and the molecular weight consequently increased (Fig. 6).

This is the main evidence for a repair system in mammalian cells which rejoins single-strand breaks caused by X rays. The rejoining

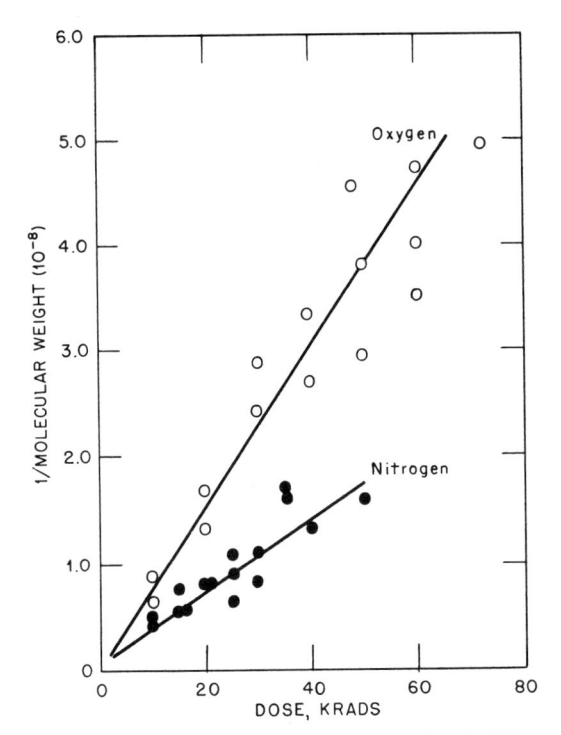

Fig. 7—Changes in the average molecular weight of DNA from mouse lymphoblasts (L5178Y) after irradiation with X rays under oxygen or nitrogen. The efficiency of breakage is 70 ev per break under nitrogen and 70 or 50 ev per break under oxygen. [From J. T. Lett, I. Caldwell, C. J. Dean, and P. Alexander, Nature, 214: 790 (1967).]

process may be complex because X-ray breaks may involve damage to the polynucleotide chain adjacent to the actual break though probably not more than one damaged base or sugar per break (Fig. 3). The least we can say is that the breaks are rejoined in some manner very soon after they have been produced by ionizing radiation. They probably have little to do with cell killing because of the efficient repair that occurs even after high radiation doses.

REPAIR THROUGH A "BYPASS" MECHANISM

Since DNA is double stranded and its information is present in duplicate, cells need not correct base damage on one strand if they can make do with information on the other strand. Such a situation may occur during DNA replication when there is base damage. The regions of interest in this process are the newly synthesized DNA strands that must be made from parental DNA containing damaged bases. These can be studied using the same alkaline sucrose gradient techniques we have discussed for X-ray damage and repair.

If we measure the molecular weight of the newly synthesized DNA strands using an alkaline sucrose gradient, the strands made immediately after irradiation appear to have a molecular weight that decreases with increasing doses of UV light (Fig. 8). If we label cells for 30 min im-

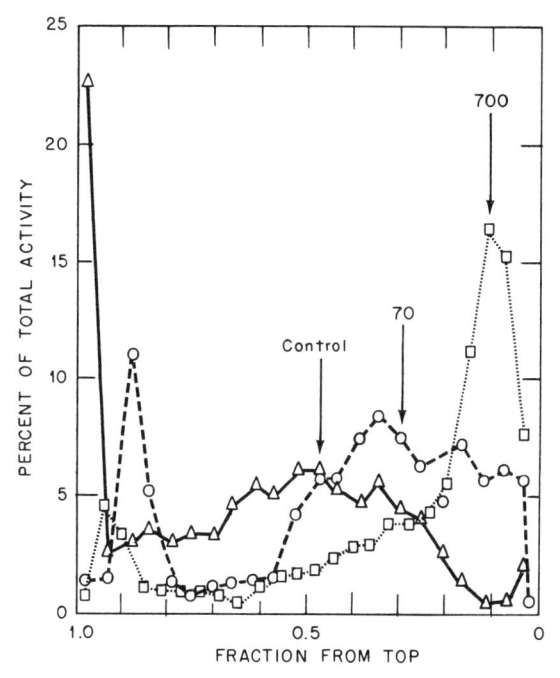

Fig. 8—Sedimentation profiles in alkaline sucrose gradients, pH 12.5, of ^{3}H-labeled DNA from Chinese hamster (V79) cells irradiated with ultraviolet light, labeled for 30 min with ^{3}H–TdR and placed on the gradients immediately. (J. E. Cleaver, unpublished experiments.)

mediately after irradiation and then allow them to grow for 6 hr in nonradioactive medium, the labeled strands all increase in molecular weight. This increase is much less in irradiated cells grown in caffeine (Fig. 9), though in control cells the increase is unaffected by caffeine.

It could be that damage to the parental DNA strands interferes with their use as templates for synthesis of new strands. Gaps are left opposite the damage, and the new strands are all in short pieces (Fig. 10). These gaps are filled, either by insertion of bases at random or with bases specified by the other undamaged strand of the parental molecule. Insertion of random bases would restore the continuity of the DNA strands but would cause a high error or mutation rate. Inhibition of this rejoining process by caffeine (Fig. 9) may be the way in

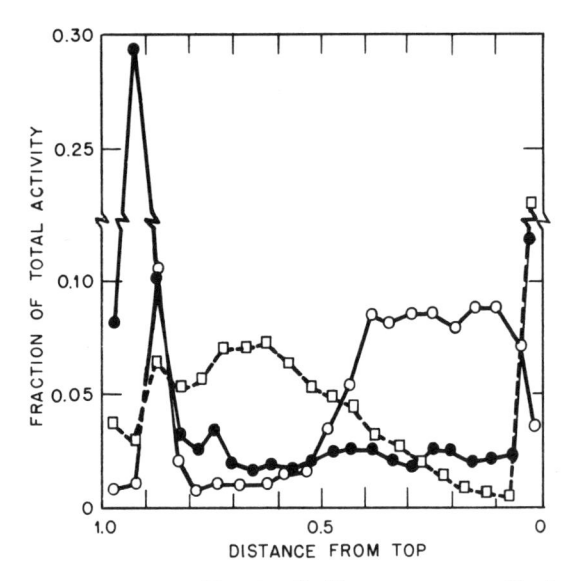

Fig. 9—Sedimentation profiles in alkaline sucrose gradients, pH 12.5, of ³H-labeled DNA from Chinese hamster (V79) cells irradiated with ultraviolet light, labeled for 30 min with ³H—TdR, and grown for 6 hr in nonradioactive medium before being placed on the gradients. (J. E. Cleaver, unpublished experiments.)

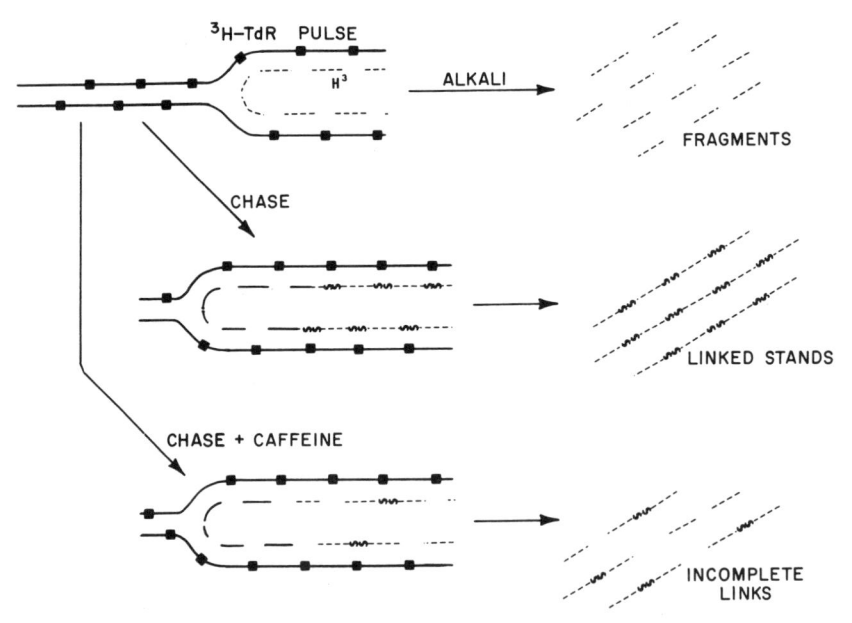

Fig. 10—Possible scheme by which DNA is synthesized in short pieces when base damage is on the parental molecule, and the intervening gaps joined later. Caffeine may interfere with the joining process. Also illustrated are the fragments observed after alkaline denaturation. (See Figs. 8 and 9.)

which caffeine kills cells irradiated with UV light. In the presence of caffeine, some gaps remain in the DNA strands with consequent lethal effects. This particular rejoining process has only recently been discovered in bacteria[26] and mammalian[27] cells, but there is a possibility it may be one of the most important processes for handling DNA damage.

REPAIR OF BASE DAMAGE

To demonstrate repair of base damage, we must show that damaged regions are removed from DNA and new regions inserted. The former is difficult unless the damage can be characterized chemically and detected easily in very low concentrations in the presence of other cellular constituents. The replacement of damage by new regions can be demonstrated fairly easily, however. This necessitates the use of a method which enables us to distinguish between a small "patch" put into preexistent DNA molecules and the synthesis of new molecules because both processes may occur after irradiation. Such a method was first devised by Pettijohn and Hanawalt[2] at Stanford. In their method, DNA is labeled by growing cells in a precursor that is both radioactive and heavier than the normal precursor and isolated on the basis of its density in an equilibrium-density gradient of cesium chloride. The most suitable heavy precursor for mammalian cells is bromouracil deoxyriboside (BrUdR: mol. wt., 308), which is an analogue of thymidine (TdR: mol. wt., 242) (Fig. 11). The principle of the method

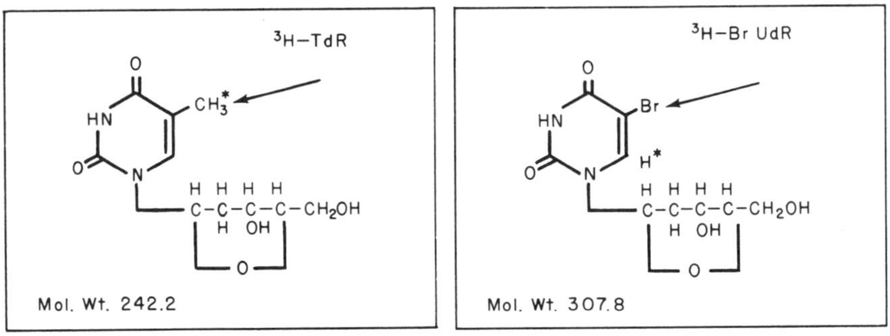

Fig. 11—*Molecules of bromouracil deoxyriboside and thymidine.*

(Fig. 12) is that normal semiconservative DNA replication in the presence of ^{3}H−BrUdR produces DNA molecules that have newly synthesized strands containing ^{3}H−BrU. These molecules will be denser than normal owing to the bromine atoms and will be ^{3}H-labeled. A repaired molecule will only have small patches of ^{3}H−BrU, which do not affect the density but do label the molecules with ^{3}H. In DNA isolated

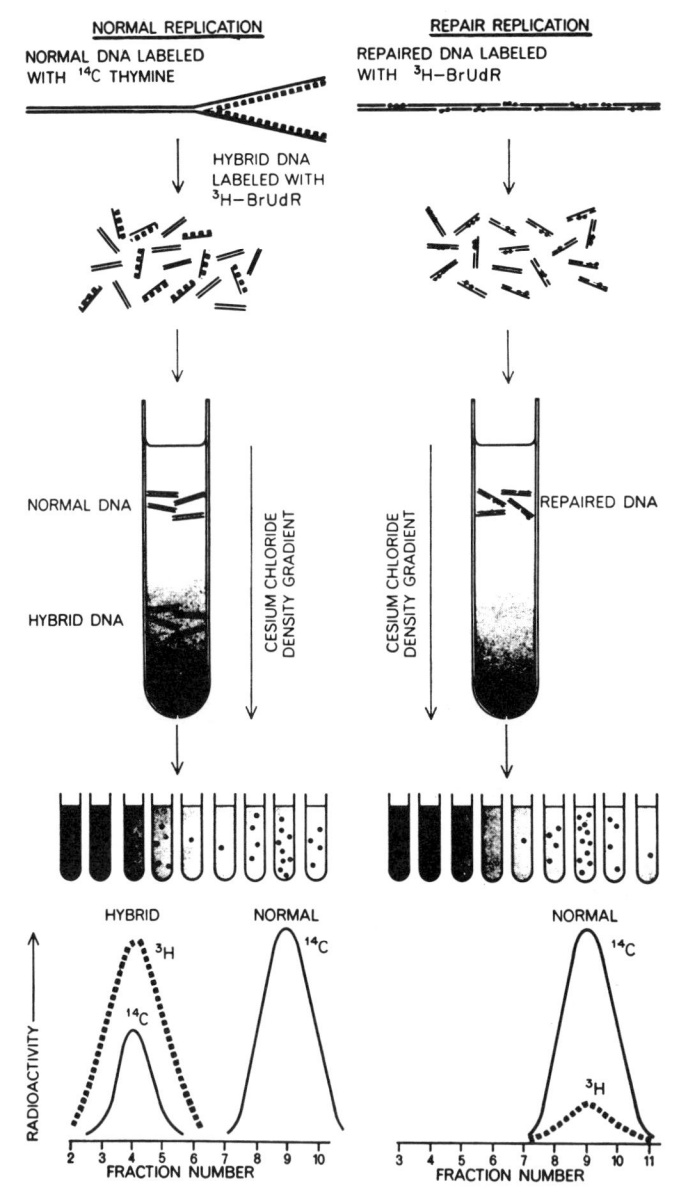

Fig. 12— *Cesium chloride equilibrium-density gradient technique used for isolated DNA labeled with $^3H-BrUdR$ by semiconservative or repair replication. Parental DNA labeled with ^{14}C, newly synthesized DNA labeled with $^3H-BrUdR$. [From P. C. Hanawalt and R. H. Haynes, Sci. Amer., 216 (2): 42-43 (February 1967).]*

from cells that were labeled with ^{3}H−BrUdR after irradiation, we can therefore say that ^{3}H-labeled molecules, which are denser than normal, represent normal semiconservative replication; ^{3}H-labeled molecules of normal density represent repair replication. Experiments[28,29] with normal and malignant cells from most mammalian species show that repair replication is widespread (Fig. 13), though it has different efficiencies in different species and saturates at a low UV dose (Fig. 14). Repair replication occurs[30] also after damage due to X rays but does

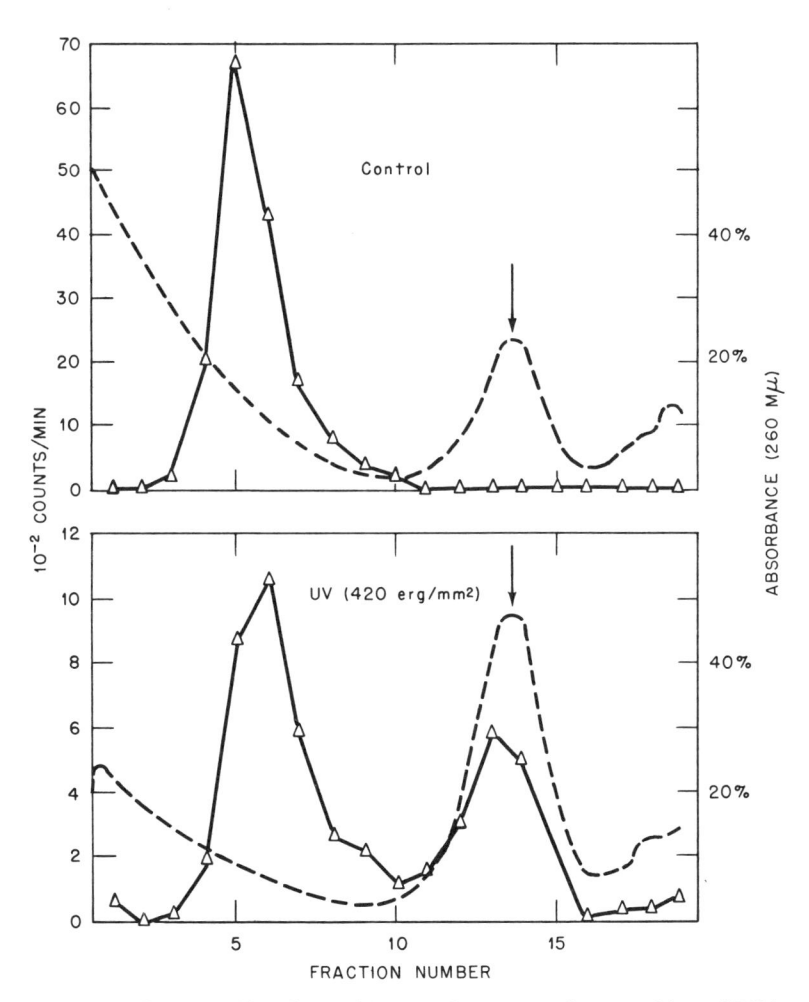

Fig. 13 — Cesium chloride equilibrium-density gradient profiles of DNA from normal human fibroblasts labeled for 1 hr with BrUdR, irradiated with UV light and labeled for 4 hr in ^{3}H−BrUdR (20 µCi/ml, 5 µg/ml). ----, absorbance 260 mµ; —▲—, ^{3}H activity. Arrows mark position of normal density DNA.

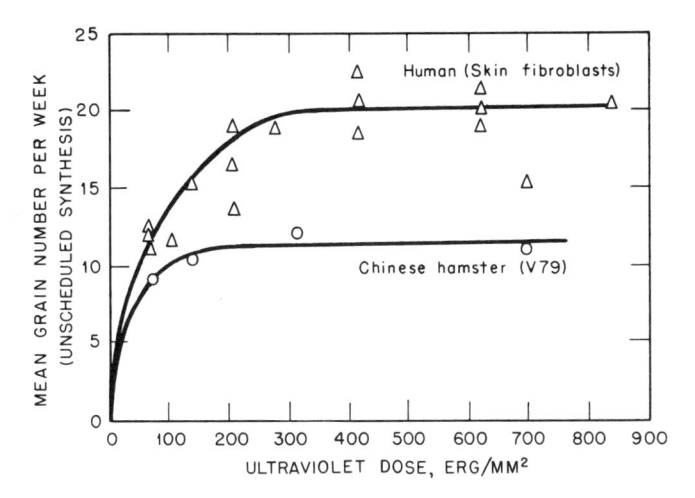

Fig. 14—*Amounts of unscheduled synthesis (an autoradiographic measure of repair of base damage) in human fibroblasts and Chinese hamster (V79) cells as a function of the dose of UV light.*

not saturate with dose up to 10^5R. The repair replication process is resistant to many drugs that inhibit normal DNA replication (e.g., hydroxyurea, fluorodeoxyuridine, and 5-aminouracil) and is only inhibited by drugs which bind to the DNA molecule or which inhibit almost every enzymatic process in the cell (e.g., high levels of actinomycin D, iodoacetate, and acriflavine).[31]

An interesting cell type[32,33] is that from human patients suffering from the hereditary disease xeroderma pigmentosum (Fig. 15). Both fibroblasts[5,30] and epithelial cells[34] from the skin of these patients are unable to perform repair replication after irradiation with UV light (i.e., they cannot repair base damage) (Fig. 16). The defect of this disease[30] probably lies at an early stage of repair because damage involving chain breaks is repaired to the same extent as in normal cells (Fig. 17). I have studied the premature-aging disease progeria and a few other genetically determined skin diseases, but none have shown qualitative defects in repair similar to xeroderma pigmentosum.[27]

DNA REPAIR AND CANCER

Xeroderma pigmentosum may hold a clue to a mechanism of carcinogenesis, since its main clinical symptom is an extremely high incidence of skin cancer induced by UV light (usually from sunlight). But we cannot say, naively, that cells which lack repair systems become malignant because many malignant cells can perform repair replication.[4,28,29] The relevance, if any, of xeroderma pig-

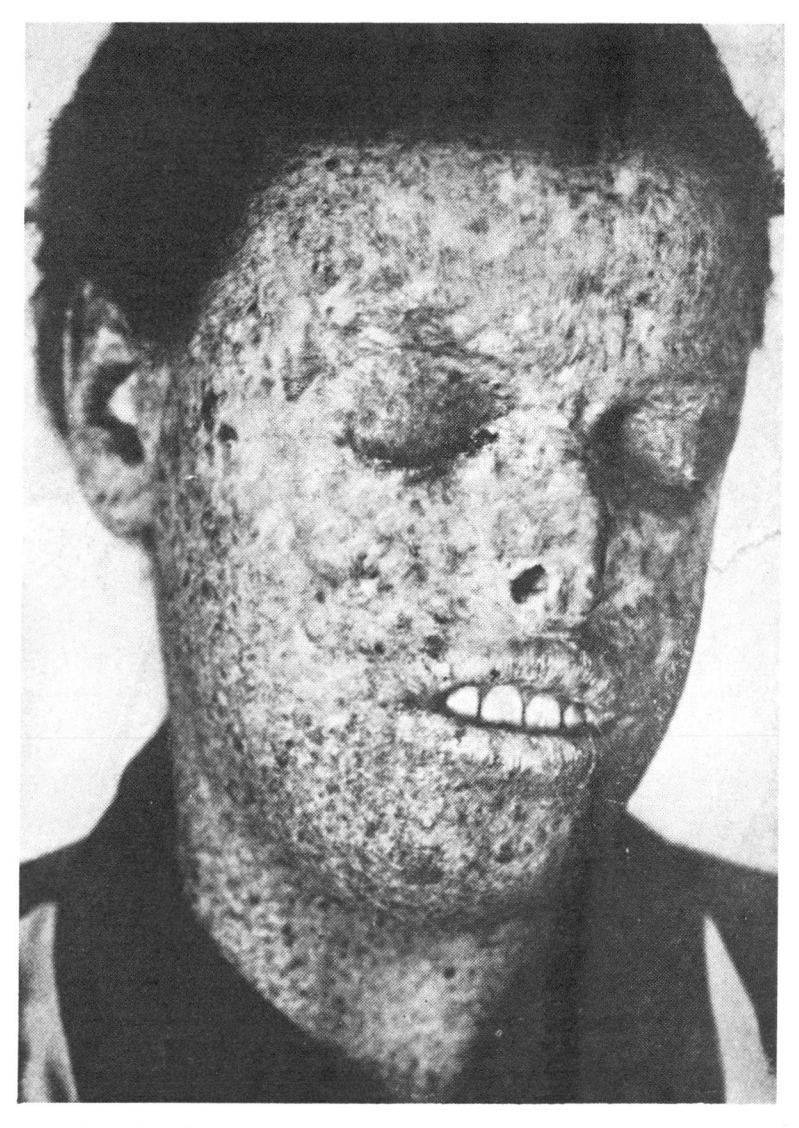

Fig. 15—*Xeroderma pigmentosum showing lentigines, atrophy, and scars due to removal of carcinomas. Tumors on the corneas have destroyed the vision. Death occurred from cancer at age 19 years. (From G. C. Andrews and A. N. Domonkas,* Diseases of the Skin, *5th ed. p. 73, Fig. 16, W. B. Saunders Co., Philadelphia, Pa., 1954.)*

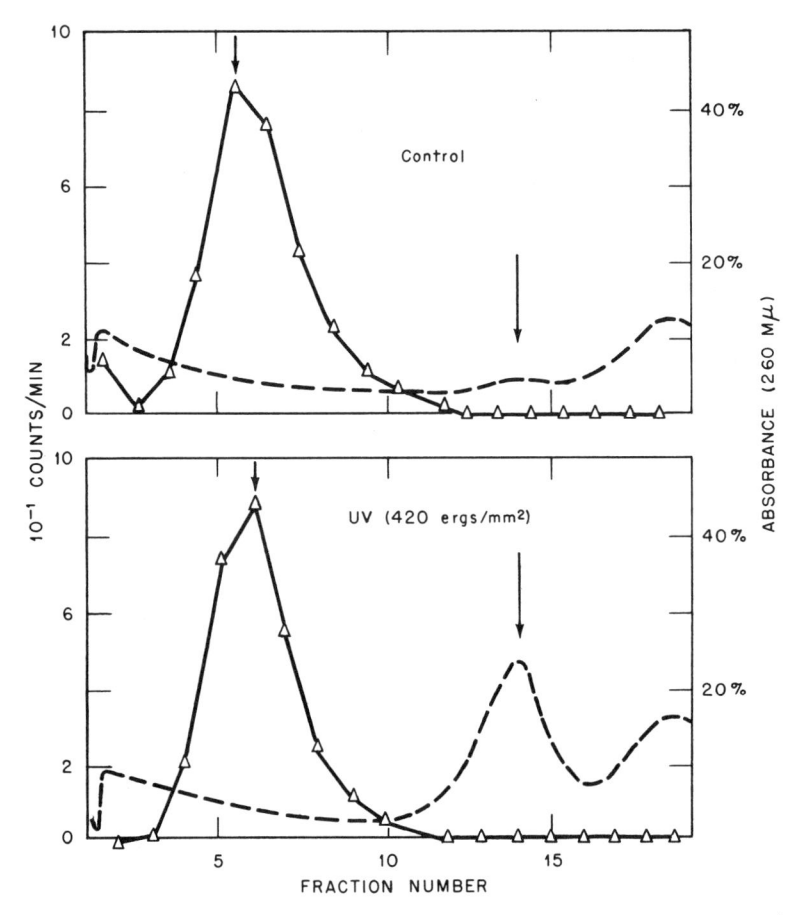

Fig. 16— Cesium chloride equilibrium-density gradient profiles of DNA from homozygous xeroderma pigmentosum fibroblasts labeled for 1 hr in BrUdR, irradiated with UV light, and labeled for 4 hr with ^{3}H—BrUdR (20 μCi/ml, 5 μg/ml). ----, absorbance 260 m; —△—, ^{3}H activity. Arrows mark positions of normal density DNA and DNA with BrU in one strand.

mentosum to a general theory of carcinogenesis is more subtle. The results at least enable us to resurrect the somatic mutation theory of cancer[35] with the possibility that somatic mutation may be produced from unrepaired base damage. I base my present thoughts on the hypothesis that the repair system detected as repair replication may be inefficient in mammalian cells. At least one form of base damage, the pyrimidine dimer, is only removed from mammalian DNA to a small extent,[36-38] and the repair system saturates at relatively low radiation doses (Fig. 14). The difference between normal cells and xeroderma pigmentosum cells may be the difference between correcting a small fraction of base damage or correcting none. In normal individuals carcinogenesis from radiations and some chemicals may perhaps be caused by somatic mutations that arise because mammalian cells have inherently inefficient repair mechanisms. But, better a low efficiency than none at all.

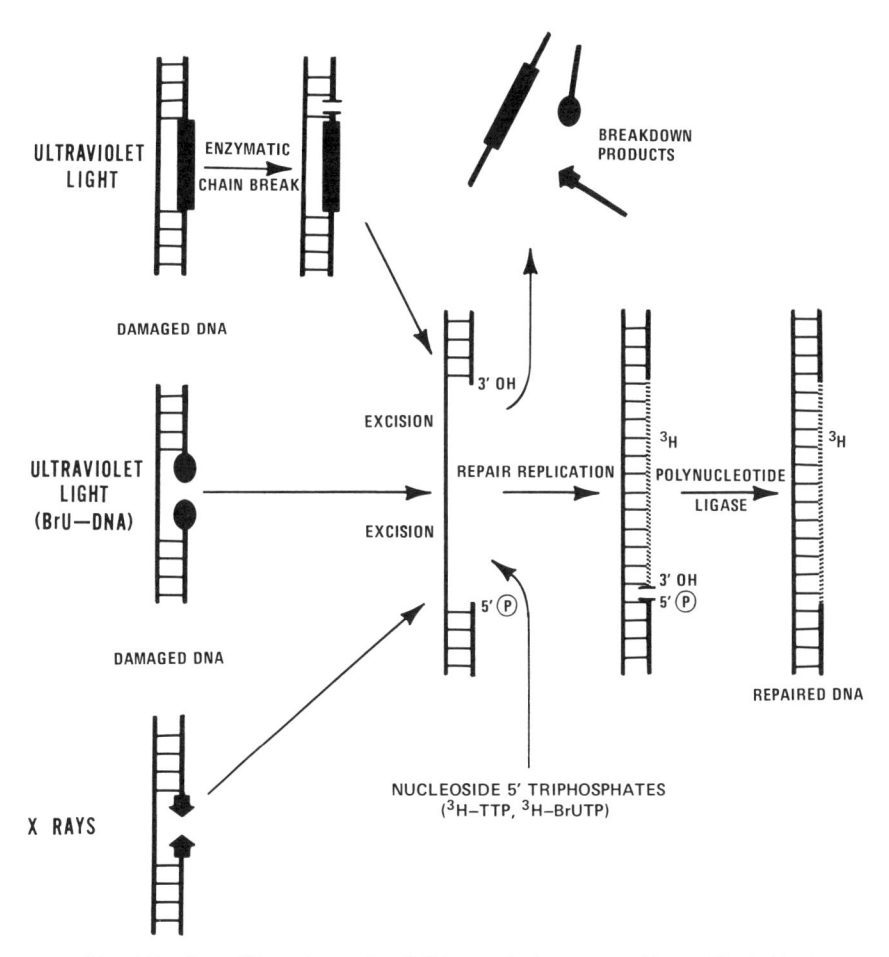

Fig. 17—*Possible scheme for DNA repair in mammalian cells indicating common pathways for repair of base damage and single-strand breaks. The scheme illustrates the necessary stages of repair but not every chemical reaction. Xeroderma pigmentosum fibroblasts are defective in the enzymatic breakage step for UV damage, but do repair both types of single-strand breakage.* [From J. E. Cleaver, Xeroderma Pigmentosum: A Human Disease Defective in an Initial Stage of DNA Repair, Proc. Nat. Acad. Sci., U. S., 63: 428(1969).]

ACKNOWLEDGMENTS

I am grateful to the U. S. Atomic Energy Commission and the scientists and staff of the Laboratory of Radiobiology for providing the support, facilities, and milieu without which this work could never have been pursued.

REFERENCES

1. D. W. Smith, Properties of the Growing Point Region in Bacteria and DNA Replication in PPLO, Ph. D. Dissertation, Stanford University, California, 1967.
2. D. Pettijohn and P. C. Hanawalt, Evidence for Repair Replication of UV-Damaged DNA in Bacteria, *J. Mol. Biol.*, 9: 38 (1964).
3. C. F. Brunk and P. C. Hanawalt, Repair of Damaged DNA in a Eukaryotic Cell: *Tetrahymena pyriformis, Science,* 158: 663 (1967).
4. J. E. Cleaver and R. B. Painter, Repair of Damaged Human Cell DNA, *Biochim. Biophys. Acta,* 161: 552 (1968).
5. J. E. Cleaver, Defective Repair Replication in Xeroderma Pigmentosum, *Nature,* 218: 652 (1968).
6. H. M. Patt, Radiobiology of Cell Renewal Systems, in *Effects of Radiation on Cellular Proliferation and Differentiation,* Symposium Proceedings, Monaco, 1968, p.3, International Atomic Energy Agency, Vienna, 1968 (STI/PUB/186).
7. W. Harm, Differential Effects of Acriflavine and Caffeine on Various UV-Irradiated *E. coli* Strains and T1 Phage, *Mutat. Res.,* 4: 93 (1967).
8. A. M. Rauth, Evidence for Dark Reactivation by UV Light Damage in Mouse L Cells, *Radiat. Res.,* 31: 121 (1967).
9. R. J. Britten and D. E. Kohne, Repeated Sequences in DNA, *Science,* 161: 529 (1968).
10. D. Freifelder, Rate of Production of Single-Strand Breaks in DNA by X-Irradiation In Situ, *J. Mol. Biol.,* 35: 303 (1968).
11. J. T. Lett, I. Caldwell, C. J. Dean, and P. Alexander, Rejoining of X-Ray Induced Breaks in the DNA of Leukemic Cells, *Nature,* 214: 790 (1967).
12. R. B. Setlow, Cyclobutane-Type Pyrimidine Dimers in Polynucleotides, *Science,* 153: 379 (1966).
13. R. B. Setlow, The Photochemistry, Photobiology, and Repair of Polynucleotides, in *Progress in Nucleic Acid Research and Molecular Biology,* Vol. 8, J. N. Davidson and W. E. Cohn, Eds., p. 257, Academic Press, Inc., New York and London, 1968.
14. H. Reiter, B. Strauss, M. Robbins, and R. Marone, Nature of the Repair of Methyl Methane Sulfonate Induced Damage in *B. subtilis, J. Bacteriol.,* 93: 1056 (1967).
15. S. Epstein, J. McNary, B. Bartus, and E. Farber, Chemical Carcinogenesis: Persistence of Bound Forms of 2-fluorenylacetamide, *Science,* 162: 907 (1968).
16. K. C. Smith, Biological Importance of UV-Induced DNA-Protein Cross-Linking In Vivo, and Its Probable Chemical Mechanism, *Photochem. Photobiol.,* 7: 651 (1968).
17. V. N. Iyer, and W. Szybalski, A Molecular Mechanism of Mitomycine Action: Linking of Complementary DNA Strands, *Proc. Nat. Acad. Sci. U. S.,* 50: 535 (1963).
18. J. K. Setlow, The Molecular Basis of Biological Effects of Ultraviolet Light and Photoreactivation, *Current Topics in Radiation Research,* Vol. 2, M. Ebert and A. Howard, Eds., p. 195, North Holland Publishing Co., Amsterdam, 1966.

19. J. E. Cleaver, Photoreactivation: A Radiation Repair Mechanism Absent from Mammalian Cells, *Biochem. Biophys., Res. Commun.,* 24: 569 (1966).
20. J. S. Cook and J. R. McGrath, Photoreactivating-Enzyme Activity in Metazoa, *Proc. Nat. Acad. Sci., U. S.,* 58: 1359 (1967).
21. B. Weiss and C. C. Richardson, Enzymatic Breakage and Rejoining of DNA. I. Repair of Single-Strand Breaks in DNA by Enzyme System from *E. coli* Infected with T4, *Proc. Nat. Acad. Sci., U. S.,* 57: 1021 (1967).
22. S. B. Zimmerman, J. W. Little, C. K. Oshimsky, and M. Gellert, Enzymatic Joining of DNA Strands: A Novel Reaction of Diphosphopyrimidine Nucleotide, *Proc. Nat. Acad. Sci., U. S.,* 57: 1841 (1967).
23. C. J. Dean, Role of DNA Damage and Its Repair in the Inactivation of Cells by Ionizing Radiations, in *Effects of Radiation on Cellular Proliferation and Differentiation,* Symposium Proceedings, Monaco, 1968, p. 23, International Atomic Energy Agency, Vienna, 1968 (STI/PUB/186).
24. R. B. Painter and J. E. Cleaver, Repair Replication in HeLa Cells after X Irradiation, *Nature,* 216: 369 (1967).
25. J. Abelson and C. A. Thomas, The Anatomy of the T5 Bacteriophage DNA Molecule, *J. Mol. Biol.,* 18: 262 (1966).
26. W. D. Rupp and P. Howard–Flanders, Discontinuities in the DNA Synthesized in an Excision Defective Strain of *E. coli* Following Ultraviolet Irradiation, *J. Mol. Biol.,* 31: 291 (1968).
27. J. E. Cleaver, unpublished observations.
28. R. E. Rasmussen and R. B. Painter, Radiation-Stimulated DNA Synthesis in Cultured Mammalian Cells, *J. Cell Biol.,* 29: 11 (1966).
29. R. B. Painter and J. E. Cleaver, Repair Replication, Unscheduled DNA Synthesis, and the Repair of Mammalian DNA, *Radiat. Res.,* 37: 451 (1969).
30. J. E. Cleaver, Xeroderma Pigmentosum: A Human Disease Defective in an Initial Stage of DNA Repair, *Proc. Nat. Acad. Sci., U. S.,* 63: 428 (1969).
31. J. E. Cleaver, Repair Replication of Mammalian Cell DNA: Effects of Compounds that Inhibit DNA Synthesis or Dark Repair. *Radiat. Res.,* 37: 334 (1969).
32. V. A. McKusick, *Mendelian Inheritance in Man,* Johns Hopkins Press, Baltimore, Md., 1966.
33. H. El-Hefnawi, S. Maynard–Smith, and L. S. Penrose, Xeroderma Pigmentosum, Its Inheritance and Relationship to the ABO Blood Group System. *Ann. Hum. Genet.,* 28: 273 (1965).
34. J. Epstein and K. Fukiyama, unpublished experiments, 1969.
35. L. Szilard, On the Nature of the Aging Process, *Proc. Nat. Acad. Sci., U. S.,* 45: 30 (1959).
36. J. D. Regan, J. E. Trosko, and W. L. Carrier, Evidence for Excision of UV-Induced Pyrimidine Dimers from DNA of Human Cells In Vitro, *Biophys. J.,* 8: 319 (1968).
37. J. E. Trosko, E. H. Y. Chu, and W. L. Carrier, Induction of T-Dimers in UV-Irradiated Mammalian Cells, *Radiat. Res.,* 24: 667 (1965).
38. M. Klimek, T-Dimerisation in L Strain Mammalian Cells After Irradiation with UV Light and the Search for Repair Mechanisms. *Photochem. Photobiol.,* 5: 603 (1966).

DISCUSSION

W. B. LANE: Would you expect a different kind of damage from beta radiation than from gamma radiation?

J. CLEAVER: I would not expect it to be different.

W. B. LANE: You did show different damage between ultraviolet and X-ray.

J. CLEAVER: Yes. Depending on the LET of a radiation, you can get different distributions of breaks on a DNA chain. Particularly when you have a high LET radiation, you get breaks that involve both strands and are very close to one another. So perhaps one difference among the whole range of different ionizing radiations may be in the distribution of breaks in DNA. It has been very difficult to characterize chemically the nature of damage from any of the ionizing radiations. The X ray, for example, is very poorly characterized.

D. BRUNER: With reference to the xeroderma cases, are you culturing the stratum germinatium of epidermis or the fibroblasts of the dermis?

J. CLEAVER: The fibroblasts. It is really a primitive experiment. We took a skin biopsy and left it in a bottle until a culture was formed. To do this type of density gradient experiment, we need a lot of DNA, a lot of cells. It has taken a long time to get just that one gradient, which shows very clearly that there is no repair. There is an autoradiographic method of seeing repair. One can see the incorporation of radioactivity from tritiated thymidine into cells that are not in a normal DNA synthesis period. By a series of inferential arguments, one can assert that one is seeing repair going on. By the autoradiographic method, people in our Dermatology Department have been able to show that repair operates throughout all the cells of the skin and is missing in xeroderma pigmentosum throughout the epidermis.

J. W. GOFMAN (LRL): In answer to your question, Dr. Bruner, it is next to impossible for anyone to tell what cells he has in a culture that is grown out of some piece of tissue.

J. CLEAVER: Everything looks like fibroblasts after a while.

J. W. GOFMAN: Occasionally fibroblasts, if they are fibroblasts, look like epithelial cells; and then they change back to look like fibroblasts in the same culture bottle.

J. CLEAVER: Our purpose was to get as many cells as possible for this experiment.

J. GILL (LRL): You told us that strand breaks are the most common type of damage due to ionizing radiation. Would you tell us what the most biologically important kinds of damage are in mammalian cells from ionizing radiation?

J. CLEAVER: From ionizing radiation I do not think anyone can make a sound suggestion. You mean the most important kind for causing cell death. I think it is quite clear from what I showed that there is such an efficient rejoining of the breaks following even enormous doses that breaks are probably trivial as far as the life of the cell is concerned.

B. ROSNYAI (LRL): Is the damage done by UV radiation exclusively due to thymine dimer formation, or are there other changes? To put it another way, is the decrease of the molecular weight proportional to the thymine dimer formed?

J. CLEAVER: The calculations have only been done properly by Rupp and Howard−Flanders for bacteria. One can measure quite accurately the number of thymine dimers and the average distance between them. The molecular weights that were found corresponded within a factor of 2 to the distance between dimers. So it does seem that this bacterial system leaves gaps opposite the dimers. I have not been able to do the calculations on the mammalian cells because the gradients are not that accurate.

B. ROSNYAI: Is DNA which has a high adenine plus thymine content more sensitive to UV radiation damage than DNA which has a high guanine plus cytosine content?

J. CLEAVER: There is a lot of information on radiation sensitivity as a function of $A + T/G + C$ ratio for X rays and ultraviolet light. The opinion on the significance of the ratio varies as the years go by. I have seen some data which show that cells with a high $A + T/G + C$ ratio are more sensitive to ultraviolet light. But it is very difficult to eliminate or control all other factors that might affect radiation sensitivity.

DELAYED RADIATION EFFECTS AMONG JAPANESE SURVIVORS OF THE ATOMIC BOMBS*

ROBERT W. MILLER
Epidemiology Branch, National Cancer Institute, Bethesda, Maryland

Since 1948 the Atomic Bomb Casualty Commission (ABCC) has been evaluating the health of survivors of the atomic bombs in Hiroshima and Nagasaki. This paper seeks to put into perspective the major findings.

GENETIC EFFECTS

In a study[1-4] of about 70,000 children conceived after the explosions, six indicators of genetic damage failed to reveal an unequivocal effect of radiation (Table 1). Furthermore, this group displayed no evidence[5-8] of cytogenetic abnormality, in contrast to the increased frequency of complex chromosomal aberrations found among those

Table 1
INDICATORS OF GENETIC EFFECTS OF RADIATION

Indicator	Result	Reference
Congenital malformations	Increase, if any, less than 2-fold*	1
Stillbirths and neonatal deaths	Increase, if any, less than 1.8-fold*	1
Birth weight	No effect attributable to radiation	1
Anthropometric values at 8 to 10 months	No effect attributable to radiation	1
Sex ratio	Small effect of uncertain significance	2,3
Childhood (F_1) mortality	No effect	4

*90% probability.

---

*A summary of paper presented. A fuller presentation is to appear in *Science*.

exposed in utero or at any time during the entire life span (Tables 2 and 3). The effect was most pronounced among persons whose exposures occurred when they were 30 years of age or older.

Table 2

FREQUENCIES BY AGE GROUP OF COMPLEX CYTOGENETIC ABNORMALITIES AMONG JAPANESE SURVIVORS OF THE ATOMIC BOMBS

	Exposed			
Age group	Min. dose, rads	Affected	Controls	Reference
≤30 years ATB*	200	34% of 94	1% of 94	5
>30 years ATB	200	61% of 77	16% of 80	6
In utero ATB	100†	39% of 38	4% of 48	7
Preconception	150†	0% of 103		8
Preconception	100‡	0% of 25		8

*ATB, at the time of the bomb.
†Maternal dose.
‡Dose received by at least one parent.

Table 3

CYTOGENETIC FINDINGS IN A-BOMB SURVIVORS WITH EXPOSURE TO 200+ RADS BY AGE ATB

	≤30 years*		>30 years†	
Cytogenetic finding	Exposed	Control	Exposed	Control
Number of persons	94	94	77	80
Number of cells examined	8283	8847	6778	7188
Single chromatid breaks or gaps	232	223	212	211
Isochromatid breaks or gaps	21	18	39	75
Rings‡	2	0	3	0
Dicentrics‡	7	0	8	1
Fragments‡	31	1	12	9
Translocations‡	10	0	72	5
Pericentric inversions‡	0	0	11	3
Others‡§	0	0	22	10

*From Bloom et al., Ref. 5.
†From Bloom et al., Ref. 6.
‡Complex chromosomal abnormalities.
§Includes deletions, chromatid exchanges, and centromere breaks.

EFFECTS ON THE EMBRYO

Although a wide variety of congenital malformations have been produced in experimental animals by irradiation of the pregnant mother,[9] the only anomaly observed among the Japanese survivors to date has been small head circumference with mental retardation, the effect[10-12] being proportionate to the radiation dose (Tables 4 and 5). The results were consistent with those of previous studies concerning infants born of women who received radiotherapy for pelvic disorders early in pregnancy.[13,14]

Table 4

EFFECTS OF INTRAUTERINE EXPOSURE TO THE HIROSHIMA ATOMIC BOMB; HEAD CIRCUMFERENCE 2 OR MORE STANDARD DEVIATIONS BELOW AVERAGE; EXPOSURE WITHIN 1800 M OF THE HYPOCENTER, REF. 12

	Gestational age	
	≤15 weeks	>15 weeks
Total exposed	57*	109
Total examined	56*	105
Small head circumference:		
With mental retardation	9	2†
With normal intelligence	14	4‡

*Excludes two with preexistent Down's syndrome.
†Exposed at 21 and 24 to 25 weeks.
‡One exposed at 16 weeks, two exposed at 32 weeks, and one at 36 to 40 weeks.

Table 5

RADIATION EFFECT ON HEAD CIRCUMFERENCE AND INTELLIGENCE FOLLOWING INTRAUTERINE EXPOSURE TO THE HIROSHIMA ATOMIC BOMB WITHIN 15 WEEKS OF THE MOTHER'S LAST MENSTRUAL PERIOD, REF. 12

Intelligence	Head circumference	Distance from hypocenter, meters			
		≤1200	1201 to 1500	1501 to 1800	1801 to 2200
Retarded	>3 standard deviations below mean	6	0*	0	0
Retarded	−2 to −3 standard deviations	2	0	1	0
Normal	>3 standard deviations below mean	1	2	0	0
Normal	−2 to −3 standard deviations	1	6	5	0
Total exposed		11	23*	23†	21†

*Excludes two with preexistent Down's syndrome.
†One not examined.

LEUKEMOGENSIS

The ABCC study[15] leaves no doubt that whole-body irradiation in sufficient dose is leukemogenic in man (Fig. 1). A similar effect following partial-body irradiation has been observed among British men given radiotherapy for ankylosing spondylitis.[16,17] In both studies the effect was proportionate to the dose, the peak occurred about 6 years after first exposure, and the increase was in acute leukemias and chronic granulocytic leukemia but not in the chronic lymphocytic form of the disease.

Recently several human attributes or exposures[18] have been associated with high risk of leukemogenesis (Table 6). Each has a genetic or cytogenetic peculiarity, though not of a uniform nature. Thus Bloom's syndrome and Fanconi's anemia are characterized by chro-

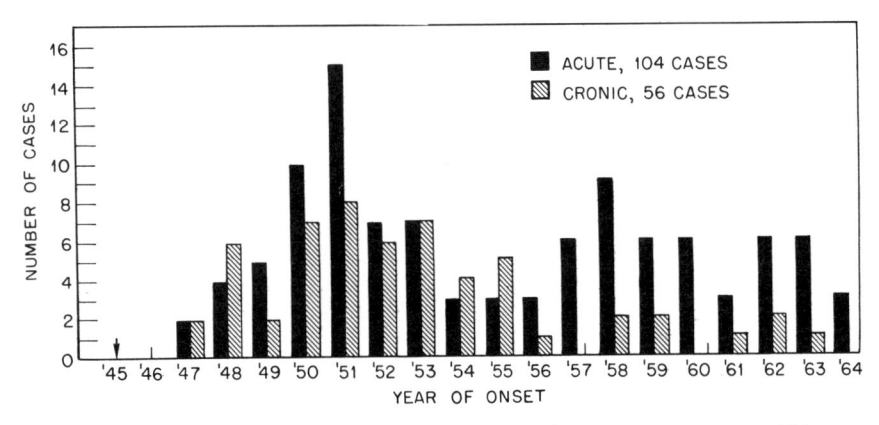

Fig. 1 — Leukemia in Hiroshima and Nagasaki among persons within 1500 m of the hypocenter. (Data from the Atomic Bomb Casualty Commission.)

Table 6

GROUPS AT EXCEPTIONALLY HIGH RISK OF LEUKEMIA, REF. 18

Group	Approximate risk	Time interval
Identical twins of children with leukemia	1 in 5	Weeks or months
Radiation-treated polycythemia vera	1 in 6	10 to 15 years
Bloom's syndrome	1 in 8	<30 years of age
Hiroshima survivors who were within 1000 m of the hypocenter	1 in 60	12 years
Down's syndrome	1 in 95	<10 years of age
Radiation-treated patients with ankylosing spondylitis	1 in 270	15 years
Sibs of leukemic children	1 in 720	10 years
U. S. white children <15 years of age	1 in 2880	10 years

Table 7

RELATIVE RISK OF VARIOUS CHILDHOOD CANCERS FOLLOWING INTRAUTERINE OR PRECONCEPTION DIAGNOSTIC RADIATION EXPOSURE

Neoplasm	Relative risk*
Intrauterine exposure:	
Stewart and Kneale, Ref. 22	
Leukemia	1.5
Lymphosarcoma	1.5
Cerebral tumors	1.5
Neuroblastoma	1.5
Wilms' tumor	1.6
Other cancer	1.5
MacMahon, Ref. 20	
Leukemia	1.5
Central-nervous-system tumors	1.6
Other cancer	1.4
Graham et al., Ref. 21	
Leukemia	1.4
Preconception exposure:	
Graham et al., Ref. 21	
Leukemia	
Mother exposed	1.6
Father exposed	1.3

*Relative risk in controls = 1.0.

mosomal fragility, Down's syndrome by aneuploidy, and radiation or benzene exposure by long-lasting chromosomal abnormalities.

In several studies[19-22] conducted in the United States and Great Britain, minimal doses of X ray were reported to be equally oncogenic whether exposure occurred before conception or during intrauterine life, whether the neoplasm studied was leukemia or any other major cancer of childhood, and whether the study was based on interviews, which are subjective, or on hospital records, which are not (Table 7). Features that argue against a causal relation are the similarity of results despite the dissimilarity of subject matter, the inability when exposures are very small to show a dose—response effect, the lack of supporting data from animal experimentation, and, with regard to preconception radiation, the failure to find an excess of leukemia in a prospective study at the ABCC of 22,400 children conceived after their parents had been heavily exposed to the atomic bomb.[23]

CANCER OTHER THAN LEUKEMIA

Increases in cancers other than leukemia have recently been reported among the Japanese survivors. The frequency of lung cancer

(Table 8) among persons exposed to 90 or more rads was said to be twice normal in a study handicapped by the failure to demonstrate specificity with regard to histologic type,[24] as in U. S. uranium miners.[25] A report of an excess of breast cancer (Table 9) was based on 6 cases observed as compared with 1.53 expected among women who were exposed to 90 rads or more.[26] In this instance it may be difficult or impossible to avoid certain biases that could produce such a small excess. Thyroid cancer, on the other hand, does appear to have been induced by radiation (Table 10) since a dose–response relation was apparent and the results are consistent with those observed following therapeutic irradiation.[27]

Table 8

LUNG CANCER* AMONG JAPANESE ATOMIC BOMB SURVIVORS (DEATH CERTIFICATE STUDY, 1950 TO 1966), REF. 24

Dose, rads	Observed	Expected	Excess
200+	6	3.68	2.32
90 to 199	11	5.27	5.73
40 to 89	9	7.43	1.57
0 to 39	5	7.66	
Other	162	171.63	

*There was no association between histologic type and radiation exposure.

Table 9

BREAST CANCER DETECTED CLINICALLY AT ABCC IN FEMALE ATOMIC-BOMB SURVIVORS* WHO HAD AT LEAST ONE PREVIOUS NEGATIVE EXAMINATION, REF. 26

Dose, rads	Observed	Expected	Excess
90+	6	1.53	4.47
0 to 89	9	10.36	
Unknown	1	0.61	

*Among all women with exposures of 90+ rads — not just those with two or more clinical examinations at ABCC, breast cancer was reported in 9 as compared with 3.7 expected.

OTHER EFFECTS

Other effects attributable to radiation but relatively small in magnitude were an increase in general mortality excluding leukemia during the first 10 years after exposure;[28] a statistically significant

Table 10

THYROID CARCINOMA BY SEX IN THOSE LESS THAN 2000 M FROM
THE HYPOCENTER AT HIROSHIMA AND NAGASAKI, REF. 27

Dose, rads	Males At risk	Males Rate†	Females At risk	Females Rate†	Total* At risk	Total* Rate†
200+	740	4.1	1100	9.1	1840	13.2
50 to 199	789	2.5	1332	6.8	2121	9.3
0 to 49	928	1.1	1806	2.8	2734	3.9

*Total thyroid carcinoma: males, 6; females, 24.
†Rate/1000.

but biologically small retardation in growth and development;[29,30] infrequent radiation cataracts, none of which greatly diminished visual acuity;[31] and a polychromatic sheen on the posterior capsule of the lens of the eye, which caused no disability but was radiation-dose related.[32]

REFERENCES

1. J. V. Neel and W. J. Schull, *The Effect of Exposure to the Atomic Bombs on Pregnancy Termination in Hiroshima and Nagasaki*, p. 241, Publication No. 461, National Academy of Sciences—National Research Council, Washington, D. C., 1956.
2. J. V. Neel, *Changing Perspectives on the Genetic Effects of Radiation*, p. 122, Charles C Thomas, Publisher, Springfield, Ill., 1963.
3. W. J. Schull, J. V. Neel, and A. Hashizume, Some Further Observations on the Sex Ratio Among Infants Born to Survivors of the Atomic Bombings of Hiroshima and Nagasaki, *Amer. J. Hum. Genet.*, 18: 328-338 (1966).
4. H. Kato, W. J. Schull, and J. V. Neel, A Cohort-Type Study of Survival in the Children of Parents Exposed to Atomic Bombings, *Amer. J. Hum. Genet.*, 18: 339-373 (1966).
5. A. D. Bloom, S. Neriishi, N. Kamada, T. Iseki, and R. J. Keehn, Cytogenetic Investigation of Survivors of the Atomic Bombings of Hiroshima and Nagasaki, *Lancet,* 2: 672-674 (1966).
6. A. D. Bloom, S. Neriishi, A. A. Awa, T. Honda, and P. G. Archer, Chromosome Aberrations in Leucocytes of Older Survivors of the Atomic Bombings of Hiroshima and Nagasaki, *Lancet,* 2: 802-805 (1967).
7. A. D. Bloom, S. Neriishi, and P. G. Archer, Cytogenetics of the In-Utero Exposed of Hiroshima and Nagasaki, *Lancet,* 2: 10-12 (1968).
8. A. A. Awa, A. D. Bloom, M. C. Yoshida, S. Neriishi, and P. G. Archer, Cytogenetic Study of the Offspring of Atom Bomb Survivors, *Nature,* 218: 367-368 (1968).
9. R. Rugh, Vertebrate Radiobiology (Embryology), *Ann. Rev. Nucl. Sci.,* 9: 493-522 (1959).
10. G. Plummer, Anomalies Occurring in Children Exposed In Utero to the Atomic Bomb in Hiroshima, *Pediatrics,* 10: 687-693 (1952).
11. R. W. Miller, Delayed Effects Occurring Within the First Decade After Exposure of Young Individuals to the Hiroshima Atomic Bomb, *Pediatrics,* 18: 1-18 (1956).

12. J. W. Wood, K. G. Johnson, and Y. Omori, In Utero Exposure to the Hiroshima Atomic Bomb, an Evaluation of Head Size and Mental Retardation: Twenty Years Later, *Pediatrics,* 39: 385-392 (1967).
13. D. P. Murphy, Ovarian Irradiation; Its Effect on the Health of Subsequent Children: Review of the Literature, Experimental and Clinical, with a Report of 320 Human Pregnancies, *Surg. Gynecol. Obstet.,* 47: 201-215 (1928).
14. L. Goldstein and D. P. Murphy, Etiology of the Ill Health in Children Born After Maternal Pelvic Irradiation. II. Defective Children Born After Postconception Pelvic Irradiation, *Amer. J. Roentgenol., Radium Ther. Nucl. Med.,* 22: 322-331 (1929).
15. O. J. Bizzozero, Jr., K. G. Johnson, and A. Ciocco, Radiation-Related Leukemia in Hiroshima and Nagasaki, 1946–1964, *New Engl. J. Med.,* 274: 1095-1101 (1966).
16. W. M. Court-Brown and R. Doll, Leukemia and Aplastic Anaemia in Patients Irradiated for Ankylosing Spondylitis, *Med. Res. Counc., Spec. Rep. Ser.,* 295: 135 (1957).
17. W. M. Court-Brown and R. Doll, Mortality from Cancer and Other Causes After Radiotherapy for Ankylosing Spondylitis, *Brit. Med. J.,* 2: 1327-1332 (1965).
18. R. W. Miller, Persons with Exceptionally High Risk of Leukemia, *Cancer Res.,* 27: 2420-2423 (1967).
19. A. Stewart, J. Webb, and D. Hewitt, A Survey of Childhood Malignancies, *Brit. Med. J.,* 1: 1495-1508 (1958).
20. B. MacMahon, Prenatal X-Ray Exposure and Childhood Cancer, *J. Nat. Cancer Inst.,* 28: 1173-1191 (1962).
21. S. Graham, M. L. Levin, A. M. Lilienfeld, L. M. Schuman, R. Gibson, J. E. Dowd, and L. Hempelmann, Preconception Intrauterine and Postnatal Radiation as Related to Leukemia, *Nat. Cancer Inst. Monogr.,* 19: 347-371 (1966).
22. A. Stewart and G. W. Kneale, Changes in the Cancer Risk Associated with Obstetric Radiography, *Lancet,* 1: 104-107 (1968).
23. T. Hoshino, H. Kato, S. C. Finch, and Z. Hrubec, Leukemia in Offspring of Atomic Bomb Survivors, *Blood,* 30: 719-730 (1967).
24. C. K. Wanebo, K. G. Johnson, K. Sato, and T. W. Thorslund, Lung Cancer Following Atomic Radiation, *Amer. Rev. Respirat. Dis.,* 98: 778-787 (1968).
25. J. K. Wagoner, V. E. Archer, F. E. Lundin, Jr., D. A. Holaday, and J. W. Lloyd, Radiation as the Cause of Lung Cancer Among Uranium Miners, *New Engl. J. Med.,* 273: 181-188 (1965).
26. C. K. Wanebo, K. G. Johnson, K. Sato, and T. W. Thorslund, Breast Cancer After Exposure to the Atomic Bombings of Hiroshima and Nagasaki, *New Engl. J. Med.,* 279: 667-671 (1968).
27. J. W. Wood, H. Tamagaki, S. Neriishi, T. Sato, W. F. Sheldon, P. G. Archer, H. B. Hamilton, and K. G. Johnson, Thyroid Carcinoma in Atomic Bomb Survivors, Hiroshima and Nagasaki, *Amer. J. Epidemiol.,* 89: 4-14 (1969).
28. S. Jablon, M. Ishida, and M. Yamasaki, Studies of the Mortality of A-Bomb Survivors. 3. Description of the Sample and Mortality, 1950–1960, *Radiat. Res.,* 25: 25-52 (1965).
29. E. L. Reynolds, Growth and Development of Hiroshima Children Exposed to the Atomic Bomb: Three-Year Study (1951–1953). Atomic Bomb Casualty Commission, Technical Report 20-59, 1954.
30. J. V. Nehemias, Multivariate Analysis and the IBM 704 Computer Applied to ABCC Data on Growth of Surviving Hiroshima Children, *Health Phys.,* 8: 165-183 (1962).
31. R. J. Miller, T. Fujino, and M. D. Nefzger, Lens Findings in Atomic Bomb Survivors: A Review of Major Ophthalmic Surveys at the Atomic Bomb Casualty Commission (1949–1962), *Arch. Ophthalmol.,* 78: 697-704 (1967).

32. M. D. Nefzger, R. J. Miller, and T. Fujino, Eye Findings in Atomic Bomb Survivors of Hiroshima and Nagasaki: 1963–1964. *Amer. J. Epidemiol.,* 89: 129-138 (1969).

DISCUSSION

TAMPLIN (LRL): I noticed in one of your earlier tables that you were looking at mothers and fathers who had been irradiated before conception. You had over 100 mothers, but you only had 25 fathers. (They received 100 to 150 r.) Do you think there was significance to the different numbers of mothers or fathers—in terms of sterility, for example?

MILLER: This was a study by A. D. Bloom, which was published in four parts; I merely put the data together in one table. He first studied cytogenetic effects in the child following maternal irradiation, and that included 103 mothers. None of the children were affected. Then for completeness he studied children of 25 irradiated fathers and again found no effects. There was no significance to the different numbers in the samples he studied.

GRAHN: What can you say about the underlying factors that have led these mothers to have X rays taken?

MILLER: There may have been a concomitant variable, such as drugs or some underlying disease. For example, if the mother has chromosomal mosaicism, it might not be clinically detectable; yet she may have some complaint for which the physician recommends pelvimetry. That is the sort of thing I meant. Or the effect may come from drugs for the complaint, perhaps interacting with the disease or with X ray. But the general idea is that there may be some other variable that explains the relation and that the X ray was an additional factor.

DUNSTER: I was a little concerned about the other point concerning the parent who is irradiated before conception in relation to this excess of leukemia. If one goes back 10 years where we are talking about a natural radiation background dose of the same order as the diagnostic dose, you could suggest that radiation is the principal cause of leukemia, which I thought was improbable.

MILLER: I agree with you. I forgot to mention previously that, with any of the data relating to preconception or intrauterine exposure, there is no dose relation demonstrable because the doses were so low.

TOTTER: Can you exclude in your head size and intelligence studies any influence of nutrition?

MILLER: Yes, I think so, for two reasons. First, the adverse social or economic effects of the bomb extended far beyond the area where the small head circumference was found; and second, the results were consistent with studies of the therapeutic X-ray exposure of women in whom the nutrition should not have been different from normal.

CLEAVER: I am interested in your comments on Fanconi's anemia and Bloom's syndrome. As far as I know, Fanconi cells repair normally; and we are doing Bloom's this week and will have the answers next week.

MILLER: We have been very much interested in the relation between cancer and congenital defects. The ABCC data reveal that in one city radiation produced both cancer and congenital defects. It produced leukemia in some people and small head circumference with mental retardation in others. Disease concurrence may be of special significance in cities, families, or individuals. We have been very much interested in quite an array of inborn defects that occur excessively in people with neoplasia.

KAPLAN: You described a number of situations in which the radiation exposure was essentially whole body. Last year I believe a large-scale study was reported on leukemia incidence in long-term survivors among women who had cancer of the uterine cervix treated with surgery or radiotherapy, which, of course, was essentially localized to the pelvic region. My recollection is that there was no excess of leukemia. Would you comment on that?

MILLER: I will, but I would rather not because it is very complicated. The study was an international one. It was made by Dr. George Hutchison, who is a very competent investigator. Women who received local pelvic irradiation in high dose to small quantities of tissues — very intensive treatment for cervical cancer — subsequently did not show an increase in leukemia frequency. I am puzzled as to why they did not, because if a large enough portion of the body is exposed to radiation there is an increase in leukemia. Dr. Richard Doll has reported a study of external radiation given to induce artificial menopause in women who had excessive bleeding at that time of life, and he did find an excess of leukemia. So when the radiation dose was lower but more tissue was involved, leukemogenesis did occur as compared with none when the irradiation was localized and intensive. The authors of the international study suggest that many cells were killed by the radiation and not enough partially damaged tissue remained to induce leukemia. One of the problems in biologic and epidemiologic research is that sometimes one comes up with quandaries like this.

KAPLAN: It is hard to see how they could kill all the cells and not kill the patient.

MILLER: Yes, it is hard to see how cells were killed without damage to the cells beyond those that were killed.

HATCH (LRL): Could I ask what the order of magnitude of peripheral dosage to the rest of the body is in therapeutic irradiation?

KAPLAN: Between 1 and 5% of the dose probably reaches most of the body.

DOBSON (LRL): The dose graded down to where about 15 r reached the neck region.

HATCH: Then you really have whole-body irradiation at moderate levels.

DOBSON: Maybe ladies with carcinoma of the cervix are not proper mosaics.

MILLER: It has been suggested that there are some diseases that protect against leukemia, but I would not want to propose that as an explanation of the data.

RADIATION AND VIRUS INTERACTIONS IN LEUKEMOGENESIS*

HENRY S. KAPLAN
Department of Radiology, Stanford University Medical Center,
Stanford, California

A study of ionizing radiation as an inducing agent for leukemia in mice has been pursued for the past 25 years. At the outset, radiation was selected as the inducing agent because its leukemogenic and mutagenic actions were better known than those of other chemical or physical agents. Radiation also had several technical advantages: (1) the dose to various tissues in the body could be determined accurately, (2) the exact period during which the agent was applied could be established, (3) the field of exposure could be the entire body of the animal or selected regions. It was found that mice of the C57 BL strain, which exhibit a very low spontaneous incidence of leukemia, are extremely susceptible to the induction of lymphatic leukemia by exposure to X rays.

The somatic mutation theory was found to be untenable for the leukemogenic action of radiation. The mutagenic action of radiation is characterized by linearity of dose response and independence of mutation yield from dose rate and dose fractionation. In contrast, there was a paradoxical increase in leukemia when the same total dose of radiation was given not as a single exposure but in several fractions separated by intervals of a few days. Second, although most of the lymphatic leukemias induced by radiation in this strain of mice originate in the thymus, radiation exposures limited to the thymic area or to the upper half of the body yielded virtually no leukemias; the somatic muta-

---
*Summary of paper presented. An extensive discussion of the subject matter summarized here and a complete bibliography will be found in the Presidential Address by Dr. Kaplan to the American Association for Cancer Research, which was published in *Cancer Research,* 27(8): 1325-1340 (1967).

tion hypothesis would have predicted a response equal to that following whole-body irradiation.

It was shown that irradiation of both the thymus and the bone marrow are essential and that protection against leukemia was afforded by shielding the spleen or the bone marrow of the legs or by injecting the irradiated animals with marrow cells from nonirradiated mice. The most conclusive evidence against somatic mutation was that susceptibility to leukemia in thymectomized irradiated C57 BL mice was partially restored by the subcutaneous implantation of isologous thymus grafts (see Fig. 1). The tumors were found to arise in the grafts

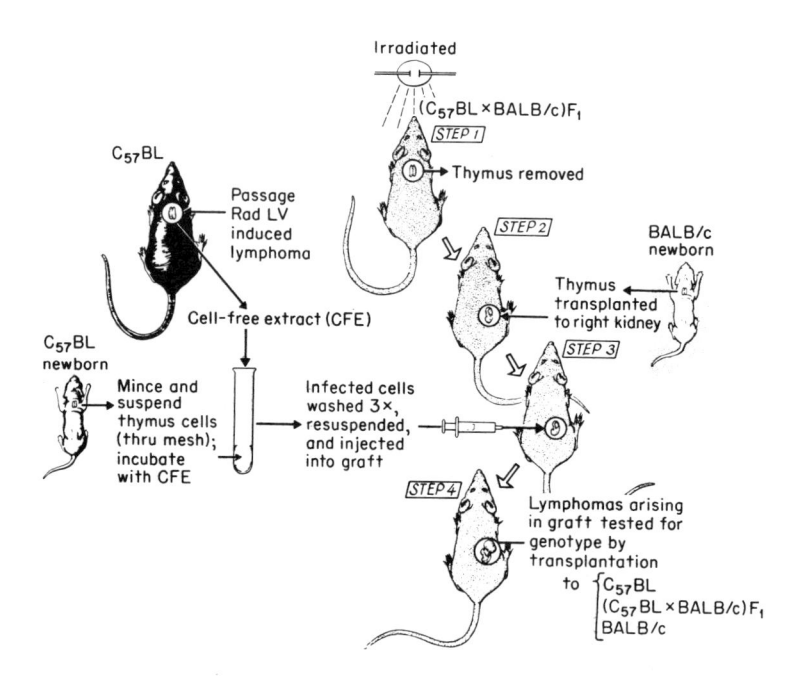

Fig. 1 — Experimental system for the demonstration of target cell, thymus graft, and systemic host contributions to susceptibility to virus leukemogensis. Rad LV, radiation leukemia virus. [From Henry S. Kaplan, Presidential Address, Cancer Res., 27(8): 1335 (1967).]

from cells originally belonging to the donor animal, which had not been exposed to irradiation. This showed a completely indirect induction mechanism. Cells of nonirradiated tissue had been induced to become neoplastic by virtue of their residence in an irradiated animal.

In parallel research, Ludwik Gross demonstrated that cell-free filtrates and extracts prepared from spontaneous lymphomas of AKR mice could induce similar lymphatic leukemias after injection into

C3H test mice. Serial passage of these extracts in newborn mice resulted in a marked increase in leukemogenic potency and in the appearance of particles in electron micrographs that were believed to represent a virus. Several other leukemogenic viruses have since been isolated. Some produce thymic lymphomas where others produce myeloid leukemia or other types of leukemia.

Nearly 15 years ago, cell-free filtrates were prepared from the thymic tumors of irradiated C57 BL mice and inoculated into newborn nonirradiated mice of several strains. Within 2 years thymic lymphomas had begun to appear in the inoculated C57 BL mice but not in mice of other strains unless they had been hybridized with the C57 BL strain. It was concluded that the mice harbor a potential leukemogenic agent that can be extracted in cell-free form from radiation-induced thymic lymphomas but not from normal tissues of nonirradiated animals. Gradually the potency of these extracts was increased by serial passage, and the latent period between injection and tumor formation was decreased. The major breakthrough in enhancement of tumor incidence during serial passage of the extracts came with injection directly into the thymus gland. The purified virus was named the radiation leukemia virus (RadLV).

Similar viruses have since been extracted from lymphomas induced by carcinogenic hydrocarbons, urethan, 4-nitro-quinoline oxide, and possibly estrogens.

A comparison of a variety of murine leukemia viruses indicates that the type of leukemia induced by a given virus depends on the state of the host and the prior passage history of the virus. Thus it is an unreliable criterion for the classification of the viruses. The Gross virus and RadLV are immunologically indistinguishable by the methods tried to date. However, the host range data strongly suggest that there are differences between these two viruses.

The AKR strain of mice, which shows high incidence of spontaneous leukemia, yields Gross virus by extraction from embryos, and it is clear that vertical transmission from mother to progeny can occur. Strain C57 BL mice, which are low in spontaneous leukemia, appear also to transmit the RadLV virus vertically from either the maternal or the paternal side.

It appears that both the RadLV and the Gross viruses are either absent, present in very low titer, or present in an inactive form in the normal thymuses of infant and young adult C57 BL and AKR mice, as long as they have not been irradiated, and that virus titer increases with age in both strains. The susceptibility of the thymus to tumor induction apparently is maximal at birth. It has been suggested that irradiation of adult mice may restore the neonatal level of susceptibility by producing a selective state of maturation arrest in the lymphoid cell population of the radiation-injured thymus. When RadLV was injected directly into the thymus of lightly irradiated C57 BL mice, lymphoma incidence in mice inoculated when 3 to 5 months old was equal to that in nonirradiated mice inoculated at birth. The same dose of radiation alone, in the absence of virus, elicited a negligible lymphoma incidence. This result provides direct experimental support for the view that an essential action of radiation in promoting lymphoma development in adult C57 BL mice is the restoration of thymic susceptibility to the neonatal level.

It has been established that lymphoid cells of the thymus separated from the epithelial–reticular elements by forcing them through a stainless-steel mesh can undergo infection by RadLV in vitro, followed by neoplastic transformation to lymphoma cells during subsequent cultivation in vivo. Thus direct experiment confirms earlier indications based on correlation analysis suggesting that immature lymphoid cells of the thymus are the actual target cells in this system. However, a thymic epithelial–reticular factor is essential for some step in the neoplastic transformation that occurs after infection of target cells by the virus.

Experimental data support the concept that one of the effects of irradiation is the release of the virus from its normal sites of residence in the animal. Cell-free extracts prepared after irradiation of mixed thymus and bone-marrow homogenates were leukemogenic when inoculated directly into thymus grafts in thymectomized irradiated C57 BL host animals. On the other hand, similar cell-free extracts from corresponding nonirradiated tissues were devoid of leukemia-producing activity. It remains to be learned whether release of the virus involves simply the killing of bone-marrow cells by radiation with disintegration of the cells and liberation of preformed virus or results from an increased rate of virus proliferation in radiation-injured cells. In any event, the net result is that radiation produces a response equivalent to an injection of virus, except that the virus is of endogenous derivation.

Is RadLV actually the proximate cause of the thymic lymphomas arising in the irradiated C57 BL mice from which it was extracted, or does the virus merely proliferate secondarily in tumors already induced by irradiation? The problem of causality is a difficult one. The available evidence strongly favors the view that the virus is the actual causative agent and that radiation (and presumably the various chemical leukemogens in other experiments) acts primarily to alter the host–virus relation, with the result that the probability of virus–target cell interaction leading to neoplasia is greatly increased.

In conclusion, the picture that emerges from this trail of research is that mice of strain C57 BL and other low leukemia strains normally harbor a latent leukemogenic virus which is probably transmitted vertically prior to the time of intrauterine implantation and which can persist in the tissues of such naturally infected strains throughout life without producing any discernable ill effects. If, however, the animals are exposed to appropriate doses of radiation or certain chemical agents, these appear to trigger a change in the host−virus relation leading to the development of leukemias. The presence or absence of virus per se does not distinguish high from low leukemia strains of mice. Indeed, it may well be that potentially leukemogenic viruses are ubiquitous among mice.

The model provided by latent, ordinarily harmless viruses, whose leukemogenic potentialities may be evoked by various physical and chemical hazards in the environment, has obvious implications for human leukemogenesis. It is not known whether leukemia in man is caused by viruses or, if so, whether they can also be propagated by vertical transmission. The high degree of natural tolerance associated with the vertical transmission of the temperate murine leukemia viruses is of great potential importance for the prospect of immunization against leukemia in man. Although it has been possible to immunize susceptible strains of mice against the induction of leukemia by some of the highly antigenic virulent viruses, this may be impossible or very difficult with the vertically transmitted viruses to which the hosts are normally tolerant.

DISCUSSION

GOFMAN (LRL): On the question of radiation dose, in any situation where you either activate or release the virus that induces leukemia, you are way above low doses such as are used in pelvimetry. I do not see why you would infer that the very low doses might operate on this type of mechanism. Is there any evidence in your own work to suggest it?

KAPLAN: No, there is not. However, I think it is important to point out that there may be a very good reason for this. Most of our studies have been made on young adult animals. We have evidence that the abundance of the specific target cells decays very rapidly after birth. One of the things radiation does is to induce a serious injury to the thymus; following this injury there is a regeneration, which recapitulates the newborn period. For a relatively brief time, the thymic cortex has a tremendous abundance of the precise target cell that the virus requires. In a sense, then, this is an artificial situation. We are starting with animals that are over the hill, so to speak, from the standpoint of target-cell susceptibility. I think that a relevant study would be a large-scale study at very low dose levels not only in newborn mice but in mice in the late stages of gestation. This is an experiment we have thought about for a number of years and have been prodded to do, but we simply do not have the facilities to carry that many animals. I would like to see such a study done. In summary, our data are in accord with what you said; but they do not rule out the possibility that very low doses would, in fact, be significant if we had the optimally susceptible system.

MILLER: I am very gratified by Dr. Kaplan's explanation of how viruses may still be implicated in human leukemia. One should always seek an explanation through animal studies that fits what one observes in epidemiologic studies. This is not the case in the conventional studies of murine or avian leukemia; also, human leukemia does not follow the transmission patterns of poliomyelitis as some investigators have suggested. But something such as Dr. Kaplan suggested is perfectly all right with us.

DOBSON: Do you have some ideas on how the virus may be transmitted to the murine population—it seems to be so widely spread. If it is not transferred horizontally, the virus must stay around a long time.

KAPLAN: This is speculation, but I think the most reasonable hypothesis is that the virus has been propagated since the primordial mouse. There are reasons to believe that we are dealing with a series of mutants in different murine leukemia viruses. For example, the antigenic characteristics of tumors induced by the Gross virus in the AKR strain and those induced by our virus are indistinguishable, using certain criteria. These viruses are thus very closely related under those terms, whereas the Friend, Moloney, and Rauscher leukemia viruses are clearly distinguishable in terms of their type-specific antigens. All these viruses, however, share a common group-specific antigen, which is revealed only when the outer coat of the virus is stripped off with agents like Tween. Despite the fact that the Gross virus and our virus yield immunologically indistinguishable tumors, nonetheless the host ranges, that is, the strains in which viral susceptibility is observed, are very different for the two viruses. The AKR mouse is highly susceptible to the Gross virus, and so is strain C3H. In contrast, the Gross virus is virtually inert in C57 black animals. Even more interestingly, in limited experiments to date, we have clear evidence that prior inoculation of Gross virus into C57 black animals will protect them against otherwise quite active leukemogenic preparations of our radiation leukemia virus. Whether or not this is by an immunological mechanism, we do not know. If it is immunological in nature, then it is interesting because it would suggest that the Gross virus (extremely close in nature to ours, but slightly different) is able to break tolerance to our virus. You would expect, since our virus is essentially inherited during in utero life, that there would be a high level of natural tolerance, and there is. But it may be that we have come upon a way to break tolerance to the virus. If that is the case, we might conceivably be able to talk in terms of the prevention of these tumors in this way. Otherwise, it is clear that vaccines would be utterly useless against this kind of system since the animals are completely tolerant already to the viral agent that induces them.

CLOSING REMARKS

JOHN W. GOFMAN
Lawrence Radiation Laboratory, University of California,
Livermore, California

I thought this was a fantastically good symposium because of the excellent presentations given by the people who came to participate in it with us. They brought us up to date on some very important issues and gave us the results of their most recent research and thoughts. Indeed, some of them really did address themselves to the "biological implications of the nuclear age." It is sometimes difficult for the papers in a symposium to add up to the title, but I think these succeeded.

As I listened to the various presentations, I alternated between the feelings of optimism and anxiety. Did we no longer need to be too concerned about low-dose radiation. Or should we be more concerned. Perhaps Mr. Parker's initial statement that we really feel that we have been very conservative and that we are on the safe side was quite right. Dr. Miller was very reassuring in his presentation on the low-dose question. Incidentally, if indeed there is something about all the people who go to physicians or clinics for whatever complaint or whatever condition that leads them to have diagnostic radiation procedures, and then their children do have a higher frequency of childhood leukemia or malignancy, it will not help us with respect to the Plowshare AEC problem. However, it will certainly be very illuminating to learn why they receive radiation exposure. I was on an upswing of optimism about low doses of radiation as a result of Dr. Miller's presentation because perhaps it really was not the low radiation dose that was responsible for the increased frequency of childhood leukemia and malignancy. With respect to the Plowshare considerations, that is extremely important. As we heard from Dr. Werth at the outset, they are really concerned about procedures that will give very low doses and usually low dose rates. But Henry Kaplan in his excellent final presentation says that radiation had better not be discounted too quickly.

I think we covered the subject quite well: the problem of setting standards, the hopeless task of ever trying to weigh biological benefits vs. risk, the whole problem of dose estimation, and finally the intricacies of not only observing but interpreting the effects. Certainly the members of the Livermore staff, biological and nonbiological, who attended the symposium learned a tremendous amount from the presentations. We are indeed grateful to the speakers. Many of the people on the Livermore staff who though they did not have a place on the program, had an intense and specific interest in one or a number of the areas covered by the speakers. You can assume that some of you will be invited to return so that we can continue our discussion on these subjects.

LIST OF ATTENDEES

ABRAHAMSON, DEAN E.
University of Minnesota
Minneapolis, Minnesota

ACEBO, ANITA
Department of Public Health
State of California Health and Welfare
 Agency
Berkeley, California

ALTER, JOHN
Department of Public Health
State of California Health and Welfare
 Agency
Berkeley, California

ANDERSON, CHARLES N.
EG&G, Inc.
Las Vegas, Nevada

BEAN, WILLARD
Department of Public Health
State of California Health and Welfare
 Agency
Berkeley, California

BLOOM, JUSTIN L.
Office of the Commissioners
U. S. Atomic Energy Commission
Washington, D. C.

BOONE, F. W.
State Office of Nuclear Energy
Sacramento, California

BOOTMANN, WILLIAM R.
Nevada Operations Office
U. S. Atomic Energy Commission
Las Vegas, Nevada

BRECHBILL, RAY
U. S. Public Health Service
Las Vegas, Nevada

BROWN, JACK
Bureau of Radiological Health
State of California Health and Welfare
 Agency
Berkeley, California

BROWN, STEPHEN L.
Stanford Research Institute
Menlo Park, California

BRUNER, H. D.
Division of Biology and Medicine
U. S. Atomic Energy Commission
Washington, D. C.

BUSTAD, LEO (speaker)
Radiobiology Laboratory
University of California
Davis, California

CAMPBELL, ERNIE D.
San Francisco Operations Office
U. S. Atomic Energy Commission
Berkeley, California

CAROLAN, JOHN J.
Veterans Administration Hospital
Livermore, California

CASSEN, BENEDICT
Laboratory of Nuclear Medicine
 and Radiation Biology
Los Angeles, California

CLEAVER, JAMES E. (speaker)
University of California Medical
 Center
San Francisco, California

COLE, RICHARD
Naval Radiological Defense
 Laboratory
San Francisco, California

LIST OF ATTENDEES

COMAR, CYRIL (speaker)
New York State Veterinary College
Cornell University
Ithaca, N. Y.

COOPER, EUGENE P.
Naval Radiological Defense Laboratory
San Francisco, California

CORNISH, AMASA
Bureau of Radiological Health
State of California Health and Welfare
  Agency
Berkeley, California

DAVIDSON, R. S.
Battelle–Columbus Laboratories
Columbus, Ohio

DE BOER, JELLE
Air Force Weapons Laboratory
Albuquerque, New Mexico

DUMMER, JEROME E.
Los Alamos Scientific Laboratory
Los Alamos, New Mexico

DUNNING, GORDON M.
Division of Operational Safety
U. S. Atomic Energy Commission
Washington, D. C.

DUNSTER, H. J. (speaker)
Radiological Protection Division
U. K. Atomic Energy Authority
Harwell, Didcot, Berks, England

EDGINGTON, DAVID
Argonne National Laboratory
Argonne, Illinois

EVANS, III, EVAN C.
U. S. Naval Radiological Defense
  Laboratory
San Francisco, California

FEINBERG, SAMUEL
Bureau of Radiological Health
State of California Health
  and Welfare Agency
Berkeley, California

FICK, T. R.
Naval Radiological Defense Laboratory
San Francisco, California

FINKLEA, JOHN F.
Medical College of South Carolina
Charleston, South Carolina

FOSTER, R. F.
Battelle–Northwest Laboratory
Richland, Washington

FOWLER, ERIC B.
Los Alamos Scientific Laboratory
Los Alamos, New Mexico

GOFMAN, JOHN W. (speaker)
Lawrence Radiation Laboratory
University of California
Livermore, California

GOLDMAN, MARVIN
Radiobiology Laboratory
University of California
Davis, California

GOULDEN, ANNE M.
Division of Technical Information
  Extension
U. S. Atomic Energy Commission
Oak Ridge, Tennessee

GRAHN, DOUGLAS (speaker)
Argonne National Laboratory
Argonne, Illinois

GRENDON, ALEX
Donner Laboratory
University of California
Berkeley, California

GROTEGUTH, WILLIAM
Bureau of Radiological Health
State of California Health
  and Welfare Agency
Berkeley, California

GUSTAFSON, PHILIP F.
Argonne National Laboratory
Argonne, Illinois

HAGUE, RICHARD S.
San Francisco Operations Office
U. S. Atomic Energy Commission
Berkeley, California

HANSEN, ROBERT H.
Veterans Administration Hospital
Livermore, California

HARDY, EDWARD
Health and Safety Laboratory
U. S. Atomic Energy Commission
New York, New York

HARLEY, JOHN (speaker)
Health and Safety Laboratory
University of California
Livermore, California

HARROWER, ROBERT
Veterans Administration Hospital
Livermore, California

LIST OF ATTENDEES

HATCH, FREDERICK (cochairman)
Bio-Medical Division
Lawrence Radiation Laboratory
Livermore, California

HAWLEY, JR., CLYDE A.
Idaho Operations Office
U. S. Atomic Energy Commission
Idaho Falls, Idaho

HOLLAND, JOSHUA Z. (speaker)
Division of Biology and Medicine
U. S. Atomic Energy Commission
Washington, D. C.

HUNGATE, FRANK P.
Battelle–Northwest Laboratory
Richland, Washington

JUNKINS, R. L. (speaker)
Battelle–Northwest
Richland, Washington

KAPLAN, HENRY S. (speaker)
Stanford University Medical Center
Stanford, California

KAYE, STEPHEN V.
Oak Ridge National Laboratory
Oak Ridge, Tennessee

KINSMAN, SIMON
Bureau of Radiological Health
State of California Health
  and Welfare Agency
Berkeley, California

KORANDA, JOHN J. (speaker)
Lawrence Radiation Laboratory
University of California
Livermore, California

LANE, WILLIAM B.
Stanford Research Institute
Menlo Park, California

LARSON, KERMIT H.
Battelle–Northwest Laboratory
Richland, Washington

LOUGH, S. ALLAN
Division of Biology and Medicine
U. S. Atomic Energy Commission
Washington, D. C.

LOWE, D.
Naval Radiological Defense
San Francisco, California

LUNT, O. R.
Laboratory of Nuclear Medicine
  and Radiation Biology
Los Angeles, California

MALIK, JOHN S.
Los Alamos Scientific Laboratory
Los Alamos, New Mexico

MARKO, A. M.
Biology and Health Physics Division
Atomic Energy of Canada Limited
Chalk River, Ontario, Canada

MASON, BENJAMIN J.
Southwestern Radiological
  Health Laboratory
U. S. Public Health Service
Las Vegas, Nevada

McEWEN, JOHN C.
Veterans Administration Hospital
Livermore, California

MEREDITH, O. M.
Naval Radiological Defense
  Laboratory
San Francisco, California

MILLER, ROBERT W. (speaker)
National Cancer Institute
National Institutes of Health
Bethesda, Maryland

MURDOCK, HAROLD R.
Veterans Administration Hospital
Livermore, California

NELSON, CLIFFORD E.
Environmental Control Administration
U. S. Department of Health,
  Education and Welfare
San Francisco, California

NELSON, NORTON (speaker)
Institute of Environmental Medicine
New York University Medical Center
New York, New York

NG, YOOK (speaker)
Lawrence Radiation Laboratory
University of California
Livermore, California

NISHITA, HIDEO
Laboratory of Nuclear Medicine
  and Radiation Biology
Los Angeles, California

O'SULLIVAN, DERMOT A.
Chemical and Engineering News
San Francisco, California

PAGLIARO, JESSE A.
Chicago Operations Office
U. S. Atomic Energy Commission
Argonne, Illinois

LIST OF ATTENDEES

PARKER, HERBERT M. (speaker)
Battelle—Northwest
Richland, Washington

PIANKA, WALLACE J.
Veterans Administration Hospital
Livermore, California

PICKLER, DAVID
Bureau of Radiological Health
State of California Health
  and Welfare Agency
Department of Public Health
Berkeley, California

RACHLIN, LILLIAN
Veterans Administration Hospital
Livermore, California

RHEUARK, ERNEST
Sanitation and Radiation Laboratory
Department of Public Health
Berkeley, California

RIVERA, JOSEPH
Health and Safety Laboratory
U. S. Atomic Energy Commission
New York, New York

ROBINSON, BOB
Mound Laboratory
Miamisburg, Ohio

RODDEN, ROBERT M.
Stanford Research Institute
Menlo Park, California

RUSSELL, WILLIAM (speaker)
Oak Ridge National Laboratory
Oak Ridge, Tennessee

SEABORG, GLENN T. (speaker)
U. S. Atomic Energy Commission
Washington, D. C.

SHORE, BARNARD (cochairman)
Bio-Medical Division
Lawrence Radiation Laboratory
Livermore, California

SHORE, MORIS L.
National Center for Radiological Health
U. S. Department of Health, Education
  and Welfare
Rockville, Maryland

SHUTE, ELLISON C.
San Francisco Operations Office
U. S. Atomic Energy Commission
Berkeley, California

SMITH, ARNOLD
Department of Public Health
State of California Health
  and Welfare Agency
Berkeley, California

SMITH, DAVID S.
Division of Radiation Protection
  Standards
U. S. Atomic Energy Commission
Bethesda, Maryland

SOUTHWICK, RODNEY L.
San Francisco Operations Office
U. S. Atomic Energy Commission
Berkeley, California

TAMPLIN, ARTHUR (speaker)
Lawrence Radiation Laboratory
University of California
Livermore, California

TELLER, EDWARD (speaker)
Lawrence Radiation Laboratory
University of California
Livermore, California

TOTTER, JOHN (speaker)
Division of Biology and Medicine
U. S. Atomic Energy Commission
Washingon, D. C.

UYESUGI, GEORGE
Department of Public Health
State of California Health
  and Welfare Agency
Berkeley, California

WARD, JOSEPH O.
Department of Public Health
State of California Health
  and Welfare Agency
Berkeley, California

WERTH, GLENN (speaker)
Lawrence Radiation Laboratory
University of California
Livermore, California

WEST, J. L.
UT—AEC Agricultural Research
  Laboratory
Oak Ridge, Tennessee

WILSON, DANIEL W.
Division of Biology and Medicine
U. S. Atomic Energy Commission
Washington, D. C.

LIST OF ATTENDEES

WOLFE, JOHN
Division of Biology and Medicine
U. S. Atomic Energy Commission
Washington, D. C.

WRIGHT, JAMES F.
Radiobiology Laboratory
University of California
Davis, California

LAWRENCE RADIATION LABORATORY, LIVERMORE

ANDERSON, RUTH N.
ANDREWS, ROBERT T.
ANSPAUGH, LYNN R.
BAGAN, CHUCK
BARR, L. K.
BARROW, NICK
BAZAN, F.
BELL, JAMES W.
BIGGS, MAX
BISHOP, STAN
BLOCK, SEYMOUR
BLOODGOOD, D.
BLUMBERG, WILLIAM A.
BOOTH, R. A.
BRANSCOMB, ELBERT
BURTON, ANN
BURTON, DONALD E.
BUTKOVICH, T.
CALDWELL, JOHN
CANE, J. W.
CARTER, ROBERT E.
CHAPIN, C. E.
CHERTOK, BOB
CHEW, MELTON H.
COHEN, JERRY
CONNELL, R. P.
CRAWFORD, TODD V.
DE LALLA, OLIVER
DOBSON, LOWRY
DOGGETT, J. N.
DORN, D. W.
DUAFALA, TOM
DULETSKI, P. S.
EVERTSBUSCH, VALESKA
FISHER, LEN
FLEMING, E. H.
FLESHMAN, DAVID
GEESAMAN, DONALD P.
GIBSON, JR., T. A.
GILL, JAMES E.
GLENN, DAVID
GOLDBERG, EUGENE

GOLDMAN, ERIC K.
GRABSKE, R.
GREENHOUSE, N. A.
GUDIKSEN, PAUL H.
HARFORD, W. B.
HARRISON, FLORENCE
HILL, JOHN H.
HOLLADAY, GALE
HORN, A. J.
HOVINGH, JACK
KASE, K. R.
KLOEPPING, ROGER J.
KNOX, J. B.
KOVICH, ERMA L.
KROTZ, STANLEY
KRUGER, P.
LAFRANCHI, E. A.
LAKE, S.
LASKARIS, M. A.
LEAHY, JOHN
LESSLER, R.
LITTLE, LARRY J.
LITTLEPAGE, LEE
LUCIDO, R. E.
MARSH, K. V.
MARTIN, JOHN R.
MAZRIMAS, JOSEPH A.
McCLELLAND, W. M.
McDONNEL, JAMES L.
McINTYRE, DAVID M.
MOORE, R. P.
MORROW, R. J.
MOULTHROP, PETER H.
MYER, DAVID S.
NELSON, GARY
NEWHOUSE, D. E.
OTT, M. JANE
PARLETT, H. W.
PERDUE, HAZEL D.
PERRY, MANUEL
PIERCE, C.
PLOTKIN, S. R.
POTTER, G. D.
PRINDLE, AUSTIN
PUCKETT, HOWARD M.
QUINN, DOROTHY
READ, ELEANOR
RICH, B.
RICKER, YVONNE
ROBISON, WILLIAM L.
ROZSNYAI, BALAZS
SATO, ELAINE
SAWYER, D.
SCHWARTZ, LARRY
SHORE, VIRGIE
SILVA, ANTHONY
SITZBERGER, EDWARD

SMITH, JR., CHARLES F.
SMITH, THELMA
SMITH, THOMAS E.
SOWERS, A. E.
STEELE, W. A.
STONE, STUART P.
STUART, MARSHALL
STUART, RICHARD N.
TAYLOR, J. C.
TAYLOR, ROBERT T.
TEWES, HOWARD A.
TIMOURIAN, HECTOR
TSCHANZ, JOHN F.
UBER, DON
VATTUONE, G.
WATCHMAKER, GEORGE
WIKKERINK, R. W.
WOODRUFF, ROY
WRIGHT, C.
YODER, ROBERT E.
YOUNG, WEI
ZESZOTEK, EILEEN
ZURAKOWSKI, PAUL R.

LAWRENCE RADIATION LABORATORY, BERKELEY

BUDINGER, T. F.
JONES, HARDIN B.

AEC-SAN FRANCISCO OPERATIONS OFFICE

BEAUFAIT, JR., L. J.
HARKER, NEIL C.
HUGHEY, ROBERT W.
JACKSON, C. D.

SANDIA LABORATORY

HELD, BRUCE J.

INDEX*

ABCC (see Atomic Bomb Casualty Commission)
Accidents, radionuclide release from reactor, 140-142
Aging and radiation, 16-17, 226
Agriculture, radiocontamination in, 95-124, 201-219
Air quality standards compared to radiation standards, 71-72
Alginates, reduction of ^{90}Sr absorption in, 212-213
Altitude, relation to infant death rate, 279
Anger camera, development of, 7
Antimony radionuclides, estimated Plowshare contribution to infant bone, 86-87
 in reactor release, 137
 soil-to-man data, 108
 30-year dose via food, 103, 109
Aquatic ecosystem, maximum dose to man from radiocontaminated, 75-94
Argon-95, estimated Plowshare contribution to infant bone, 86
Arsenic-76, release from reactors, 134
Atomic Bomb Casualty Commission, studies on delayed radiation effects, 17, 307-317
Atomic Energy Commission, role of in radiation protection, 27, 64
Auto fluoroscope, development of, 8

Background radiation levels, 67
Barium-140, estimated Plowshare contribution to infant bone, 86
 from reactor release, 137
 30-year dose via milk, 104
Benefits vs. risk concept in Plowshare programs, 63-65, 68
Biochemistry, AEC sponsored studies in, 26
Birds, tritium uptake at Sedan site, 173
Bismuth-210, estimated Plowshare contribution to infant bone, 87
Blood, effects of ^{226}Ra and ^{90}Sr on, 237-240
Blood flow rate, measurement of, 9-10
Bone, dose from aquatic ecosystems, 75-94
 effects of ^{226}Ra and ^{90}Sr on, 235-247
Bone-marrow transplantation, 14-15, 25, 26
Brachytherapy, development and use of, 12
Breast cancer in atomic bomb survivors, 312
Bromine-82, 30-year dose via milk, 105

Cabriolet crater, radionuclide inventory of, 182, 184-185

---

*Prepared by Charlie M. Pierce, Technical Information Division, Lawrence Radiation Laboratory, Livermore, California.

335

INDEX

Cadmium radionuclides, estimated Plowshare contribution to infant bone, 86
  soil-to-man data, 108-109
Caffeine, enhancement of radiation damage by, 284-285
Calcium-45, 30-year dose via milk, 105
Californium-252 in brachytherapy, 12
Canal construction, Plowshare project, 49
  radionuclide dose to man from, 75-94
Cancer (see type of tumor)
Cancer induction, 227-228, 311
Cancer therapy, use of ^{67}Ga in, 5
Carbon-14, on Pacific Atolls, 161-162
  reactor release of, 140
Carcinogenesis, relation to unrepaired DNA damage, 298-301
Centrifuge, zonal, development and use of, 17-18
Cerium radionuclides, concentration by edible seaweed, 149
  estimated Plowshare contribution to infant bone, 86
  on Pacific Atolls, 161
  soil-to-man data, 108, 112
  30-year dose via soil—root path, 109
Cesium radionuclides, estimated Plowshare contribution to infant bone, 86
  food content, 151, 190, 192, 196
  means of reducing in food chain, 203, 213, 215
  on Pacific Atolls, 161
  reactor release of, 140
  soil-to-man data, 108
  30-year dose via food, 104-105, 109, 112
  use in teletherapy, 11
Chalk River accident, 141
Chapelcross, waste discharge at, 151
Chlorine-36, 30-year dose via soil—root path, 112
Chromium-51, release from reactors, 134-135, 137, 138
  use in brachytherapy, 12
Chromosome analysis, use of electronic scanners in, 18
Chromosomes, atomic bomb survivor studies, 308
Cobalt radionuclides, estimated Plowshare contribution to infant bone, 87
  on Pacific atolls, 161

release from reactors, 134-135, 137
  30-year dose via food, 103, 112
  use in teletherapy, 11
Columbia River, radionuclide release into, 133-143
Contamination (see Pollution)
Copper ore, Plowshare projects, 39-41
Cosmic rays, relation to infant death rate, 279

Dam construction, Plowshare project, 49-51
Diet (see Food)
DNA, repair of radiation damaged, 283-305
Dogs, effects of bone-seeking radionuclides on, 235-247
  effects of single or fractionated doses on, 231-235
DOPA, therapeutic use of, 18-19
Dounreay, waste discharge at, 151
Dragon Trail project, 39
Drugs, effects of radiation on metabolism of, 225-226
  enhancement of radiation damage by, 284-285
Ducks, concentration of radionuclides in, 137
Dysprosium-159, estimated Plowshare contribution to infant bone, 87

Ecology, AEC sponsored studies in, 26, 28
  radionuclide persistence in, 159-187
  studies of reactor-produced radionuclides, 137
Ecosystems, aquatic, radionuclide contamination and man, 75-94
Embryo, effects of atomic bomb on, 308-309
Europium radionuclides, estimated Plowshare contribution to infant bone, 86-87
  soil-to-man data, 108, 112
Extra-corporeal irradiation, immunological suppression by, 13
  leukemia management by, 12-13

Fallout, agricultural land, dose to man from, 95-124
  from Plowshare projects, 56-59
Fast-neutron reactors, potential problems with, 141-142

INDEX

Federal Radiation Council, role in Plowshare activities, 64-72
Fetus, effects of atomic bomb on, 308-309
Fish, radionuclide concentration in, 150-151
(See also Food)
Food, combating radiocontamination in, 201-219
fallout in, 95-124
Forage, radionuclide contaminated milk from, 98-106, 201-219
Fruit (see Food)
Fuel-reprocessing plants, radionuclide release from, 151
Fusion devices, radionuclides from, 162-163

Gadolinium-162, soil-to-man data, 108
Gallium-67, therapeutic use of, 5
Gamma rays, genetic effects of, 262-263
Gamma spectrometry, nuclides at Sedan site, 181-182
Gasbuggy project, 37-39, 54-57
tritium production by, 54-56
Gas storage, Plowshare cavern production, 40, 42
Geese, concentration of radionuclides by, 137
Genetic damage, radiation protection guidelines, 66, 71
Genetic repair of radiation damage, 283-305
Genetics, AEC sponsored studies of, 25-26, 28
effects of low-level radiation on, 255-267
offspring of atomic bomb survivors 307-317
Grass, tritium levels at Sedan site, 174
(See also Forage)
Ground squirrels, tritium levels at Sedan site, 173

Hafnium-181, soil-to-man data, 112
Heart, artificial, radioisotope power source of, 15-16
radioisotope-powered pacemaker, 15-16
Hiroshima survivors, delayed radiation effects in, 307-317
Hodgkin's disease, therapy with ^{67}Ga, 5

Horned toad, tritium levels at Sedan site, 178
Human (see Man)

Immunogenetics, AEC sponsored studies of, 25-26
Indium-114, estimated Plowshare contribution to infant bone, 87
30-year dose via soil—root path, 112
Infant bone dose from Plowshare canal, 75-94
Infant death rate, United States, 278-279
Insects, tritium levels at Sedan site, 178
Insulin assay, technique of, 9
International Atomic Energy Agency, radiation protection guides, 64
International Commission on Radiological Protection, role in Plowshare activities, 64-72
Iodine radionuclides, blocking uptake of, 207-208
ecology studies at Sedan crater, 164
in vitro diagnostic procedures with, 9
means of reducing in food chain, 201, 203-208, 215, 216
reactor produced, 126, 128, 140
30-year dose via food, 104
Iridium-192, estimated Plowshare contribution to infant bone, 87
soil-to-man data, 112
30-year dose via food, 103, 112
Irish Sea, waste discharge into, 145-155
Iron radionuclides, on Pacific atolls, 161
reactor produced, 134
use in iron metabolism studies, 11

Japanese survivors, delayed radiation effects in, 307-317

Kangaroo rat, tritium levels at Sedan site, 173-179
Karotype analysis, electronic scanner for, 18
Krypton radionuclides, reactor produced, 125-126, 128, 130-132, 139, 140
use in blood-flow measurement, 10

Lawrence Radiation Laboratory Biomedical Division, origin of, 23
Lead-205, 30-year dose via milk, 103
Leukemia, in atomic bomb survivors, 310-311
  radiation and virus interactions in, 319-325
  radioinduction of, 238-239, 273-275
Life-span, effects of radiation on, 16-17, 70-72, 269-281
Linear hypothesis, application to radiation protection, 69-70
Liver cancer, radioinduction of, 274
Lizards, tritium levels at Sedan site, 178
Low-dose radiation, genetic effects of, 255-267
  late effects of, 269-281
Low-dose-rate facility, development and use of, 13-14
Lung cancer, radioinduction of, 273-274, 277, 311, 312

Man, fallout and agriculture, 95-124
  radionuclide contaminated aquatic ecosystem, 75-94
Manganese-54, estimated Plowshare contribution to infant bone, 87
  on Pacific atolls, 161
  production of, 128, 134, 137
Marmosa, laboratory-animal potential, 247-249
Meat (see Food)
Medicine, atomic energy application to, 1-19
Mercury-197, 30-year dose via milk, 103
Mice, effects of low-level radiation on, 255-267
  radiation and viral interactions in leukemogenesis in, 319-325
  tritium levels at Sedan site, 173
Milk, methods of reducing radionuclide contamination in, 204-211, 213-216
  radionuclide contamination of, via forage, 98-106
  (See also Food)
Mining, Plowshare ventures in, 39-41, 43, 47
Molecular biology, AEC sponsored studies in, 26
Molybdenum-99, 30-year dose via milk, 104
Monitoring, environmental, 148-151, 160
Mutagens, radiation and other, 223-230
Mutations, effect of low-level radiation on, 255-267

Nagasaki survivors, delayed radiation effects to, 307-317
National Advisory Committee on Radiation, functions of, 202
National Committee on Radiation Protection and Measurements, role in Plowshare activities, 64-72
Neptunium-239, release from reactors, 134
Neutrons, genetic effects of, 262, 263
Nickel-59, 30-year dose via milk, 103
Niobium-95, concentration by edible seaweed, 149, 150
  reactor release of, 137
Nuclear explosions, effect on aquatic ecosystem and man, 75-94
  planned Plowshare activities, 31-61
  protection guidelines for, 63-72
  thermonuclear, radionuclides from, 162-163
Nuclear reactors, radionuclide release from, 125-143

Ocean, disposal of waste into, 145-155
Oil shale, Plowshare projects with, 40, 43-45
Ore bodies, Plowshare projects with, 39-41, 43, 47
Organ transplantation, effect of radiation on, 14
Ovarian cancer, radioinduction, 273, 274, 276
Oysters (see Shellfish)

Pacemaker, miniature radioisotopic powered, 15-16
Pacific Proving Grounds, ecological study at, 161-162
Palladium-112, 30-year dose via milk, 104
Parkinson's disease, DOPA therapy for, 19
Pesticides, testing of, 226-227
Phosphate gels, reduction of ^{90}Sr absorption in, 212
Phosphorus-32, biological concentration of, 137
  estimated Plowshare contribution to infant bone, 87
  release from reactors, 134-135, 137
  30-year dose via milk, 103, 105

INDEX 339

Pi-mesons, application to tumor therapy, 11
Plants, tritium levels at Sedan site, 173-177
Plowshare, benefits vs. risk concept, 63-65, 68
 canal construction, 49
 dam construction, 49-51
 ecology at shot sites, 159-187
 explosion, depth vs. effect, 32-36
 fallout from projects, 56-59
 LRL biomedical program, 23
 mining ventures, 39-41, 43, 47
 production of gas-storage caverns, 40, 42
 quarrying project, 43, 48, 49
 radiation protection guidelines and, 63-72
 techniques for gas stimulation, 37-39, 54-57
 techniques for oil-recovery enhancement, 40, 43-45
 transisthmus canal, radionuclide dose to man from, 75-94
 tritium production, 54-56
Plutonium toxicity studies, 24
Pollution, radiation and other, 71-72, 223-230
Polonium-210, food content, 190, 196
Population exposure, guidelines and Plowshare events, 63-72
Potassium radionuclides, concentration by fish, 151
 30-year dose via milk, 105
Power reactors, atmospheric pollutants, 125-132
Power sources, miniaturized radioisotope, 15, 16
Promethium-147, estimated Plowshare contribution to infant bone, 86
 soil-to-man data, 108
Prussian blue, reduction of ^{137}Cs absorption by, 213, 214
Public Health Service, role in Plowshare activities, 64

Quarrying project, 43, 48, 49

Radiation, detectors, miniaturized, 9
 effects on life-span, 70-72
 effects of low level, 255-267, 269-281
 effects relative to other agents, 223-230
 effects of single and fractionated doses of, 231-235
 interaction with virus in leukemogenesis, 319-325
 (See also specific radiation)
Radiation damage, repair of, 66
Radiation repair, cellular, 283-305
Radiation standards (see Standards)
Radioimmunoassays, use of, 9
Radionuclides, atmospheric pollution by, 125-132
 bone seeking, effects on dogs, 235-247
 cyclotron produced, 6, 7
 diagnostic scanning techniques with, 7-9
 dose to man from aquatic environs, 75-94
 estimated Plowshare canal contribution to infant-bone dose, 75-94
 in food, 190-200, 210, 211
 long-term-effect studies, 24-26
 marine disposal of, 145-155
 medical applications of, 1-19
 persistence at detonation sites of, 159-187
 protection guidelines for, 67-68
 reduction of environmental contamination by, 201-219
 release from fuel-reprocessing plants, 151
 release from reactors, 133-143
Radium-226, effects on bones of dogs, 236-240, 242, 244-247
 in food, 190, 192, 193, 196, 197
Reactors, atmospheric pollutants from power, 125-132
 potential problems from fast neutron, 141, 142
 radionuclide release from, 133-143
Repair mechanisms and radiation protection criteria, 66
Rhenium radionuclides, presence in plants at Sedan site, 180
 30-year dose via milk, 103
Rhodium-105, 30-year dose via milk, 104
Risk vs. benefit concept, Plowshare programs, 63-65, 68
Rubidium radionuclides, 30-year dose via food, 105, 112
Rulison project, 39
Russian thistle, tritium levels at Sedan site, 173-177, 182
Ruthenium radionuclides, concentration by edible seaweed, 149, 150
 concentration by fish, 151
 estimated Plowshare contribution to

INDEX

infant bone, 86
on Pacific atolls, 161
reactor release of, 137
soil-to-man data, 108
30-year dose via soil—root path, 109
Salmon, uptake of radionuclides by, 137
Saltbush, tritium levels at Sedan site, 173-177
Samarium-151, soil-to-man data, 108
Scandium-46, estimated Plowshare contribution to infant bone, 87
reactor release of, 137
soil-to-man data, 112
Scanning devices, chromosome analysis with, 18
Scanning techniques, medical diagnosis by, 7-9
Seaweed, edible, radionuclide concentration of, 148-150
Sedan site, ecological studies at, 163-182
radionuclides present at, 181, 182
Shellfish, concentration of radionuclides in, 137, 155
(See also Food)
Silver-111, estimated Plowshare contribution to infant bone, 86
30-year dose via milk, 104
SL-1 reactor accident, 141
Smoking, lung cancer from, 228
SNAP program, biomedical research associated with, 24, 25
Sodium radionuclides, release from reactors, 134
30-year dose via food, 103, 105, 112
Soil—milk path, reducing radionuclide levels in, 201-219
Soil—root path, entry of fallout into, 106-113
Soil-water movements, studies of tritium in, 169-173
Springfields, waste discharge at, 151
Standards, application to Plowshare, 63-72
effects on reactor programs, 126-132
UKAEA, 146
Strontium radionuclides, concentration by edible seaweed, 149
ecology studies at Sedan crater, 164
effects on bones of dogs, 235-244, 245-247
estimated Plowshare contribution to infant bone, 86
food content, 190-193, 195-198
leukemia induction in dogs, 238-239

means of reducing in food chain, 203, 208-213, 215, 216
on Pacific atolls, 161
reactor release of, 140
soil-to-man data, 108, 109
30-year dose via food, 104, 109
Sulfur-35, 30-year dose via soil—root path, 112
release from reactors, 135
Systems for Nuclear Auxiliary Power, biomedical research associated with, 24, 25

Tantalum-182, estimated Plowshare contribution to infant bone, 87
soil-to-man data, 112
Technetium-99, diagnostic use of, 5, 6
Teletherapy devices, development and use of, 11
Tellurium radionuclides, estimated Plowshare contribution to infant bone, 86
soil-to-man data, 108, 109
30-year dose via food, 103, 104, 108, 109
Terbium-160, soil-to-man data, 112
Thallium-204, 30-year dose via soil—root path, 112
Thermonuclear explosions, radionuclides from, 162, 163
Thulium-170, soil-to-man data, 112
Thyroid gland, imaging techniques for, 8
Thyroid cancer in atomic bomb survivors, 313
Thyroxine, serum, measurement of, 9
Tin radionuclides, estimated Plowshare contribution to infant bone, 86
soil-to-man data, 108
30-year dose via food, 103, 109
Triiodothyronine binding test, 9
Tritium, at Cabriolet site, 182, 184, 185
dose from Plowshare canal, 86, 87
ecological studies at Sedan crater, 165-182
origin of, 162-163
on Pacific atolls, 161
produced in Plowshare gas wells, 54-56, 68
release from reactors, 126, 135, 140, 142, 143
Tumors (see specific tumor)
Tungsten radionuclides, production of, 128

INDEX

at Sedan crater, 163, 164
30-year dose via soil—root path, 112

United Kingdom Atomic Energy Authority, waste discharge by, 145-155
Uranium, food content, 190, 194, 196
  reactor activated and release of, 134
U. S. Atomic Energy Commission (see Atomic Energy Commission)
U. S. Public Health Service, role in Plowshare activities, 64

Vaccines, purification using zonal centrifuge, 17, 18
Vegetables (see Food)
Virus, interaction with radiation in leukemogenesis, 319-325
  isolation using zonal centrifuge, 17, 18

Wagon wheel project, Plowshare, 39
Wasp project, Plowshare, 39
Waste disposal, at marine environs, 145-155
  fuel-reprocessing plants, 151
Whole-body counters, development and applications of, 10, 11

Windscale, waste discharge from, 146-151
Windscale incident, 140

Xenon-133, reactor produced, 126
  use in blood-flow measurement, 10
Xeroderma pigmentosum, carcinogenesis mechanism, 298-301
X-ray fluorescence, thyroid imaging technique of, 8
X rays, genetic effects of, 262, 263
  medical, population exposure levels, 67

Yttrium-91, estimated Plowshare distribution to infant bone, 86
  soil-to-man data, 108

Zinc-65, biological concentration of, 137
  concentration by oysters, 155
  estimated Plowshare distribution to infant bone, 87
  on Pacific atolls, 161
  release from reactors, 134, 135, 137, 138, 143
  30-year dose via soil—root path, 112
Zirconium-95, concentration by edible seaweed, 149, 150
  reactor release of, 137
Zonal centrifuge, development and use of, 17, 18

LEGAL NOTICE

This book was prepared under the sponsorship of the U. S. Atomic Energy Commission. Neither the United States, nor the Commission, nor any person acting on behalf of the Commission:

A. Makes any warranty or representation, expressed or implied, with respect to the accuracy, completeness, or usefulness of the information contained in this publication or that the use of any information, apparatus, method, or process disclosed in this book may not infringe privately owned rights; or

B. Assumes any liabilities with respect to the use of, or for damages resulting from the use of any information, apparatus, method, or process disclosed in this publication.

As used in the above, "person acting on behalf of the Commission" includes any employee or contractor of the Commission, or employee of such contractor, to the extent that such employee or contractor of the Commission, or employee of such contractor prepares, disseminates, or provides access to, any information pursuant to his employment or contract with the Commission, or his employment with such contractor.

NUCLEAR SCIENCE ABSTRACTS

Nuclear Science Abstracts, a semimonthly publication of the U.S. Atomic Energy Commission, provides comprehensive abstracting and indexing coverage of the international literature on nuclear science and technology. It covers (1) research reports of the U.S. Atomic Energy Commission and its contractors; (2) research reports of other government agencies, universities, and industrial research organizations on a worldwide basis; and (3) translations, patents, conference papers and proceedings, books, and articles appearing in technical and scientific journals.

INDEXES

Indexes covering subject, author, corporate author, and report number are included in each issue. These indexes, which are cumulated and sold separately, provide a detailed and convenient key to the world's nuclear literature.

EXCHANGE

Nuclear Science Abstracts is available on an exchange basis to universities, research institutions, industrial firms, and publishers of scientific information; inquiries regarding the exchange provision should be directed to the Division of Technical Information Extension, U.S. Atomic Energy Commission, P.O. Box 62, Oak Ridge, Tennessee 37830.

SUBSCRIPTIONS

Nuclear Science Abstracts is available on subscription from the Superintendent of Documents, U.S. Government Printing Office, Washington, D.C. 20402, at $42.00 per year for the semimonthly abstract issues and $38.00 per year for the cumulated-index issues. Subscriptions are postpaid within the United States, Canada, Mexico, and most Central and South American countries. Postage is not paid for Argentina, Brazil, Guyana, French Guiana, Surinam, and British Honduras. Subscribers in these countries and in all other countries throughout the world should remit $52.50 per year for the semimonthly abstract issues and $47.50 per year for the cumulated-index issues.